CAREGIVING
AND
CARE SHARING
A LIFE COURSE PERSPECTIVE

ROBERTA R. GREENE AND NANCY P. KROPF

NASW PRESS

National Association of Social Workers
Washington, DC

Darrell P. Wheeler, PhD, MPH, ACSW, *President*
Angelo McClain, PhD, LICSW, *Chief Executive Officer*

Cheryl Y. Bradley, *Publisher*
Julie Gutin, *Project Manager*
Julie Kimmel, *Copyeditor*
Wayson R. Jones, *Proofreader*
Laurie Graulich, *Indexer*

Cover by Britt Engen, Metadog Design Group
Interior design and composition by Cynthia N. Stock, Electronic Quill
Printed and bound by P. A. Hutchison Company

First impression: November 2014

Library of Congress Cataloging-in-Publication Data

Greene, Roberta R. (Roberta Rubin), 1940–
    Caregiving and care sharing: A life course perspective / Roberta Greene and Nancy P. Kropf.
      pages cm
    Includes bibliographical references and index.
    ISBN 978-0-87101-456-6—ISBN 0-87101-456-4 1. Caregivers. 2. Caregivers—Family relationships. 3. Care of the sick. 4. Older people—Care. 5. Human services. I. Kropf, Nancy P. II. Title.
    HV65.G74 2014
    362'.0425—dc23
                                                                    2014027208

Printed in the United States of America

We dedicate this book to all of the families who are in caregiving roles. Through their important work, children, adults, and older adults are able to remain in their homes and communities. In addition, we pay our respect to the social workers who have devoted their professional lives to sharing care provision tasks with these families. Finally, we honor the future generation of social workers as they begin their careers helping families with responsibilities of care.

✳ Contents

✳
About the Authors

Roberta R. Greene, PhD, was professor and the Louis and Ann Wolens Centennial Chair in Gerontology and Social Welfare at the School of Social Work, University of Texas at Austin. She served as a clinical social worker at Jewish Federation of Greater Washington, where she counseled Holocaust survivors and their families. She also resettled refugees who came to the United States from around world.

Dr. Greene has authored more than 100 publications in the areas of aging, human behavior, and social work. Her books include *Social Work Practice: A Risk and Resilience Perspective, Resiliency Theory: An Integrated Framework for Practice, Research, and Policy, Human Behavior Theory and Social Work Practice,* and *Social Work with the Aged and Their Families.*

Nancy P. Kropf, PhD, is associate dean at Andrew Young School of Policy Studies and professor, School of Social Work, Georgia State University. She is a John A. Hartford Geriatric Social Work Scholar and fellow of the Gerontological Society of America. As a practitioner, she was a therapist with families who have members with disabilities, and worked with grandparents who are raising grandchildren.

Dr. Kropf has more than 100 publications in social work and aging, with the majority in the area of older adults in caregiving roles. Her books include *Social Work & Restorative Justice: Skills for Dialogue, Peacemaking, and Reconciliation* (coedited with Elizabeth Beck and Pamela Blume Leonard), *Handbook of Psychosocial Interventions with Older Adults: Evidence-Based Treatment* (coedited with Sherry M. Cummings), *Competence: Theoretical Frameworks* (cowritten with Roberta R. Greene), and *Human Behavior Theory: A Diversity Framework* (cowritten with Roberta R. Greene).

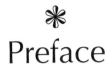

Preface

Recent decades have brought significant changes in family form and function, as well as new service delivery models that promote health and well-being for people with various disabilities within their own homes and communities. Nevertheless, providing care to family members continues to be part of family life across the life course. This text discusses select caregiving situations that illustrate traditional models and emerging social work practice trends. These models may be used in a wider array of caregiving situations than is presented here.

This book was inspired by evolving caregiving theoretical approaches. For example, caregiving has usually been thought of as a family matter, often involving the care recipient and one primary caregiver. This text suggests a different point of view proposed by Daatland, a Swedish scientist who studied the life course and social welfare services for older adults. Daatland (1983) suggested that "caregiving be seen as a form of social organization that includes the interpersonal relationships and the division of practical tasks: a truly collective action, depending upon direct and indirect contributions from a number of actors, including the cared for himself" (p. 1). That is, all activities of family and friends, state programs, and services should come together to form a coherent whole. Daatland also extended the caregiving concept to include the idea of *social care,* a network of formal and informal services that support care provision.

The term "social care" takes social workers back to their roots, when we were part of the fabric of the social welfare system, taking action to ensure that people's basic needs were met. Practitioners worked closely with the client and client system to improve social functioning. This was a collective action—whether formal or informal—encompassing complex social relationships. This broad definition included practice methods as well as policy and programs to improve the well-being of people at risk and in need of care.

Still another influence was Stanley's (2007) work on risk management in New Zealand's child welfare system. Using a narrative perspective, Stanley described the social worker's role as facilitating discourse among families, practitioners, and policymakers in order to reach an understanding of the level of risk for children and who is chosen to give care. Care sharing is another concept that gave rise to the approach taken in this book. *Care sharing* was coined by Covan (1998) to describe a type of care collective, a communal effort that organizes a combination of strategies to maximize pleasure and minimize losses that might otherwise be associated with the aging process.

This book aims to provide a fuller context for caregiving practice situations, "continuously discovering, appraising, and attending to changing locales, populations, scientific and technological developments, and emerging societal trends to provide relevant services" (Council on Social Work Education [CSWE], 2008, p. 6). Because of rapidly emerging caregiving innovations, such as those prompted by the Affordable Care Act, readers are encouraged to seek out new care strategies as they become available.

CHAPTER ONE

Introduction to Care Provision

[Social welfare is] all social interventions intended to enhance or maintain the social functioning of human beings. . . . Social workers deliver social welfare services.

—Dolgoff & Feldstein (2008, p. 4)

This book explores the experiences of families that provide care for family members with extended care needs. Reading it will give you the opportunity to examine several caregiving configurations—from parents caring for sons or daughters with disabilities to families caring for military veterans with physical and psychiatric conditions. As social work practitioners, many of you will be working with families in caregiving roles. Thus, you will need to understand family-related issues and dynamics. At the same time, your knowledge and skills must extend beyond family life. You will need to understand the social conditions of caregiving, including the services, programs, supports, policies, and cultural assumptions and expectations surrounding care. Assisting people and designing and advocating for caregiving programs are key responsibilities of social workers.

To promote this type of understanding, this book describes various caregiving situations. You will find that although the initial focus of assessment and intervention is on the person in need, approaches to these tasks ultimately include the identification and involvement of families, significant others, and relevant societal institutions. The following are examples of questions that will guide your work in caregiving situations:

- What are the basic components of the social welfare program in this practice arena?
- Who is eligible for these programs or benefits?
- What policies and funding sources are pertinent?
- What current research is germane to this area, and are there evidence-based practice approaches to guide practice?

- What ethical dilemmas and values may need to be resolved in this practice setting?
- Are innovative methods of providing care emerging and available to the clients?
- Can I, as a social worker, contribute to these innovations?

These are just some of the relevant questions you will address as you explore caregiving and care-sharing experiences within families.

Covan (1998) coined the term *care sharing* to describe a care collective that organizes multiple strategies for maximizing pleasure and minimizing loss associated with the aging process. In other words, care sharing is a conscious attempt to support those in the community who are frail. The title of this book, *Caregiving and Care Sharing: A Life Course Perspective*, is significant. It includes the idea of care sharing because families do not provide care in isolation. Mutual aid approaches to care are emerging as a result of changing demographic trends.

Although Covan's original work focused on older adults, caring in fact takes place across a family's entire life course. The initial chapters of this book provide a historical context for care and describe how family life and caring have evolved over time. Although caring is a fundamental experience in the lives of contemporary families—that includes, for example, raising children and caring for aging parents—it can also be stressful and difficult. Programs and institutions that exist to support caregivers may unintentionally add to the stress with cumbersome intake processes, inaccessible services, or a lack of attention to the needs of the family. This book will help you analyze how services, programs, policies, and cultural issues support or challenge families providing care.

The social care approach works at both a micro level (representing the most personal, immediate interactions that affect a client) and a macro level (representing more distant interactions). This context brings together elements of both direct and indirect practice. Whereas *direct practice* attends to the situations of the caregiving family, *indirect practice* necessitates consideration of the cultural milieu, worldview, and historical times that affect both you and your client (Greene, 2007). This integrated perspective will require you to think holistically, taking into account such issues as how the structure of the U.S. and global economies influences a caregiving family. This approach to social work delivery has been called "social care."

The social care approach also highlights practitioners' concern with enhancing the social functioning of all people. Competent and effective practice begins with a person-in-environment perspective and underscores the client's human dignity and self-worth. At the same time, the ability to adapt these concepts to changing contexts is the foundation of effective social work practice in caregiving situations. Contemporary social factors influence the nature and experience of care and include escalating violence in neighborhoods, communities, and the world; increasing receipt of information from social media and expanded global television coverage; and increasing stress in the family as a result of enhanced technology and changing labor force conditions. Other contributing factors include changes in U.S. demographics, such as the growth of the aging population and the number of new Americans; these factors are also important for understanding caregiving and care sharing.

Historical Social Construction of Direct Social Work Practice

The concept of social functioning distinguishes social work from other helping professions. Sheafor, Horejsi, and Horejsi (2012) devoted their practice text to this vision of social care. They suggested that effective *social functioning* is an individual's ability to meet basic needs and perform major social roles successfully. This involves positive interdependence and interactions among people in all social systems, and it applies in particular to family caregiving roles. Ultimately, the purpose of social work from this perspective is to match the fit between people's capacities, actions, and demands with the resources and opportunities of the environment.

When we examine the history of social work practice, we see long-standing attention to social functioning. Since the inception of the profession, pioneers, educators, and theorists have contributed ideas that suggest social workers should ensure that clients have the basic life necessities and should promote resilience and quality of life. To help us begin to think about which social work practices might be most relevant today, let's take a quick journey back in time through the changing landscape of care provision.

Boards of Charity Initiate Care

In the beginning, the social work profession imported Elizabethan Poor Laws from England and informally began its activities in large U.S. cities, where friendly visitors went to the homes of poor families to assess their needs. Boards of charity then determined who would receive financial aid and other types of assistance. In addition, community centers were established to provide instruction for Americanizing new immigrants. These centers also produced the *Settlement Cookbook*. Early social work practitioners had a hands-on approach that gave them an understanding of a family's everyday needs and the community-based services available to address them.

This type of approach exists today in community partnerships designed to provide public services, such as the Charlotte-Mecklenburg Schools' Parent University, which offers courses in English and Spanish, including Your Mental Health Matters, Using an E-Reader to Promote Literacy, and Self-Esteem and Its Impact on Academic Development. This public service resembles the social care provided today in countries such as Great Britain and Scandinavia, where local councils are the primary source of immediate care, often through public education.

Pioneers Define Our Work

Another way to decide which social work practice strategies might be useful in caregiving situations today is to revisit the ideas of founding pioneers such as Mary Richmond and Bertha Reynolds. Mary Richmond (1917) believed that people should be understood within their social environment, which included their closest social ties: families, schools, churches, jobs, and so forth. She was one of the early *friendly visitors*, who made home visits to explore how families dealt with everyday concerns. She placed an emphasis on "social diagnosis." From an assessment perspective, this process individualizes the client. In the context of caregiving, it allows practitioners to become familiar with their caregiving clients' day-to-day needs, coping capacities, and social support networks.

Bertha Reynolds (1935) characterized casework as a form of social work that assists the client with "a problem which is essentially his own" (p. 235). Ann Weick (1993) revisited the idea of allowing clients to speak to their own issues when she said that people are more likely to grow and develop when their stories and strengths, rather than their problems, are emphasized. Families in caregiving situations often express their burdens, but a strengths-based philosophy can help social workers reframe the burden of caregiving to explore the rewards.

Educators Define Our Purpose

Another way to think about helping caregivers is to refer to the curriculum study groups that defined the domain and purpose of the social work profession. In 1959, the Council on Social Work Education (CSWE) conducted a curriculum study and adopted the enhancement of social functioning as the profession's major goal (Boehm, 1959). *Social work* was defined as "a profession concerned with the restoration, maintenance and enhancement of social functioning. It contributes, with other professions and disciplines, to the prevention, treatment and control of problems in social functioning of individuals, groups and communities" (Boehm, 1959, p. 1). Because of its dual focus on individuals and society, the definition remains important to a social care model today. This focus allows the practitioner to seek out multilevel interventions that may enhance or maintain social functioning.

Defining Social Care in Direct Practice

Every society has a means of caring for its members. In fact, caregiving is at the heart of family, community, and societal functioning. Care provision is organized differently in every society depending on the roles of various institutions, individual and family responsibility, values and ethics, and economic and political considerations. As you read each chapter, you will see how the provision of care varies depending on such influences as family role allocation, societal epoch, and historical and economic factors.

Care is sometimes given without our even knowing it; at other times, giving care requires a great deal of effort and support and can cause considerable stress. Social workers generally see caregivers and their care recipients at times of distress—when people and institutions seem to be failing and caregivers are not receiving the support they need. The term "social care" is used during these times when social workers become part of the fabric of the social welfare system, taking action to ensure that people's basic needs are met. Therefore, social workers must be knowledgeable about the distinct systems that address client care needs—mental health, aging, and so forth—within the general social welfare system.

In Europe, Australia, and New Zealand, social care has various definitions, and it is sometimes seen as a profession distinct from social work (Lalor & Share, 2013). For example, the Irish Association of Social Care Educators defines social care as "a profession committed to planning and delivery of quality care and other support services for individuals and groups with identified needs" (Irish Social Care Gateway, 2005). The association's Web site goes on to state that social care workers give emphasis to those who have been marginalized—those who receive unequal resources or are the recipients of discrimination by society. Moreover, social care workers, often working in conjunction with social workers, advocate for interventions based on established best practices as well as knowledge of life-span development.

Social care is composed of those actions designed to provide people in need with access to the basic necessities of life. Social care workers offer clients, such as children and people who are dying, belonging, acceptance, and comfort in times of distress. They are also part of the health care delivery system, including midwifery. Social care workers take preventive actions as they work to improve social conditions and strive for social and economic justice (Sheafor et al., 2012) (see "Social Work as Social Care: A Micro Perspective" on page 6).

Work with Clients in Distress

Social care is suitable for people in distress; for those dealing with the effects of a natural disaster, such as Hurricanes Sandy and Katrina; and for veterans returning from war with adjustment issues (see chapter 7). In these cases, practitioners attempt to foster resilience by engaging in many strategies common to social care, including providing for basic needs, such as safety, food, water, and electricity; helping clients access their own resources; tapping the intrinsic worth and ability of each individual; offering group support; and engaging in community renewal strategies (Greene & Livingston, 2012).

Social care workers in the United Kingdom have taken a rights-based and solution-focused approach to meeting the social care needs of refugees and asylum seekers under duress. Their principles for practice include respect for cultural identity and the experience of migration, nondiscrimination and the promotion of equality, decision making that is timely and transparent and that involves the client,

Social Work as Social Care: A Micro Perspective

Social workers who emphasize the social care purpose of the profession are more likely to do the following:

- Reflect on their own ability to give care
- Encourage the client to express his or her own needs
- Work toward a client's positive social functioning
- Provide for basic needs
- Work at the center of a client's life space
- Research the needs of marginalized groups
- Advocate for caregiving policy
- Seek economic and social justice
- Attend to vulnerable populations
- Coordinate efforts with other agencies and professionals

and the promotion of social inclusion and independence (Department of Health, n.d.). Community-based meetings are held, as are individual counseling sessions.

Self-Reflection

Although it is beyond the scope of this chapter to distinguish social work from social care, two major elements of social care derived from postmodern theory are especially important:

1. The need for the practitioner to be self-reflective
2. The importance of interventions being pertinent and taking place in the client's day-to-day shared life experiences or space

What do postmodern thinkers mean when they ask practitioners to be self-reflective? A self-reflective stance involves critical thinking and the interpretation of complex situations (CSWE, 2008; Laird, 1993; Schon, 1983). Using this approach, knowledge is gained from clients' "lived experience" and from master practitioners (Weick, 1993). Therefore, reflective practitioners can learn at the local level, think within the larger sociopolitical context, and engage in lifetime learning (Schon, 1983).

Postmodern thinkers have proposed that individuals gain knowledge through social discourse within a particular historical and sociopolitical context (Greene, 2008a, 2008c). In addition, the postmodern practitioner's goal is to obtain client-generated meaning to enable a positive reframing of events (Duncan, Solovey, & Rusk, 1992). Clients' ability to re-create their life story or rename their problem is empowering (White & Epston, 1990). Thus, learning how the caregiving family perceives its own needs is paramount.

For example, Tony Stanley, a social worker from New Zealand, said that he had to deal with the discourse of risk with children every day (Stanley, 2007). He thus wanted to better understand how other social workers perceived and talked about the risks they faced in their work in child protection. What risks were children exposed to in abusive or neglectful families? How could practitioners determine a family's readiness to resume raising a child after the child had been in foster care?

To look into this dilemma, Stanley (2005) chose to conduct research for his doctoral dissertation, "Making Decisions: Social Work Processes and the Construction of Risk(s) in Child Protection." His findings were then taken to the Department of Child, Youth and Family Services, Aotearoa—New Zealand's statutory body of child protection—to help it legitimize its assessment decisions. Thus, self-reflection built knowledge to address everyday professional concerns as well as the well-being of individual clients.

Defining Community Practice in Care Provision

At the micro, or direct, level of care, interventions in a social care model emphasize the profession's central purpose of supporting social functioning and quality of living. Hands-on concern may be combined with efforts to advocate for just social service delivery systems (see "Social Work as Social Care: A Micro Perspective" on page 6 for a summary). The use of macro level principles is also warranted and is aimed at creating more comprehensive, accessible, and effective experiences within health and social programs and within the natural environments of families, such as neighborhoods and communities (see "Social Work as Social Care: A Macro Perspective" on page 8 for a summary).

Families live and function within the context of their neighborhoods and communities, and they integrate local resources into their caregiving responsibilities. Although the intervention approaches discussed previously are helpful in direct work with caregivers, the use of macro-focused interventions is also necessary. In addition, case management is an important social work role in care provision and is a practice intervention that includes both micro- and macro-focused approaches.

Building and Sustaining Community Partnerships

Because many systems are involved in the lives of caregivers, one important macropractice approach is linking together these disparate entities (Kropf, 2006). These community partnerships need to involve not only those who are in professional services, but also other groups, such as faith communities, businesses that want to retain employees who are providing care, and related organizations or services involved with individuals with disabilities or older adults (for example, funeral directors and public transportation services). Successful community partnerships have the following characteristics (Mizrahi & Rosenthal, 2001):

- *Conditions.* Partnerships need to focus on the right issues at the right time. Do any current issues hold a great deal of attention in the media? Are families concerned enough about particular issues to rally together for a united agenda?
- *Commitment.* Partnerships often involve a broad scope of interests. The people involved must be able to compromise and work together toward outcomes that are feasible, not simply ideal.
- *Contribution.* Those entities involved in the community partnership need to have a sense of how resources can be combined to attain goals. Some partners may have financial resources, whereas others may have social connections that can provide resources in the community and beyond.
- *Competence.* Although partnerships involve a shared sense of responsibility, there also needs to be leadership to handle internal dynamics and maintain goal direction.

Social Work as Social Care: A Macro Perspective

Social workers who emphasize the social care purpose of the profession are more likely to do the following:

- Focus on community capacity building:
  - What resources are available to families in caregiving roles?
  - What untapped or potential resources (for example, religious congregations or volunteer and civic organizations) are available?
  - What environmental opportunities (for example, good public transportation systems or good seasonal weather) are available to families?
- Partner with
  - local businesses to support the workforce with caregiving responsibilities
  - intergenerational programs to support caregiving across the generations (for example, through the Retired and Senior Volunteer Program and service learning projects in schools)
  - universities for demonstration projects and the evaluation of innovative practices
- Create linkages to
  - community coalitions to support care provision initiatives
  - public–private initiatives
  - media sources to raise awareness of local caregiving issues
- Seek funding and resource development
  - as joint collaborations across agencies that support family care
  - from local foundations and businesses that have a philanthropic mission compatible with care
  - to enhance the volunteer segment of caregiving and care sharing

Communication and facilitation skills are important in helping social workers develop and maintain effective community partnerships in caregiving.

Advocacy

According to the *Code of Ethics of the National Association of Social Workers* (NASW, 2008), one responsibility for ethical social work practice is to engage in social and political action. These efforts are aimed at providing access to rights and resources for those who are disenfranchised and expanding choice and opportunity for all. Because of conditions that precipitate the need for care provision, all social work practitioners must be involved as advocates in this area. Although evidence-based practice approaches are becoming a more central aspect of teaching practice skills, few studies have researched the effectiveness of macropractice skills (McNutt, 2011; Ohmer & Korr, 2006). Nevertheless, practitioners need to be able to advocate for individual clients within their practice. Through involvement in organizations such as NASW and similar professional societies, social workers can also participate in collective forms of advocacy that deal with policy-related issues.

Like direct practice interventions, advocacy practice involves particular skills and orientations. In their analysis of social advocacy roles, Schneider and Lester (2001) summarized the characteristics of advocacy practice. Working as advocates, practitioners are the following:

- *Action oriented.* Advocacy requires that social workers take action to bring about change. Advocacy is behavior, not simply an attitude.
- *Opposed to injustice.* Advocates are involved in promoting justice principles in meeting human needs.
- *Not neutral.* The values of the social work profession compel practitioners to side with those who are in disadvantaged, vulnerable, marginalized, or at-risk situations. The primary principle of social work is to enhance human well-being and promote the basic needs of all individuals.
- *Able to link policy to practice.* Clients' lives are directly related to decisions that are made at policy levels. Practice to address the immediate needs of clients is insufficient if broader social issues are not addressed.
- *Patient and hopeful.* According to Schneider and Lester (2001), drawing on Freire's (1990) principle of "impatient patience," advocates should be patient enough to sustain change but impatient enough to initiate movement. In this role, social workers' steady efforts in advocacy and activism provide a message of hope and involvement for their clients.
- *Empowering.* In their role as advocates, social workers try to develop the leadership and problem-solving capacities of their clients. They work to help clients develop roles that allow them to communicate for themselves as much as possible.

As this summary suggests, the primary role of most social workers may not be to serve as advocates for clients. However, all social workers should develop advocacy skills, as social justice issues are part of all practice contexts.

Case Management: Bridging Micro- and Macropractice

As an integrated practice approach, case management bridges micro- and macropractice roles. Case managers provide services to many types of caregiving families and often are the first point of contact for families as they enter service systems. Often case managers provide many different types of services, including linking families to resources, being the primary contact for families in interdisciplinary team approaches to treatment, and evaluating and measuring the success of treatment goals. Although case managers come from many backgrounds (for example, nursing and finance), their background in social work, with its person-in-environment framework, provides the requisite foundation for them to function effectively in their role (Rothman, 1994).

The aspect of case management that makes this role exciting also makes it challenging—it involves a broad spectrum of skills. To be competent in this role, case managers must be able to work directly with individuals, families, and the community and be competent advocates and change agents in social policy arenas. Several skills are important for effective case management practice (Greene, Cohen, Galambos, & Kropf, 2007):

- *Engaging in sensitive relationship building.* Case managers may intervene with clients during times of stress or transition. Regardless of the specific caregiving issue, case managers should assess what is happening with the client and family and determine the most effective way to build trust.
- *Delivering appropriate resources and services.* Beyond referring clients to existing programs, case managers must help motivate client involvement in services. In addition, they must be aware of barriers that may prevent clients from accessing services and work to eradicate these conditions.
- *Having a network of alliances.* Case managers need to have positive and extensive relationships with colleagues within the service system. Especially in areas where services are limited, such as rural communities, case managers need to go beyond the usual suspects in identifying potential resources (Myers, Kropf, & Robinson, 2002). They must investigate and approach nontraditional partners as possible collaborators in service delivery in these areas.
- *Constructing service plans.* Social workers in all roles are increasingly accountable for delivering cost-effective services. Case managers must be able to determine the needs of families and provide a plan to address these needs in an efficient manner.

- *Evaluating service delivery.* Case managers are pivotal in determining how changes in service delivery and policy affect the lives of clients. In this role, they can determine where gaps in services are and what changes need to be made to services to make them more effective and accessible for caregivers.
- *Acting as an advocate.* As previously discussed, advocacy is part of social work with caregivers. Within case management, advocacy roles are primary, as practitioners often act on behalf of clients who have limited skills or ability to act on their own (Frankl & Gelman, 1998).

Case management has been part of social work practice since the beginning of the profession. Because caregiving families often have multiple service needs, case managers are frequently involved in helping them access needed services. In this way, families receive the assistance and support they need to navigate disparate programs and service networks.

Application to Social Work Practice

Many social work practitioners are involved with families in their caregiving roles. Yet social workers are also involved as administrators of programs that serve caregiving families and promote mutual aid interventions in care provision. In addition, some social workers rise to the challenge of working to change social policy. For example, NASW (n.d.) lists 165 elected officials who hold a social work degree. Because of this breadth and scope of practice, social workers in various professional roles will face families in care provision situations.

Social Work Competencies Applied to Family Care

Regardless of one's level of practice (direct or indirect), CSWE has mandated a set of competencies that are the foundation for curricula in social work programs (CSWE, 2012, pp. 3–7). The following are the 10 competency statements as they apply to caregiving circumstances:

1. *Identify as a professional social worker and conduct oneself accordingly.* When working with families in vulnerable states, social workers need to maintain professional roles, boundaries, and standards of practice. Practitioners might experience countertransference and should seek appropriate supervision or consultation to remain effective. While reading this book, you will be able to identify the issues in family caregiving that may present difficulties using experiences from your family life.
2. *Apply social work ethical principles to guide professional practice.* Care provision often involves various ethical issues, as often no ideal standard or outcome is possible. For example, consider the out-of-home placement decisions that child protective services workers have to make. Although the

family is the best place for a child, child protective services workers must be able to assess the family environment and make decisions about whether this situation is adequate for children. Adult protective services workers make similar decisions about adults with disabilities. In their work with families, social workers must be able to engage in appropriate decision making in planning interventions and services. This book highlights various professional and ethical dilemmas to demonstrate the practice considerations in family care situations.

3. *Apply critical thinking to inform and communicate professional judgments.* Social workers need to have good communication skills in order to relate to diverse family systems. In addition, practice in this area is inherently multidisciplinary, and social workers need to be able to practice and communicate with colleagues of other professions. Critical thinking is vastly important, as practitioners will need to assess individuals within the family as well as the family as a functioning whole. Thus, knowledge and understanding of various theoretical perspectives is required. Theories and models of family and individual functioning are part of this book.

4. *Engage diversity and difference in practice.* Families have particular cultural and value perspectives. In addition, cultural contexts also affect caregiving within the family. Because caregiving involves personal decisions within families, practitioners will need to assess and intervene in culturally competent ways. The situations presented in this book include multicultural issues within family life.

5. *Advance human rights and social and economic justice.* As discussed, caregiving is a shared experience, as health and social programs, policies, and resource allocation affect the ability of families to provide care. Oppressive structures and regulations hinder this ability and create stress in the family. One example is the current health care structure in the United States, which saddles families with many of the costs of care. This book considers these situations and discusses possible roles for social workers advocating for economic and social justice in these areas.

6. *Apply knowledge of human behavior and the social environment.* The person-in-environment framework provides the lens through which family caregiving is presented here. Family care includes a number of subsystems as well, such as the caregiver–care recipient dyad, couple and marital relationships, and relationships with children and grandchildren. In addition, it is critical to understand the relationships of the family to other systems in the environment. The chapters in this book highlight these connections and provide knowledge about family care at different times in the life course.

7. *Engage in research-informed practice and practice-informed research.* In this book, evidence-based practice interventions are included for areas with a

sufficient literature on interventions and programs. To be an effective practitioner, you need to know which interventions are effective in addressing
issues of family care.

8. *Engage in policy practice to advance social and economic well-being and to
deliver effective social work services.* Policies can either support families in
their caregiving roles or create challenges for them. This book includes
examples of contextual issues that affect family care experiences.

9. *Respond to contexts that shape practice.* Social conditions affect care provision and the impact of care on families. For example, the number of military veterans returning from combat with physical and emotional wounds
has created a new context for care provision. Likewise, the prominence of
grandparent-headed families, another care configuration, has increased
over recent years. These types of care arrangements have prompted new
social policy and practice methods to be more responsive to the needs of
these families.

10. *Engage, assess, intervene, and evaluate with individuals, families, groups, organizations, and communities.* To be an effective practitioner, you must analyze
various assessment and intervention approaches for work with diverse family forms. Practice at different system levels, from the individual level to the
community level, is explored and discussed.

These competencies are addressed throughout this book. Across the life course,
people will need assistance from social workers in making decisions, dealing with
stressful situations, and accessing appropriate resources. In addition, practitioners
will need to assume more macro-focused roles to advocate for resources and to
address gaps in health and social welfare policies. Finally, practitioners also need
skills in researching effective interventions, as well as constructing well-designed
needs assessments.

Specialized Curriculum Content

To be effective in working with caregiving families, social workers should be
exposed to specialized content that will help broaden their perspective on caregiving and care sharing. For example, they will need to become cognizant of medical
terminology in their specific area as well as of biomedical concerns. They also need
to be aware of palliative care opportunities (Chang et al., 2012). *Palliative care* is
relieving the symptoms of an illness, pain, and stress rather than using aggressive
treatments. Patients who are informed may choose the palliative care option at any
time in treatment, not only at the end of life (personal communication with A. L.
Greene, MD, St. Vincent Anderson Regional Hospital, Anderson, IN, April 2013).
Palliative care is one type of care-sharing service that assists families with health
and end-of-life issues.

End-of-life issues may present challenging circumstances within family care-giving. When care providers reach the end of their lives, questions emerge about future care arrangements and needs. If the person needing hospice or palliative care is the care recipient, additional complexities arise. For example, end-of-life care for adults with severe mental illness is often difficult to access owing to a lack of coordination between health care and mental health programs (Cummings & Kropf, 2011). Certainly, end-of-life situations demand family resources and can dramatically affect the future structure of care.

In addition, social care workers may need training for working on multidisci-plinary teams. A *multidisciplinary approach* to health care involves an integrative team of medical and allied health professionals who work together to create and advance a patient's care plan. A team may be involved, for example, in planning a patient's treatment and quality of life following a breast cancer diagnosis. The social care worker in this case would focus on the psychosocial factors that accompany health concerns. Other examples of social workers' participating in multidisci-plinary teams are discussed in the following chapters.

A final area of specialized content in this book is caring for the caregivers them-selves. Although social work services may be focused on the person with the illness or functional limitation, caregiving itself can also be stressful and require a tre-mendous amount of energy. Learning about caregiving must include understand-ing how to support the care providers. Depending on the context of care and the circumstances of the care provider, supports may take quite different forms and focus on different aspects of care. For example, older care providers of adults with lifelong disabilities may find the transition out of their care provision role stressful (see, for example, Kelly & Kropf, 1995). In this circumstance, a social worker must help the care providers create new opportunities and connections as they transition away from their caregiving role.

In sum, we have presented all of the CSWE (2012) competencies to be used in conjunction with our caregiving model. These competencies constitute the domain of social work and address all of the knowledge and skills needed for effective social work practice. The ultimate goal of this all-encompassing model is to encourage interventions that enhance social functioning (Dolgoff & Feldstein, 2008; Sheafor et al., 2010; see also chapter 2).

CHAPTER TWO

Changing Families

Chapter 1 introduced you to the assumptions of social care, an approach to social work in which the social worker assesses the context of practice, enhances social functioning, uses a more hands-on approach, and integrates micro and macro levels of practice. This chapter explores the changing nature of family life and shifting patterns of family structure and organization, communication, socialization, and belief systems. It introduces societal and institutional transformations that accompany everyday family circumstances and necessitate the evolution of professional social work tasks related to care provision. Current research and media commentary inform our understanding of the changing society in which we live and deliver services. These complex familial and societal transitions are examined as they relate to fostering positive day-to-day caregiving situations.

Overview of Changing Family Caregiving Configurations

As we begin the journey to explore family caregiving and care sharing, it is helpful to look at some examples of experiences in care provision. The experiences of various families are discussed in greater detail in the following chapters. As a starting point, however, this section provides a brief overview to help you begin to conceptualize the experience of care across a variety of historical contexts and family configurations.

Nurturing and Caring

Regardless of the culture, one of the common functions of the family is to provide nurturing and caring for its members. In the contemporary United States, we often think about caring from an emotional perspective; that is, we care about those we love. Traditional wedding vows embody this concept, as spouses-to-be pledge to love and cherish each other in good times and bad and declare their devotion for better or for worse, for richer or for poorer, in sickness and in health. In other words, these partners for life proclaim both love and care for each other. Models of care would be shallow if they did not address the family as both a "social and emotional unit" (Ackerman, 1970, p. 14).

Yet family life was not always based on the emotional bonds of love and affection. In *Marriage, a History*, Stephanie Coontz (2006) traces the evolution of marriage from ancient to modern times. Her narrative discusses the varied reasons why marriages have happened, including to merge families' resources for economic gains, to keep peace among warring tribes, and to create labor through bearing children. Although these earlier motivations for marriage were not based on romantic love, a sense of care was embedded in marital decisions. The joining of husband and wife functioned to meet the needs of families based on the needs of the society at the time. In other words, the man and woman were taking care of their families by partnering and joining together in marriage.

In current American society, people typically choose to marry or live together because of romantic love. However, family forms continue to evolve and change, and as a result, the aspect of caring within family life has also shifted. Several significant trends are creating different caregiving roles within families, as well as new configurations to meet the care needs of family members. Many times, families come to the attention of social work practitioners because of issues or needs related to support and care provision.

It is important that social workers know about needs, resources, and cultural values when working with diverse families; sometimes advocacy may come into play. For example, although same-sex marriage remains a controversial issue in some states, many other states have given legislative approval to these diverse family forms following years of advocacy by gay rights activists. Older lesbian, gay, bisexual, and transgender (LGBT) individuals may have extensive care-sharing networks that include individuals who are not related by blood (Hash & Netting, 2009). Examples of these individuals include friends, ex-partners, and other LGBT individuals. Although some LGBT individuals do receive care from family members, a high level of mutual aid exists in these care networks.

Demographic Shifts

Another trend in care is the ever-shifting demographic makeup of the population as a result of extended life expectancies. In 2010, 13 percent of the population was 65 or older (U.S. Census Bureau, 2010a). With the aging of the baby boom generation (that is, those individuals who were born between 1946 and 1964), this number is expected to double in the coming decades. It is estimated that by 2050, individuals older than 65 will make up 25 percent of the U.S. population. In addition, life spans are increasing, which means that older adults will live longer. The fastest growing segment of the 65-plus population is individuals older than 85 (Federal Interagency Forum on Aging Related Statistics, 2012).

Shifting Family Structure

Yet another population trend involves the changing structure of family life. Birth and pregnancy rates have changed, and this has resulted in different generational configurations within families. Baby boomer families tended to have a pyramid shape; that is, there were many children, two parents, and perhaps a grandparent or two. An issue of the *National Vital Statistics Reports* (Ventura, Curtin, Abma, & Henshaw, 2012) summarizes several changes in pregnancy and birthrates from 1990 to 2008. Except among women in their 30s and early 40s, pregnancy rates have decreased among all races, ethnicities, and age groups. In addition, the teenage pregnancy rate is the lowest it has been since 1976. This report indicates that these changes are associated with changing patterns in sexual activity; differences in marriage, divorce, and cohabitation; changes in contraceptive methods and their effectiveness; and changing social and economic decisions about childbearing. These factors influence the shape and dynamics of contemporary family life.

Diverse Composition

The current family is also diverse in its composition and characteristics (for example, in terms of stepparents, single parents, blended families). Instead of a pyramid, the family of today looks more like a beanpole: fewer children, variability in the number of parents (for example, a single parent, a couple, stepparents), grandparents, and quite possibly, great-grandparents (see Bengtson, Rosenthal, & Burton, 1990). Over the past few decades, the shape of family systems and membership within those systems has changed dramatically.

From a caregiving perspective, these changes mean that families are facing ever more complex issues. With the greater number of older adults, families can expect to assume some amount of care for older members. In some cases, members of more than one generation are in late life at the same time, which creates multiple caregiving situations. Furthermore, there are fewer members of younger generations to assume the tasks associated with care. Finally, diversity in family forms is a part of caregiving. Diversity might yield resources for the family, such as a greater number of people who are part of a care team. However, it can also result in complexities, such as adult children having to negotiate with a new spouse or partner of their older parent.

Communal Care

In the United States, most care is provided within the family. Although some cultures raise children more communally (Ochs & Izquierdo, 2009), the family is the source of nurturing and guidance for most children. In addition, gerontologists have long held the view that the long-term care system in the United States is one of family, friends, and other informal supports (Greene, 2005a). That is, the majority of older adults receive assistance from these individuals and not from those in professional helping roles.

As already noted, caregiving is inherently a shared responsibility. To provide care, families must interface with various social systems. For example, children attend school, join scout troops and clubs, go to day care, and participate in religious activities. In all of these situations, parents place their trust in other adults to uphold the welfare of their children. Although families have primary responsibility for caring for children, numerous social institutions are involved in care-sharing roles.

This is also true for adult care, as families have connections with agencies and staff that are part of a care management system. For some adults, the need for care is based on physical, emotional, or cognitive challenges. In these situations, families will have relationships with health and social welfare services. Unfortunately, these networks are often quite different from one another, which can be complicated and frustrating for families. Consider the situation of a person with a chronic mental illness. In addition to the mental health system, the family may have to be involved with health care providers, the Social Security Administration (for disability payments), and possibly residential service staff. Research on family connection with these services indicates that working with disparate staff and professionals is a significant source of stress for families (Cummings & Kropf, 2011). This is in addition to the stress of dealing with the challenges of the mental illness itself.

Caring across the Life Course

This book addresses numerous issues involved in caregiving and care sharing across the life course. Many social work roles deal with issues of caregiving and care sharing, and practitioners in multiple service sectors are involved in this work. The purpose of this book is to provide a framework for understanding caregiving and care sharing and to offer the perspectives of several configurations of families as they interface with health and social service agencies and other social systems. Although the focus is on caregiving within families, the person-in-environment perspective is used to look contextually at families and their responsibilities and to develop practices based on the family–health–social services interface.

Parenting Situations

Being a parent can be stressful, regardless of the specific circumstances. Bringing home a newborn changes a family's life and experience in many ways. Parents have to revise their expectations for how they spend time, money, and energy. During parenthood, energy that once flowed outside the family to leisure pursuits, employment, and other activities is needed inside the family. Parents are required to attend to frequent feedings, soothe crying spells, and spend time getting to know their baby. In addition, changes also take place as other family members, such as siblings and grandparents, accommodate the new addition to the family system. Even the joy of having a new child precipitates a series of changes within families.

Some families experience additional responsibilities and transitions as a result of child care. Families that have a child with a disability often must interact with additional service providers. A child with medical needs, for example, may need to be hospitalized or have medical procedures, which creates emotional and financial stress for families. Caring for children with intellectual disabilities or psychiatric conditions can also be challenging for families and parents. The following is an example of a family that includes a young child with a disability:

> Mr. and Mrs. H have three children. Their youngest child, Jason, is three years old and has been diagnosed with intellectual disability. Jason is nonverbal and does not interact with the Hs' other two children. Mr. and Mrs. H have always considered Jason to be a "difficult" baby. He did not begin to make sounds (for example, gurgling and cooing) like their other children. In addition, he would cry for extended periods and could not be comforted. Mrs. H has had to quit her job as a teacher because the family has not been able to find acceptable day care to meet Jason's needs. Jason's care has created additional stress within the family, and the other children have started acting out at school. Mr. and Mrs. H's marriage has also become more stressful, as the financial strain of raising three children on one income has increased the tension in the household.

The H family faces numerous challenges as a result of Jason's diagnosis. Part of an effective social work assessment of the family is taking note of at what point in the life course caregiving is taking place. This family is in the process of re-creating a family structure, adding a child who has particular care needs. The experience of this young family is different from the experience of a family later in the life course, for whom services and social and cultural assumptions about disabilities are vastly different.

In this example, the social worker needs to be aware of changes that have taken place in medical technology and service delivery for children with disabilities. Years ago, children with disabilities often did not live past childhood, and if they did, medical professionals commonly advised parents to have the child reside in an institution. Often the residents lived in horrific conditions, as chronicled in the seminal photographic essay "Christmas in Purgatory" (Blatt & Kaplan, 1966). The atrocities (for example, cramped living spaces, lack of stimulation and interaction, and poor quality of care) pictured in this work were credited with raising awareness of the conditions in institutional settings and helping to bring about changes in disability services. Although significant improvements, such as implementing a more consumer-oriented and community-based approach to services, have since been made, these changes did not take place overnight. Many families today have members with disabilities who have spent time living in institutional settings. Knowing about this changing context is important for understanding the experiences and care needs of this population.

In connecting the example of the H family to practice competencies, a social worker would need to have skills to

- assess the family situation by listening to its story, including the level of change and transition that has taken place as a result of having a child with a disability
- identify and help the family access needed resources
- be an advocate for programs and policies that provide families raising children with disabilities the services they need to function
- assist the family with developing caregiving competencies for a child with special needs

These examples show how some competencies match with the special transitions that the H family is experiencing as they raise a child with an intellectual disability.

Midlife Caregiving Issues

Whereas for some families midlife is a time to relinquish responsibilities for caring for children who are approaching adulthood, other families continue or assume new caregiving tasks. For families with sons and daughters with disabilities, midlife is a time when qualitative shifts in care may require additional resources and tasks. For example, children with disabilities are entitled to educational services but may have few program options when they graduate from school. If they are unable to find or retain employment, they have few other possibilities to pursue. In these cases, families may be the primary or sole source of care and social contact. This situation can limit opportunities pursued by other family members, such as accepting more responsibility at work.

At midlife, families potentially face other situations that require that they care for one of their members. For example, trauma from violence, auto or other accidents, or military service can render adults in need of support and care. At this point in the life course, families have to deal with the experience of the changed member; for example, someone who was previously independent in activities of daily living may now need assistance in a variety of functions. One high-profile example of this is the experience of Gabrielle Giffords, a congresswoman from Arizona who was critically wounded in an assassination attempt in 2011. The resulting injuries had marked effects on her physical and functional abilities, and as a result, she was forced to relinquish her elected position in Congress. She and her astronaut husband, Mark Kelly, have talked candidly about some of the challenges that their family has faced with her convalescence and changes in abilities.

As another example, soldiers who return from military duty may have physical and emotional wounds that require care and support. In 2012, the number of U.S. soldiers who were wounded in Iraq and Afghanistan totaled more than 49,000 (Iraq Coalition Casualty Count, n.d.). These men and women often return home with physical and emotional wounds, and spouses, partners, parents, and siblings must become acquainted with the changes in their loved one. This task can be complex, as functional and personality changes can accompany scars from military combat. In many cases, families must establish a new relationship with an individual who has changed physically or emotionally.

Care needs are different for today's returning military because of the nature of wounds caused from explosions. Although service personnel may be very seriously injured, they are likely to survive from wounds that would have been lethal in previous conflicts. However, less is known about the care of service members. The need for social workers in this practice area has increased dramatically, as evidenced by the NASW collaboration with the Joining Forces initiative. Started by Michelle Obama and Jill Biden, Joining Forces aims to provide more care for veterans, with NASW offering free online courses on military culture, advocacy, direct practice, cultural competency, and standards review (Clayton, 2012). Consider the following example:

> Private M, a veteran of the Iraq War, was deployed to active combat on two missions. During his second mission, he was severally wounded by a grenade and lost both of his legs. After a lengthy stay in a Department of Veterans Affairs facility, he was fitted with prostheses and returned to his home in a southern state. Private M is 27 years old and the father of a young daughter who was born during his second tour. His wife, age 24, has a high school education and works as a beautician in their small town. She has filed for divorce, as she is unable to handle his volatile mood swings. As a result, he has been living with his parents in a basement apartment of their house in a small rural community with few services for veterans. Private M's parents have become increasingly worried about him, as they hear loud music at all hours of the night and are aware that he is drinking heavily. More than his physical condition, the family is very concerned about his emotional state and his inability to retain employment.

This case exemplifies the complexity of physical and emotional trauma that results from military service. At this point, Private M's psychological needs are more extensive than the physical challenges he has faced. The family has lost the young soldier who went off to war and is now struggling to accept the one who has returned; the returning soldier himself may have lost his sense of identity. Often it is harder for families to face the emotional scars than the physical ones, especially when there are few avenues for help.

In Private M's case, the social worker has to integrate several practice competencies, including the ability to evaluate, if not resolve, the complex ethical dilemma involved in a case resulting from a client's voluntary military service and subsequent lack of access to comprehensive behavioral health services. How would you as a social worker resolve your frustrations about the dearth of available medical and behavioral resources?

Family of Later Years

The aging of the baby boom generation and the expected increase in the number of older adults create additional concerns about the availability of sufficient caregiving resources. Adults older than 65 are expected to represent 19.3 percent of the U.S. population by 2030; at the same time, there will be 70 million older adults, more than twice the number in 1999 (Administration on Aging [AOA], 2011).

Greene (2005a) described how family characteristics differ among the baby boomer generation and noted that these changes may influence caregiving patterns:

> Baby boomers have the highest rates of postponing marriage, a smaller family size, more dual-career marriages, and higher rates of preventing pregnancy and getting divorced. In addition, there are more single parents and blended households. Furthermore, baby boomers will have a smaller pool of family members due to falling birth rates. These changes will require a reexamination of caregiving distributions to meet the changes in household, family, and kinship arrangements. (p. 112)

Most families can expect to assume care for an older family member at some point in the life course. However, a common myth about social policy is that Medicare and Social Security cover the majority of care costs during later life. The reality is that even with these entitlement programs, the costs of care are great for families. The lifetime income-related losses sustained by family caregivers 50 and older who leave the workforce to care for a parent are estimated at $115,900 in wages, $137,980 in Social Security benefits, and conservatively $50,000 in pension benefits (MetLife Mature Market Institute, 2011). Clearly, families absorb much of the cost of care and, in so doing, decrease their own stores of resources for later life.

Because the population is aging so rapidly, the number of older adults who are frail and in need of support may outpace the number of formal professional care providers available. This means that social workers will have to modify their services with a form of triage, assessing which older adults have the least and the greatest functional capacity (Vourlekis & Greene, 1992). They would also have to provide or help access wellness programs, preventive services, and care-sharing arrangements.

Although they themselves may need assistance, significant numbers of older adults provide care to younger family members. With the help of community-based services, family members may provide care to adults with intellectual and psychiatric conditions across the life course. Some grandparents also provide care for their grandchildren (see chapter 9). About 4.9 million grandparents are responsible for raising one or more grandchildren within the same household (Goyer, 2010). In addition, about 15 percent of grandparents in a custodial role are older than 70 (Fields, O'Connell, & Downs, 2001), meaning they are raising children significantly beyond the usual time frame for this role. As the following case study illustrates, the responsibility of raising grandchildren is challenging, especially when one is also facing physical and functional age–related changes:

> Mrs. W is a 67-year-old widow who is raising two of her grandchildren, ages five and seven. Her daughter is addicted to drugs and alcohol and has not been in contact with her children in about two years. Although Mrs. W. loves her grandchildren, they both have special needs that resulted from her daughter's substance abuse during pregnancy and neglect during their first few years of life. This situation makes Mrs. W's single grandparenting quite challenging, and her own health has worsened since she assumed care. Mrs. W cannot imagine having her grandchildren go into foster care, and kin keeping is a major motivating factor for her. However, her most recent checkup indicated that her blood pressure has increased and that she is a Type II diabetic. She tearfully confessed to her physician that she had no idea what would happen to her grandbabies if something happened to her.

This situation exemplifies the complexities faced by custodial grandparents. Often the grandparent will sacrifice his or her own health to care for the children. In addition, the family dynamics are usually complex, as illustrated by this situation with an addicted parent.

With regard to the practice competencies, practitioners need to have several skills to work with these types of caregiving families. These include the ability to

- listen to the family's story a propos to their life course development
- assess the intergenerational issues that are part of the family constellation
- advocate for intergenerational programs and services to support older care providers, including custodial grandparents, in their roles
- establish linkage and referral services to appropriate health, educational, and aging services

As the number of older adults continues to increase, more and more caregivers will be in later life themselves. In addition to understanding how caregiving affects younger generations who care for older adults, social workers need to have a greater awareness of the roles assumed by older adults who provide care.

Creating Your Caregiving Model

The following chapters present current challenges facing social workers who are providing help to increasingly vulnerable populations that require care. As we describe these various caregiving situations, it is important that we consider which theoretical frameworks need to be emphasized and which newer ideas, concepts, and research need to be explored.

There is an abundance of social work practice theories from which to draw a caregiving model (see chapter 3). Of course, whenever possible, we want to use theories that are supported by empirical findings. But how will we come to an individualized client-centered approach? In general, some theories suggest that problems are related to emotional difficulties in the individual, necessitating intrapsychic or cognitive interventions, whereas others imply that problems reside within the environment, requiring institutional reform and adequate resources.

Moreover, there is still another debate about which practice settings are clinical in nature (that is, which client populations should receive counseling or therapy and which should be given supportive, concrete, or tangible services). For example, revised instructions for clinical supervision and clinical supervision plans from the Texas Social Work Licensing Board dated March 1, 2012, contained information that inappropriately generalized the following settings as nonclinical: schools, medical venues, and employee assistance programs. In a document titled "A Review of Clinical Supervision Plan Approval Criteria" authored by Carol Miller and obtained via Open Records Request, additional settings are indicated as "generally not considered clinical," including child placement agencies, adoption services, and nursing homes (Texas Department of State Health Services, 2012).

As social workers decide on the most promising theory base, it is best that they not debate these false dichotomies. Rather, practitioners will want to develop an integrated approach based on client-centered assessment. They and the client must consider their course of action and philosophy of practice. As we review caregiving models, we will ask the following:

- How do we define the purpose of our profession as it relates to caregiving needs?
- What theoretical constructs remain constant and applicable to caregiving models?
- Can we retain our core professional values that seek social and economic justice, the prevention of conditions that limit human rights, the elimination of poverty, and the enhancement of the quality of life of all people even as they come to need care?
- Can we ease the telling of the client's story?
- How do we involve our clients and empower them in their own care?
- How do we create practice strategies that recognize, support, and build on the strengths and resiliency of all human beings, especially those who are vulnerable or in need of our assistance?

- What caregiving strategies are useful? Are certain interventions most pertinent to current caregiving needs?

In summary, this chapter has explored why we need to revisit and redefine some of our professional tasks so that we can remain grounded and ready to serve clients during turbulent times. Furthermore, it has suggested that social workers continue to use select tried and true constructs while reclaiming or adopting elements of social care, an emerging approach to service delivery and care in Europe, Australia, and New Zealand.

Finally, we suggest you use this book to create your own model of care that stems from a strengths-based, resilience perspective. To construct your own resilience-enhancing model, do the following:

- Consider the current cultural milieu, including the historical time, government policy, and worldview. What will influence our ability to support those who need our help? How have these factors influenced family configurations (see chapter 1)?
- Build on social work's core principles of respect for diversity, appreciation of values and ethics, and commitment to professional purpose. Can we successfully translate our models to serve diverse populations? With increased demands on families and their social workers, will we be true to our mission?
- Understand risk and resilience research, which provides empirical support and practice implications. Are we proficient at understanding and applying research?
- Appreciate the assumptions of risk and resilience theory, which augments the theoretical context for the practice models. Will we master the knowledge and skills to make us competent in the helping relationship?
- Decide what best practices you want to adopt. Can we attain a sense of self-efficacy about our own professional decision-making capabilities?
- Select various change strategies, engaging multiple schools of thought and associated techniques. Have we become critical thinkers who can select interventions that match the client's self-identified needs?
- Choose methods that enhance resilience. Will we be able to appreciate client strengths?
- Review existing programs and learn about current interventions. Can we affect formal policy initiatives so that they support informal care?

The next chapter provides further information on theoretical assessment and intervention strategies to help you create your model.

CHAPTER THREE

Theory for Care:
Integrating Your Caregiving Model

This chapter presents concepts that will help you construct an integrated model in which the social worker enhances social functioning, uses a more hands-on approach, and integrates micro and macro levels of practice. Such a model synthesizes multifaceted theoretical frameworks of human behavior and practice from the structural and postmodern points of view (see Greene, 2008a). It assumes that caregiving *structures* allow the social worker to act as a case manager to coordinate care. At the same time, the social worker influences dialogue, attending to meaning making in participants' collective narratives. In this way, the voices of all care participants are heard and the meaning of care is uncovered.

This approach involves the use of two *paradigms*, or perceptions of reality. *Modernists*, or *positivists*, emphasize the scientific method, whereas *postmodernists* give less credence to scientists' ability to discover the ultimate truth. Rather, postmodern theorists discuss art, intuition, spirituality, and the creation of meaning in a cultural, historical, and sociopolitical context (Weick, 1993). Consequently, the social worker may consider using both traditional structural theories and postmodern narrative techniques.

The model of practice presented here brings together the historical elements of case management: direct and indirect practice. In addition, the social care approach to caregiving is distinguished by its attention to the social, cultural, political, historical, and geographic narrative of each participant included in the sphere of care. That is, the key to the model is the social worker's ability to collect each participant's narrative or story. In this way, the practitioner learns about the strengths and challenges faced by all participants and develops a plan of action, providing for a rich assessment and intervention arrangement with individuals, families, and communities engaged in care provision.

The emphasis is on family-centered assessment and interventions and their augmentation by community assets and collective efficacy. Emerging caregiving strategies to complement the model are discussed. A case study is presented so that you can envision working with theories at the micro, meso, and macro levels.

The Ecological Perspective

Ecological theory relevant to caregiving situations begins with the concepts of person-in-environment, the flow of stress through the family, person–environment fit, and the life course. Knowledge of these concepts allows the social worker to understand and assess clients from a holistic point of view.

Bronfenbrenner: A Human Development Model

Bronfenbrenner's (1979) model of human development depicts the multiple levels of the ecological environment and is conceived as "a set of nested structures, each inside the next, like a set of Russian dolls" (p. 22) (see Figure 3.1).

FIGURE 3.1
Bronfenbrenner's Model of the Ecology of Human Development

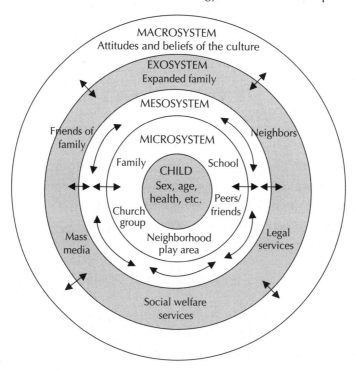

Source: Adapted from *Children and Families in the Environment* (p. 648), by J. Garbarino, 1982, New York: Aldine de Gruyter.

Bronfenbrenner (1990) identified four levels of systems, all of which concern different aspects of social care:

1. A *microsystem* is composed of a pattern of activities and roles and interpersonal face-to-face relations in the immediate setting, such as the family. Micro level family caregiving, often called "informal care," is the most prevalent type of care. It may include shopping for or bathing family members or trying to ensure their physical safety within the home. A family member or friend may search for programs or benefits that an individual is entitled to receive.

2. A *mesosystem* encompasses the linkages and processes that occur between two or more settings containing the (developing) person, such as schools and the family. Schools increasingly supply meals for children living in poverty as well as before- and after-school care for children with working parents, and teachers often identify vulnerable children. School programs are often shaped and funded by federal mandates.

3. An *exosystem* involves the linkages and processes that occur between two or more settings, at least one of which does not ordinarily contain the developing person, such as the parents' workplaces. Many workplaces now offer employee assistance programs and benefits for child care and eldercare. Evolving federal laws and regulations can require workplace equity and address disparities between the labor force experiences of members of designated groups (for example, women, minorities, and people with disabilities).

4. A *macrosystem* consists of the overarching patterns of a given culture or a broader social and political context, such as an ethnic group system. Social welfare policy is framed at the macro level and shapes much of the assistance available at the local level.

Consequently, it can be said that many societal institutions—hospitals, nursing homes, day care centers—are concerned with providing social care. The social worker's task—in collaboration with the client—is to assess where the best interventions to improve social functioning may be carried out.

Flow of Stress through the Family

Families face different challenges and experience stress in different ways as they interact with other social systems. This is important to remember when you are providing social care; you must understand what contributes to a particular family's challenges. To better explain the stress families may experience, Carter and McGoldrick (2005) developed a schema based on an ecological design—an ever-widening environment of concentric circles that surround the individual, moving from the nearest to the most remote (see Figure 3.2). The schema shows the horizontal and vertical stressors that can negatively affect individuals, the extended family, the community, and the larger society.

FIGURE 3.2
Flow of Stress through the Family

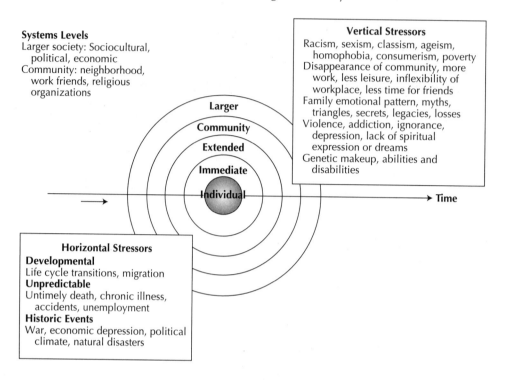

Systems Levels
Larger society: Sociocultural,
   political, economic
Community: neighborhood,
   work friends, religious
   organizations

Vertical Stressors
Racism, sexism, classism, ageism,
   homophobia, consumerism, poverty
Disappearance of community, more
   work, less leisure, inflexibility of
   workplace, less time for friends
Family emotional pattern, myths,
   triangles, secrets, legacies, losses
Violence, addiction, ignorance,
   depression, lack of spiritual
   expression or dreams
Genetic makeup, abilities and
   disabilities

Larger

Community

Extended

Immediate

Individual

→ Time

Horizontal Stressors
Developmental
Life cycle transitions, migration
Unpredictable
Untimely death, chronic illness,
   accidents, unemployment
Historic Events
War, economic depression, political
   climate, natural disasters

Source: Adapted from *The Expanded Family Life Cycle: Individual, Family, and Social Perspectives,* 3rd ed. (p. 27), edited by B. Carter and M. McGoldrick, 1999, Boston: Allyn & Bacon.

The schema in Figure 3.2 can be understood by tracing the horizontal axis (representing time) and the vertical axis (representing social systems of various size). Horizontal stressors depicted on the schema include

- developmental events, such as life-cycle transitions and migration
- unpredictable events, such as the untimely death of a friend or family member, chronic illness, accident, and unemployment
- historical events, such as war, economic depression, political climate, and natural disasters

Vertical stressors include

- racism, sexism, classism, ageism, consumerism, and poverty
- the disappearance of community, more work, less leisure, the inflexibility of the workplace, and lack of time for friends
- family emotional patterns, myths, triangles, secrets, legacies, and losses

- violence, addictions, ignorance, depression, and lack of spiritual expression or dreams
- genetic makeup, abilities, and disabilities

You can use the schema in Figure 3.2 to examine issues in your own family that may stand in your way of providing care. Or it may help you ask the following assessment questions about a client: Does the caregiver face poverty or unemployment? Is the care recipient a member of a stigmatized group? How has the family coped with additional caregiving responsibilities? Identifying the family's experience of stress is essential to social care.

Stress Research

A great deal of attention has recently been paid to the reasons for and consequences of stress on individuals, families, and communities. The American Psychological Association (APA, 2010) surveyed more than 1,000 people about family stress. Causes of stress mentioned by respondents (in descending order) included work (74 percent), money (73 percent), the economy (69 percent), family responsibilities (60 percent), relationships (59 percent), personal health concerns (55 percent), health problems affecting one's family (55 percent), housing costs (51 percent), job stability (42 percent), and personal safety (31 percent) (p. 8; see also APA, 2012).

The report *Stress in America*

> paints a picture of an overstressed nation. Feeling the effects of prolonged financial and other recession-related difficulties, Americans are struggling to balance work and home life and make time to engage in healthy behaviors, with stress not only taking toll on their personal physical health, but also affecting the emotional and physical well-being of their families. (APA, 2012, p. 5)

A review of online resources indicates the extent to which all Americans live in relatively stressful environments. For example, the *New York Times* (n.d.) has created a health guide to stress and anxiety, and the Mayo Clinic (2013) has a Web page titled *Stress Management: Know Your Triggers*. Bear in mind that we as social workers may experience and need to attend to our own life stresses. In addition, we may have to teach caregivers self-care practices.

Person–Environment Fit

Because families experience stress from multiple sources, a caregiving model must include an evaluation of person–environment fit. Assessing a family's person–environment fit over time allows the social worker to determine *goodness of fit*, or the extent to which there is a nurturing or positive match between an individual's adaptive needs and the qualities of the environment. Goodness of fit provides insight into the structural reasons for a sense of well-being or lack thereof. Multilevel interventions may be required for those living in harsh or oppressive environments.

Appraisal of Life Stressors

Social workers must consider the client family's point of view when determining whether an environment is nurturing. A person's individual appraisal of an event determines whether it is a *life stressor*, or something perceived to potentially trigger harm or loss. Stress is not simply a matter of responding to negative environmental stimuli. Rather, people determine stressors through a subjective, cognitive process of appraising stimuli, including caregiving.

The first step in this process is *primary appraisal*, or an evaluation of the potential threat. What is the significance of the event? Is it controllable or challenging? The *secondary appraisal* involves thinking about the coping mechanisms and resources available to deal with the situation. At this point, the person decides what is at stake and what can be done. This appraisal involves the way the person construes the event. What does he or she make of it? The meaning of the event shapes the emotional and behavioral response to it (Lazarus & Folkman, 1984).

An assessment of caregiver burden is an evaluation of the extent of emotional stress brought about by caregiving or the degree of strain on the caregiver. For example, caregivers may feel resentful of the many demands placed on them or may experience a loss of friends and leisure time (Zarit, Reever, & Bach-Peterson, 1980). Stressors may also include the fear of losing employment or missing days at work or the feeling of being trapped by the relative's illness.

In addition to stresses, caregiving includes rewarding aspects. A *caregiver reward* is the value the caregiver sees in caregiving. Caregivers may develop more effective problem-solving skills, emotional coping skills, and personal competence (Garity, 1997). The social worker can help caregivers see the rewards in caregiving, including the good feeling they derive from helping (Farran, Miller, Kaufman, Donner, & Fogg, 1999). In reality, most families experience a mix of caregiver burden and rewards. When the social worker sorts this out with the caregiver, intervention strategies become more apparent.

Life Course

Taken in conjunction with the person-in-environment perspective on stress, an examination of an individual's and a family's life course allows the social worker to take into account the timing of life events in relation to social structures and historical happenings (Greene, 2008a) (see Figure 3.3). Did the client live through the Great Depression or experience (through television) the attack on the World Trade Center? Listening to the client narrative will help answer such questions.

Figure 3.3 shows both *normative events*, which are considered typical at certain times in life, and *nonnormative events*, which are individualized occurrences

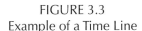
FIGURE 3.3
Example of a Time Line

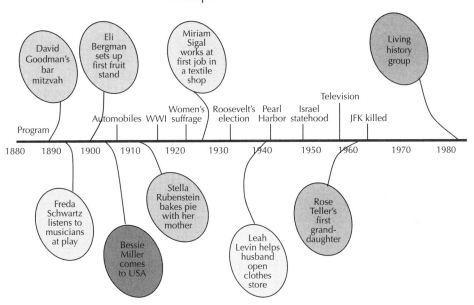

Note: WWI = World War I; JFK = John F. Kennedy.
Source: Adapted from *Tips for Getting the Best from the Rest* (p. 13), by C. Frank, J. Kurland, and B. Goldman, 1978, Baltimore: Jewish Family & Children's Service.

that may be unexpected. Nonnormative events are sometimes called "off-time" transitions. The line between typical and atypical events is increasingly becoming blurred. Grandparents may raise grandchildren, and a woman may act as a surrogate mother. Another example is how one military family has dealt with years of war and its effect on their marriage and children (Zoroya, 2009). This experience is anything but typical and may require coaching in life transitions.

Other examples of the changing configuration of life course events have appeared in the *New Yorker* and *NASW News*. In the *New Yorker*, Marx (2012) proposed that the baby boomers not only are delaying retirement but are not retiring at all. Rather, they are constructing new careers, often with the help of retirement coaches at firms such as Encore Career (http://www.encore.org). In *NASW News*, Pace (2012) suggested that a master's-level social worker is quite prepared for launching a career in life coaching. Life coaches help clients identify life development goals and guide them to actualization. Information about starting new careers is available on various Web sites, including YouTube.

Life course development is a series of transitions, both individual and collective, some of which require both informal and formal caregiving. Family development, as described in the case studies in this book, involves the family as a unit. Each critical life event affects the adaptability of the whole family, challenging its ability to function successfully. In the following chapters, you will learn more about how family members adjust their respective roles to maintain a functional system.

The Martinez Family: Facing Diabetes

Before you begin constructing your caregiving model, you should understand the extent to which context, family configurations, neighborhoods, and social care institutions may vary. Read the following case study. Would you be ready to help the Martinez family using your assessment and care planning model?

Diabetes and Family Caregiving

According to the Centers for Disease Control and Prevention (CDC) (2011c), 26 million Americans now suffer from diabetes. This translates to about 8.3 percent of the U.S. population. Some areas of the country have disproportionately high rates. For example, rates of diabetes are higher in the southern United States, with California, Texas, and Florida having the most new diagnosed cases (CDC, 2008).

When a person has diabetes, his or her body is unable to produce insulin, and this condition can lead to high or low levels of glucose (sugar) in the blood. That is, diabetes involves an imbalance between amounts of insulin and glucose in the body. People with diabetes may experience symptoms that include frequent urination, unusual thirst, extreme hunger, unusual weight loss, or extreme fatigue and irritability (American Diabetes Association, 2014).

Individuals diagnosed with diabetes may have to make extensive modifications to their lifestyle or diet to manage their health. This may require buying cookbooks, planning menus, and tracking their blood sugar levels (see National Diabetes Education Program, n.d.). Those who are diabetic are encouraged to limit their intake of foods high in sugar, eat smaller portions spread out over the day, monitor when and how many carbohydrates they consume, eat a variety of whole-grain foods and fruits and vegetables daily, eat less fat, limit their consumption of alcohol, and use less salt. These changes in food choices and preparation can affect not only the individual with the diagnosis but the entire family.

When the social worker initiates an assessment of a caregiving family, his or her first priorities are to (1) provide information about medical conditions, functional ability, limitations, and prognosis; (2) foster stress reduction; (3) offer concrete guidelines for sustaining care, problem solving, and optimal functioning; and (4) make available linkages to supplemental services to support the family's efforts (Walsh, 1998).

Case Study

The Martinez family is facing the numerous changes that accompany a family member's diagnosis of diabetes. The family consists of nine members: Mr. and

Mrs. Martinez, the grandparent generation; Mr. and Mrs. Alvarez, their daughter and her husband; and the Alvarez's three children. They live together in a modest home just outside the colonias in Texas. Mr. and Mrs. Martinez also have a son and daughter-in-law who live in Houston.

Colonias were developed in Texas around the 1950s from land considered worthless for farming or ranching. Developers sell these low-income homes as unincorporated subdivisions, and the property may lack electricity, plumbing, and other basic amenities. Unemployment is high and loans difficult to obtain (see Federal Reserve Bank of Dallas, 2008). However, the Martinez family, which includes three employed adults, was able to move out of the colonia to an incorporated suburb nearby. They still keep contact with their friends from the colonia through their church support group.

Mrs. Martinez, the matriarch of the family, babysits for the three children so the other adults can go to work. She told the social worker that she was frequently tired and experienced a significant weight loss. She initially thought that her symptoms were caused by the stress of her best friend's death in a car accident. But at her daughter's insistence, she went to the local clinic and was diagnosed with Type II diabetes. Since her diagnosis, she has been taking herbal cures—nopal (cactus), sabila (aloe vera), and nispero (Chinese plum)—and her blood sugar level has not been checked in two months. She continues to think, "I really miss my friend."

The family is accustomed to eating the large Mexican-style meals Mrs. Martinez prepares. She does not believe that she should make the family eat "those special foods" required for her to control her diabetes. She says, "They are too expensive, and I cannot buy them nearby." When she attends a wedding or fiesta in the church in the colonia where they used to live, she does not see foods on her diet there.

As a result of Mrs. Martinez's diagnosis, several changes have taken place in the family. Mrs. Alvarez, the adult daughter, is worried about her mother and has been hypervigilant about her mother's diet. This has created friction in the family, as mother and daughter often have heated discussions. Because food preparation and meals are such important components of life in the colonia, Mrs. Martinez has been reluctant to attend church, and Mr. Martinez will not attend without her. As a result, they both have become more isolated, socially withdrawn, and lacking traditional spiritual support. Although the family is aware that dietary changes need to be made, no one knows what or how much needs to be done.

Applying the Functional-Age Model in Assessment

The functional-age model (FAM) is a family-centered social work model of human behavior theory and practice. FAM begins with an assessment of the individual care recipient and proceeds to an assessment of family functioning (see Table 3.1). It then considers community-level care issues.

TABLE 3.1
Assessment in Caregiving Situations

FAM (individual)	Identify the role of biological factors in client functioning
	Examine client psychological well-being and adaptation
	Explore client social relationships and support networks
	Attend to client spirituality as a source of life satisfaction
	Determine client's level of functionality and need for intervention
FAM (family)	View the family as a caregiving system
	Explore the development of family care over time
	Examine the role(s) that family members play in caregiving activities
	Recognize how diverse family forms provide care
	Determine a family's caregiving capacity and need for intervention
	Evaluate the family's relationship to other social systems
REM (individual and family)	Address risk factors, source of stress, sense of loss, vulnerability, and grief
	Identify protective factors
	Determine the goodness of fit between an individual and family and the environment
	Examine a client's competence across the life course and the effect of sociopolitical change on his or her generation
	Individualize a client's biopsychosocial and spiritual functioning
	Explore the extent of a client's support system
	Learn what culturally sound solutions are acceptable to the client (system)
	Understand the client belief system
	Arrive at the meaning of an adverse event
	Examine societal and collective well-being, including social and economic justice
	Determine the degree of resilience and need for intervention
Life stressors	Identify the major life stressor
	Examine the significance of the event to the client
	Explore the client's coping mechanisms and resources
	Determine what the client thinks about the event
	Learn how the client construes or makes meaning of the event
	Identify what responses have been made to the stressor
	Develop an awareness of one's own cultural limitations
	Be open to cultural differences
	Use a client-oriented learning style
	Develop cultural awareness
	Acknowledge cultural integrity

TABLE 3.1
Assessment in Caregiving Situations *(continued)*

Collective efficacy	Examine the relational, collective capacity of formal and informal systems of care in care delivery
	Evaluate the ability of the community's belief systems to provide a care system
	Determine the levels of connection among various contingencies within the community
Human capital	Determine the effectiveness of the physical and social environment in building human capital
	Consider the level of collective investment among members of the community
	Examine the strengths of network bonds within the community
	Evaluate the relationship between traditional and nontraditional systems involved in care provision
Coalitions and community partnerships	Determine the level of cooperation among services that provide support to caregiving families
	Evaluate the motivation for shared resources among service providers

Note: FAM = functional-age model; REM = resilience-enhancing model.

Source: Steps for FAM assessment from *Social Work with the Aged and Their Families,* by R. R. Greene, 2008, New Brunswick, NJ: Aldine Transaction Press; REM assessment from *Social Work Practice: A Risk and Resilience Perspective,* by R. R. Greene, 2007, Monterey, CA: Brooks/Cole; life stressor assessment from *The Expanded Family Life Cycle: Individual, Family, and Social Perspectives* (3rd ed.), by B. Carter and M. McGoldrick (Eds.), 2005, Boston: Allyn & Bacon; and *Stress, Appraisal, and Coping,* by R. S. Lazarus and S. Folkman, 1984, New York: Springer; cultural sensitivity assessment from *Cultural Awareness in the Human Services: A Multi-Ethnic Approach* (3rd ed.), by J. W. Green, 1999, Boston: Allyn & Bacon; collective efficacy assessment from "Self-efficacy Mechanism in Human Agency," by A. Bandura, 1982, *American Psychologist, 37,* pp. 122–147; and "Exercise of Personal and Collective Efficacy in Changing Societies," by A. Bandura, 1995, *Self-efficacy in Changing Societies,* edited by A. Bandura, pp. 1–45; human capital assessment from "Building Community Capacity: A Definitional Framework and Case Studies from a Comprehensive Community Initiative," by R. J. Chaskin, 2001, *Urban Affairs Review, 36,* pp. 291–323; and *Guide to Sustainable Community Indicators* (2nd ed.), by M. Hart, 1999, North Andover, MA: Hart Environmental Data; and coalition and community partnership assessments from *Strategic Alliances among Health and Human Service Organizations: From Affiliations to Consolidations,* by D. Bailey & K. M. Koney, 2000, Thousand Oaks, CA: Sage Publications.

Biopsychosocial and Spiritual Functioning

FAM (Greene, 2008c) is based on the notion of functional age (Birren, 1969), which suggests that people's capacity to perform rests on their ability to manage or operate effectively in their environment (see Figure 3.4). Application of the model at the micro level begins with an exploration of individual biological, psychological, social, and spiritual functioning, all of which interact with one another.

Biological age refers to changes over time to the structure and functions of body organs and systems. These physiological aspects of functioning affect people's

FIGURE 3.4
Functional-Age Model of Intergenerational Treatment

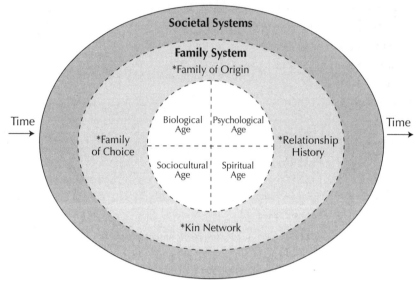

Functional-Age Model of Intergenerational Treatment
Modified by Eunkyung Kim

Source: Adapted by Eunkyung Kim from *Social Work with the Aged and Their Families* (p. 17), by R. R. Greene, 2008, New Brunswick, NJ: Aldine Transaction Press.

vulnerability to disease and disability but may also positively influence such things as energy levels. Daily living habits, mobility, safety, and home management fall under the rubric of biological age.

Psychological age involves the ability to adapt to or modify the environment across the life span. It includes what we often think of as personality, the affective aspect of our behavior, or coping styles. In addition, psychological age may be thought of as the ability to find meaning in life. *Social-cultural age* encompasses the roles that people play based on the expectations of family and society. The final dimension, *spiritual age*, may involve religion or transcendence, which are often drawn on in times of crisis.

By applying the concepts of biopsychosocial-cultural and spiritual age to Mrs. Martinez, the designated care recipient in our case study, we can see how these components are intertwined. When the social worker first visits Mrs. M, she takes along the nurse on her team. The nurse is concerned about whether Mrs. M is measuring her blood sugar level with the device the health care agency gave her. What is her present blood sugar level? Is she experiencing sweating, palpitations, hunger, confusion, blurred vision, dizziness, or fainting—all of which are warning signals of the progression of diabetes? The social worker also inquires about the family of Mrs. M's best friend, who died three months ago. (There is a belief in some Latino cultures that a shock can set off an illness.) When the social worker learns that there has been no memorial for Mrs. M.'s friend, she encourages Mrs. M to ask her friend's family whether they would like to plan an activity with the priest.

Family as a Social System

Families are the primary source of caregiving. In this section, we outline elements of FAM that provide insight into the family caregiving process and establish how the family may maintain or regain its equilibrium during caregiving (Bertalanfy, 1968). These elements may be incorporated into your caregiving model. FAM assumes that the family functions as a *social system*, or a structure of interacting and interdependent people. By using a systems model, social workers are able to learn how structure, communication patterns, and belief systems vary from one family to the next and what each family's caregiving needs may be.

During assessment, the social worker first wants to learn how the family defines its membership or boundaries. Who does the family say is in the family system? Then he or she wants to determine whether the family is relatively open or closed. An open family uses energy—resources and communication—well and is goal oriented; thus, it is more adaptive. Families that are adaptive seek out resources and try many problem-solving strategies. Families that are closed to solutions may be coached in this area. That is, the social worker wants to know how adaptive a family is so that its capacity can be fostered. The more adaptive a family, the more it will be able to grow and change when necessary to complete its caregiving tasks.

The Martinez family appears to have both open and closed structural elements. They have used their energy well to overcome extreme poverty by moving out of the colonia, and they have also accepted home services to aid their matriarch. However, they are somewhat reluctant to accept health education about diabetes.

Another assumption of FAM is that the family consists of a set of roles with reciprocal expectations and responsibilities (Parsons, 1951). Roles in a family are patterned with each family member in mind. Namely, an obligation is established by virtue of the role a person plays. For example, as grandmother, Mrs. M is expected to babysit for the three children. When the roles of grandchildren and grandmother complement each other, the family functions more successfully. If Mrs. M's disease goes unchecked, she may be less able to perform her role effectively, leading to role strain. Then how will the breadwinners continue to work? What will be the responsibilities of Mr. and Mrs. M's son and daughter-in-law, who live 50 miles away?

Roles develop over the family life course and are associated with a family's culture and values (Rhodes, 1980). Exploring with the family how these roles are transmitted from generation to generation allows the social worker to understand the family as a developmental unit encompassing interconnected life tasks. If the social worker can facilitate the process of role enactment in the Martinez family, especially given the added strain of caregiving, the family will remain a functional unit.

As the social worker goes out for her second visit, she is interested in obtaining an intergenerational picture of how the family functions. She may address some of the following questions:

- What does the family believe is the caregiving issue?
- Does each family member have a different view of the situation?
- What role does each member play? Who is in charge of family decisions?
- What solutions have been tried?

The social worker extends the scope of her assessment to understanding the family beyond simply Mrs. Martinez's condition. That is, she gathers information about how the diagnosis affects the family as a system. In addition, she focuses on subsystems, such as the relationships between members of various generations (for example, Mrs. Martinez and Mrs. Alvarez as mother and daughter) and vertical linkages (for example, marital relationships and relationships between siblings).

When the social worker arrives for her second visit, she finds that Mrs. Alvarez has stayed home from work to care for her mother, who was feeling dizzy that day. Even though Mrs. A earns the most money as a factory supervisor, the men have gone to work because "caregiving is not a man's job." The men are said to be annoyed with the small dietary changes that the family has made recently.

Mrs. A says that she loves and wants to help her mother, but she is feeling stressed out and is afraid of losing her job. The family is barely paying its bills.

Mrs. M is encouraged to measure her blood sugar with the device provided by the home health care agency. When she does, she finds that it is too low. To remedy this, she takes the last glass of orange juice left in the tiny refrigerator (because the budget did not allow for a larger bottle).

The social worker praises Mrs. M and Mrs. A for the changes they have made to address Mrs. M's diabetes. She asks them whether the men will accept enrolling in a family education program before the stress in the family escalates further.

Community-Level Factors

FAM also addresses how caregiving relationships are integrated into the larger sociocultural environment. Caregiving relationships take place in the context of a macroenvironment that includes physical aspects (such as buildings, roads, and weather conditions) as well as political, social, and cultural aspects. Unfortunately, little caregiving research has focused on community-level factors of care (Robert, 2002). Yet the conditions in which a caregiving system, such as a family, lives have a tremendous impact on the quality of care provided and overall quality of life. As stated by Robert and Lee (2002), "Living in socioeconomically disadvantaged communities exposes residents to greater environmental pressure—more challenging social, service, and physical environments. Older adults may be more vulnerable to the health effects of these challenging environments" (p. 658).

In addition to assessing the functioning of the individual and family, the practitioner will also need to be aware of environmental factors that support or challenge caregiving. Hart (1999) developed a model that delineates three different strata of community (see Figure 3.5). Similar to Maslow's (1968) hierarchy of conditions necessary for human functioning, this model depicts community-level factors that represent natural, human, and constructed capital. At the base is natural capital, including natural resources, such as food, energy, and water; ecosystem services, such as water filtration and fisheries; and the beauty of nature, such as mountains, seashores, and forests, which can enhance the quality of life.

✳

FIGURE 3.5
Hart's Community Capital Triangle

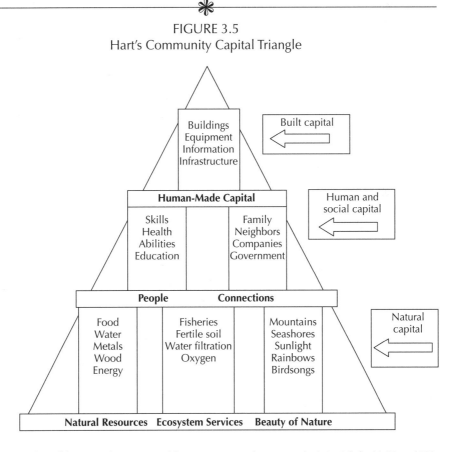

Source: Adapted from *Guide to Sustainable Community Indicators,* 2nd ed. (p. 16), by M. Hart, 1999, North Andover, MA: Hart Environmental Data. Retrieved from Sustainable Measures Web site: http://www .sustainablemeasures.com/node/32

The middle stratum, human and social capital, includes individuals within the community and their skills and resources, as well as the connections among individuals, families, organizations, and social institutions. The top stratum, built capital, is the human-made environment. This aspect of the environment rests on the other strata in the model and includes the production of goods and services and community infrastructure, such as roads, sewage systems, information systems, and government. This model presents a framework for understanding which environmental factors support or challenge caregiving systems.

As the social work practitioner views a caregiving situation, the following questions about the family environment provide a focus for understanding the environmental issues involved:

- How does the natural environment promote or create stress for families? For example, what is the air quality? Are there extreme weather conditions, such as significant snowfall? Do unstable energy sources create power outages in the home?
- What resources exist within the environment for care provision? What formal care resources can be accessed to support caregivers? What formal and informal services exist within the community to help these families?
- What care policies in the local environment support the family or create challenges? For example, some states have passed same-sex marriage legislation, which aids same-sex couples in making decisions about care. However, the majority of states have not passed this legislation, which makes planning and caregiving more difficult.
- How is the built environment conducive to care? Are there adequate transportation options? Are resources (such as shopping, medical personnel, and health care resources) close to caregivers?

Applying FAM in Intervention

FAM offers individual-, family-, and neighborhood-level interventions. At the individual level, interventions are aimed at maintaining and enhancing biopsychosocial and spiritual functioning.

Family Interventions

Whatever the assessment indicates, family-focused interventions generally view the family as adaptive and able to generate its own coping strategies (Greene, 1986).

The social worker has choices to make when it comes to family-focused social work interventions. For example, some families have unsettled debts and conflicts that can possibly be resolved. It may be helpful for such families to discuss these emotional issues in order to better proceed with caregiving responsibilities (Ackerman, 1958). Conflicts may present as family structural issues, such as disagreements between siblings or marital discord. The social worker may want to use strategies to realign relationships so that these difficulties do not interfere with caregiving tasks (Minuchin, 1974). For example, does Mrs. Alvarez resent her brother's absence in the caregiving process? How do the emerging caregiving tasks for Mrs. Martinez affect the marital relationships in the family?

The FAM family-focused treatment approach includes overlapping phases for working with caregiving families (see Table 3.2). In the case of the Martinez family, the social worker has started to learn how Mrs. M's diagnosis of diabetes has changed the system. Mrs. Alvarez fears losing her job, and Mr. M and Mr. A resent the attempts at dietary changes. Finances are now further strained. Child care arrangements that have worked well are now precarious as a result of Mrs. M's health status. The social worker believes that the next step in the intervention could involve family education that will help members reframe the problem. Will she be able to arrive at family-focused interventions and goals?

Applying the Resilience-Enhancing Model in Assessment

The resilience-enhancing model (REM) (Greene, 2007) is based on risk and resilience theory, which provides an increasingly popular mode of postmodern intervention. This approach is compatible with social care and can also be used to help the Martinez family. Risk and resilience is a multitheoretical framework for understanding how people individually and collectively maintain well-being despite adversity (Fraser, 1997; Greene, 2002, 2007). The theory is designed to help people cope, reduce stress, and foster strength. It also offers ideas for providing client care in a stressful environment, fostering adaptation, healing, and self-efficacy. For these reasons, it offers a philosophy and core concepts that can assist in care planning.

Resilience is not a single concept but instead encompasses coping, self-efficacy, and competence (Gordon & Song, 1994). Definitions include markedly successful adaptation following an adverse event (Rutter, 1987); the continuity of a personal narrative or life story (Borden, 1992); and a developmental process linked to demonstrated competence, or the learned capacity to interact positively with the environment and to complete tasks successfully (Masten, 1994).

Addressing Risk

In caregiving situations, social work assessment and practice must include attention to those junctures or situations that create particular risk, such as sources of stress and a sense of loss. In this way, the social worker knows ways to enhance the resilience of the individual and family. *Risk* is a factor that influences or increases

TABLE 3.2
Intervention in Caregiving Situations

FAM (individual)	Work to reintegrate and optimize biopsychosocial and spiritual client functioning
	Connect with the client system
FAM (family)	Call on the family's adaptive strategies
	Determine what issues are disrupting or enhancing family functioning
	Reframe the issue to arrive at a family-focused mutually acceptable description of the problem and possible solution
	Assist the family in performing its basic functions
	Address poor communication and organizational patterns that are not sufficient to carry out family tasks
	Mobilize the family's strengths and accomplishments as a resource
	Set mutual (reachable) goals with the care recipient and family
	Evaluate, provide feedback, and terminate (how did the family meet its goals?)
REM (individual)	Listen to client stories
	Acknowledge client loss, vulnerability, and future aspirations
	Alleviate the source(s) of stress and support responses
	Stabilize or normalize the situation
	Help clients take control
	Provide resources for change
	Promote self-efficacy
	Collaborate in self-change
	Strengthen problem-solving abilities
	Address positive emotions
	Reach for creative expressions
REM (family)	Focus on the collective
	Build on family's prior success
	Develop a shared view of the situation
	Reframe, when necessary, the meaning of an adverse event
	Work out a shared solution
	Adopt culturally sensitive adaptive strategies
	Evaluate progress
Life stressors	Help client develop meaning of life events
Therapeutic conversations	Discover historical, sociocultural, and political and policy contexts of caregiving
	Allow clients to speak to their own issues
	Attend to meaning making within participants' collective narratives
	Enhance growth and resilient functioning with helping strategies

TABLE 3.2
Intervention in Caregiving Situations *(continued)*

Cultural sensitivity	Aim for client problem recognition when a difference in usual functioning is acknowledged
	Have clients label their problem according to their everyday knowledge, cultural experience, and opinions from their social network
	Include indigenous help providers, such as folk doctors or herbalists
	Achieve problem resolution by helping clients shape their use of help providers
Collective efficacy	Develop and strengthen trust and safety among community members
	Promote levels of care sharing and advocacy to enhance caregiving experiences
Human capital	Advocate for community-level resources that promote care provision
	Enhance social network functioning among informal and formal sources of support
Coalitions and community partnerships	Strengthen coordination between organizations involved in care provision
	Create or support community coalitions for care provision
	Involve nontraditional partners in care provision

Note: FAM = functional-age model; REM = resilience-enhancing model.

Source: Steps for FAM intervention from *Social Work with the Aged and Their Families,* by R. R. Greene, 2008, New Brunswick, NJ: Aldine Transaction Press; REM intervention from *Social Work Practice: A Risk and Resilience Perspective,* by R. R. Greene, 2007, Monterey, CA: Brooks/Cole; life stressor intervention from *Symbolic Interactionism: Perspective and Method,* by H. Blumer, 1969, Englewood Cliffs, NJ: Prentice Hall; therapeutic conversation intervention from *Therapeutic Conversations,* by S. G. Gilligan and R. Price, 1993, New York: Brunner/Mazel; cultural sensitivity intervention from *Cultural Awareness in the Human Services: A Multi-ethnic Approach* (3rd ed.), by J. W. Green, 1999, Boston: Allyn & Bacon; collective efficacy intervention from *Self-efficacy: The Exercise of Control,* A. Bandura, 1997, New York: Worth Publishers; human capital intervention from "Building Community Capacity: A Definitional Framework and Case Studies from a Comprehensive Community Initiative," by R. J. Chaskin, 2001, *Urban Affairs Review, 36,* pp. 291–323; and *Guide to Sustainable Community Indicators* (2nd ed.), by M. Hart, 1999, North Andover, MA: Hart Environmental Data; and coalition and community partnership intervention from *Strategic Alliances among Health and Human Service Organizations: From Affiliations to Consolidations,* by D. Bailey and K. M. Koney, 2000, Thousand Oaks, CA: Sage Publications; and "Complexities of Coalition Building: Leaders' Successes, Strategies, Struggles, and Solutions," by T. Mizrahi, and B. B. Rosenthal, 2001, in *Social Work, 46,* pp. 63–78.

the (statistical) probability of the onset of *stress* or a negative outcome following adverse events. Risk factors that the Martinez family faces include controlling Mrs. M's disease, maintaining employment and finances, and bolstering family function.

In the Martinez family, fiestas and other cultural celebrations are times of particular risk, as the traditional Mexican diet is so interwoven into the festivities. At these times, it might be important for the social worker to check in with Mrs. Martinez to help her retain her commitment to her health and embrace ways in which she can participate in the festivities without deviating from her diet.

Discovering Protective Factors

Another term pertinent to risk and resilience theory is "protective factors." *Protective factors* are situations or conditions that help individuals to reduce risk and enhance adaptation. They may be internal personal characteristics, such as good problem-solving skills, or external environmental factors, such as viable support networks that modify risks (Rutter, 1987). An important protective factor in the Martinez family is the family members' love and nurturing of each other. Another protective factor is the family's support network.

As can be seen in Table 3.2, many of the assessment factors found in FAM are included in REM. An important difference is drawing a conclusion (with the family) about the meaning of an adverse event, such as a diabetes diagnosis, and how resilient they believe they are. Knowledge of a family's belief system will lead to potential resilience-enhancing strategies.

Applying REM in Intervention

Individual Interventions

REM presents individual interventions "to form a therapeutic alliance with clients that facilitates the self-healing process" (Greene, 2007, p. 73) (Table 3.2). REM is in the postmodern tradition, in which "the therapeutic conversation is the primary vehicle for helping the client become more efficacious" (Greene, 2007, p. 28). That is, the client–social worker conversation begins a helping process that reframes a problem-laden client narrative with little or no sense of agency as a new story with a sense of empowerment (McNamee & Gergen, 1992). Client-centered therapies help the client formulate "competing experiences—[those] that compete in some way with the client's actual experiences of the presenting problem" (Duncan et al., 1992, p. 92).

Many steps in REM were carried out with the Martinez family, such as stabilizing the situation and providing resources for change. Because of the primacy of the extended Martinez family system, conversations were personal, yet family focused. The social worker engaged Mrs. M by exploring ways in which her strong attachment to family and the importance of traditions (including food) could be used creatively. Complimenting and acknowledging Mrs. M's strong beliefs were important in establishing a working relationship. Advocating the belief that she could do something about her diabetes was a hopeful and optimistic approach to a difficult situation—it reframed her story.

To create competing experiences, the practitioner adopts a nonpathological posture and focuses on client resources, learns client goals or what the client wants, collaborates with the client in the description of the problem and selection of solutions, interrupts negative solutions or counterproductive behavior, helps seek new meaning of events, and validates client experiences.

Meaning making, therefore, is a communal process that depends on people's understanding of themselves and interaction with others. Language is the vehicle for this natural or innate process (Greene & Kropf, 2011). The social worker could ask questions to discover what new meanings diabetes has in Mrs. M's life and in the life of her family. Perhaps Mrs. M's knowledge of traditional foods could help her create meals to maintain her diet and at the same time maintain traditions for her family members. Thus, the challenge for Mrs. M becomes maintaining her family traditions as well as providing a better diet for herself. This becomes a personal challenge and desired outcome for her. Rather than being seen as resistant and needing confrontation, she is now being asked to find an answer to what might be her wish to live to see her family grow.

Family Resilience

The family may also be treated using a risk and resilience approach. The concept of family resilience is relatively new and builds on the strengths-based therapy movement (Walsh, 1998). It complements FAM, which mainly focuses on structural issues within the family. Theorists interested in family resilience emphasize a family's natural resources, patterns of functioning, and capabilities that enable family members to deal with—and even thrive in the face of—a crisis (see Table 3.2).

Because they value keeping challenges to themselves, the Martinez family members are reluctant to seek help and support from other sources. A social worker might engage with this family using a strengths perspective, in which he or she listens to the solutions the family has tried. Given that the family was able to move out of the colonia and extreme poverty, a resilience approach may be helpful.

Community Resilience

For Latino families, the connections among individual, family, and community resilience are particularly strong (Cardoso & Thompson, 2010). These connections need to be considered holistically in social work assessment and practice. The concepts of family and community resilience can be applied to the Martinez family. Numerous social relationships exist within the family and colonia, and these are important ties for Mrs. Martinez. In addition, she continues to hold a valued role in her family and community, as her contribution in terms of caring for her grandchildren is significant for the family's economic health. These relationships are important sources of support for Mrs. Martinez. Although difficult lifestyle changes are necessary as a result of her health crisis, she has many sources of potential support within her family and community.

The concept of community resilience can also be applied to the relationships that exist between individuals and families, social institutions, and government. Components of community resilience are often keys to individual resilience (Greene & Livingston, 2012). Community capacity is also important to resilience at the community level. *Community capacity* is "the interaction of human capital, organizational resources, and social capital within a given community that can be leveraged to solve collective problems and improve or maintain the well-being of that community" (Chaskin, 2001, p. 295).

The connections that exist within the community provide a framework for social work interventions that can enhance overall community resilience. These include the connections among community members, skills and resources that can be mobilized for social change, and the sense that the community has attained a higher level of positive outcomes in particular areas such as health and well-being (Greene & Kropf, 2011). As social entities, communities are dynamic and changing and adapt to new conditions and opportunities.

Several environmental challenges are present for the Martinez family. In addition to understanding the dynamics of the family, the social worker assesses what available resources could be a source of caregiving support. In addition, she notes the gaps or challenges that create stress and need to be addressed at an advocacy or political level.

The soil surrounding the colonia is of poor quality, so the Martinez family could not plant or maintain a garden, even though this would provide some healthy and affordable food. However, the social worker approaches the priest at the local church, a key figure within the community who holds a great deal of social capital, about a possible solution. The priest is able to recruit several men in the colonia to construct raised beds for planting. In her role as an advocate, the social worker also approaches a Texas foundation that promotes health and wellness. This foundation provides $10,000 for a community garden. This effort increases access to healthy food throughout the colonia and decreases the stigma Mrs. Martinez feels for requiring a special diet.

Next, the social worker partners with a university nutrition department to provide nutrition courses at the church in the colonia. Graduate students receive course credit to provide general nutrition courses to raise awareness of healthy eating. Included in these courses are cooking demonstrations in the church kitchen, and those in attendance are able to share a meal after the class. Part of the curriculum concerns conditions such as hypertension and diabetes, and the information provided is helpful for Mrs. Martinez and Mrs. Alvarez, who attend the classes.

From a strengths perspective, Mrs. Martinez's health issues may have potential benefits for others in her family and community. Some of the community-level interventions (for example, the community garden, nutrition and cooking classes, access to culturally and linguistically specific health information) are helpful and healthful for others who may be at risk for suffering from health problems of their own.

Cultural Sensitivity in Assessment and Intervention

In the case of the Martinez family, the social worker should be active in searching out information on diabetes that is both culturally and linguistically appropriate for the community. Spanish-language recipe books and pamphlets on diabetes are provided to the local clinic. Although information is available in Spanish online (for example, National Institute of Diabetes and Digestive and Kidney Diseases, 2013), many households near the colonia do not have access to a computer or do not have the skills to do research on the computer. To accommodate these households, the social worker prints out the brochures and makes a few spiral notebooks that can be easily checked out from the clinic and read.

Families and other care providers construct responsibilities and caregiving tasks within their particular cultural framework. Because social workers serve caregiving families and care recipients of different cultures, a sensitive help-seeking model should be integral to their work. In addition, because U.S. society has become increasingly diverse, social workers must consider whether they engage in culturally sensitive practice, which considers "the intersectionality of multiple factors including age, class, color, culture, disability, ethnicity, gender, gender identity and expression, immigration status, political ideology, race, religion, sex, and sexual orientation" (CSWE, 2012, pp. 4–5).

Therefore, the next concept in our social care model is adopted from Green (1999), who created a schema of help-seeking behavior that clarifies the client–provider relationship as a cross-cultural experience (see Figure 3.6). In Green's depiction, a distinction is made between the client culture and the professional subculture. The *client culture* includes problem recognition, problem labeling and diagnosis, indigenous help providers, use of help providers, and problem resolution.

Client problem recognition takes place when the client acknowledges a difference in his or her usual functioning. Can Mrs. M and her family acknowledge her diagnosis of diabetes and the changes required in the family system? The client labels the problem according to his or her everyday knowledge, cultural experience, and opinions from his or her social network. How does Mrs. M's social network begin to tackle the disease as a community issue? Indigenous help providers may include folk doctors, herbalists, or other significant healers. In the example of the Martinez family, the priest played a critical role in getting support for community interventions in the colonia. Can other indigenous helpers become part of the collaborative effort to educate the community about blood sugar control? Together these factors shape a client's use of help providers. Can the social worker mobilize the social network to work together to share information about care? This intended

FIGURE 3.6
Green's Help-Seeking Model

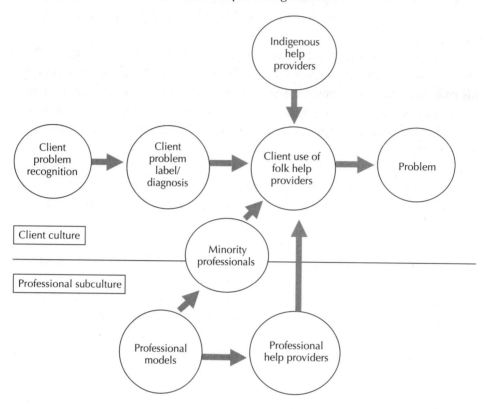

Source: Adapted from *Cultural Awareness in the Human Services: A Multi-ethnic Approach* (p. 33), by J. Green, 1999, Boston: Allyn & Bacon.

result is problem resolution. How can collective efforts that are culturally sensitive assist the Martinez family?

Because cross-cultural social work involves interacting with clients who are ethnically distinct and serving communities that are culturally unfamiliar, the practitioner must be willing to learn about the culture from the client and to respond appropriately in such encounters. Green (1999) has delineated five steps for achieving such culturally competent practice (see Table 3.2).

Intervention as Case Management: Bridging Micro- and Macropractice

In the example of the Martinez family, case management was used to bridge micro- and macropractice roles. The social work case manager provided various services to the family, starting with the first point of contact. These included linking the family to resources, being the primary contact for the family in the interdisciplinary team, and evaluating and measuring the success of treatment goals. In this example, the social worker not only worked with the family, but also implemented community helping strategies.

The aspect of case management that makes this role exciting also makes it challenging—the fact that it involves a broad spectrum of skills. To be competent in this role, case managers must be able to work directly with individuals, families, and the community and be competent advocates and change agents in social policy arenas. Several skills are important for effective case management practice (Greene et al., 2007):

- *Engaging in sensitive relationship building.* Case managers may intervene with clients during times of stress or transition. Regardless of the specific caregiving issue, case managers should assess what is happening with the client and family and determine the most effective way to build trust. As can be seen in the Martinez family, building trust may take time and resolve. Praising family members for the steps they have taken may aid in this regard.

- *Delivering appropriate resources and services.* Beyond referring clients to existing programs, case managers must help motivate client involvement in services. In addition, they must be aware of barriers that may prevent clients from accessing services and work to eradicate these conditions. With this in mind, Mrs. M's social worker began her interactions with the family by ensuring that the family members had the equipment necessary to measure Mrs. M's blood levels.

- *Having a network of alliances.* Case managers need to have positive and extensive relationships with colleagues within the service system. Especially in areas where services are limited, such as rural communities, case managers need to go beyond the usual suspects in identifying potential resources (Myers, Kropf, & Robinson, 2002). They must investigate and approach nontraditional partners as possible collaborators in service delivery in these areas. In Mrs. M's case, the social worker developed a network of gardeners to supplement the community food supply. This is an example of traditional case management and care-sharing activities.

- *Constructing service plans.* Social workers in all roles are increasingly accountable for delivering cost-effective services. Case managers must be able to determine the needs of families and provide a plan to address these needs in an efficient manner. In the case of the Martinez family, the inclusion of a nurse on the interdisciplinary team brought a more efficient approach to the service plan.

- *Evaluating service delivery.* Case managers are pivotal in determining how changes in service delivery and policy affect the lives of clients. In this role, they can determine where gaps in services are and what changes need to be made to services to make them more effective and accessible for caregivers. The social worker who assisted the Martinez family was effective because she understood how family culture and living environment affected the use of service delivery systems.

- *Acting as an advocate.* As discussed in chapter 1, advocacy is part of social work with caregivers. Within case management, advocacy roles are primary, as practitioners often act on behalf of clients who have limited skills or ability to act on their own, as in the case of obtaining and accessing information on managing diabetes (Frankl & Gelman, 1998).

Case management has been part of social work practice since the beginning of the profession. Because caregiving families often have multiple service needs, case managers are frequently involved in helping them access needed services. In this way, families receive the assistance and support they need to navigate disparate programs and service networks.

CHAPTER FOUR

Caring for Older Adults:
Functional Capacity and Health Status

This chapter is the first in the book to discuss how to implement the various theoretical assumptions and practice models introduced in chapters 1, 2, and 3. It begins with a fuller explanation of the development and implementation of theory relevant to family caregiving.

Older adults are understood on the basis of the individual, family, community, and societal contexts in which their functional capacity and health status play pivotal roles in influencing caregiving and care-sharing arrangements. That is, the ways in which older adults are able to navigate their environments as well as the care systems available to them shape their quality of life in old age. In this chapter, the case of Gerald illustrates the use of FAM for assessing the appropriate level of care, the case of Rachel shows how REM can be used in dealing with bereavement, the case of Mario highlights multigenerational caregiving and its cultural variations, and the case of Elaine's community-based program demonstrates a practice approach that builds community assets and collective efficacy. Comparisons of international social service design systems show how policies affect care.

Using a Social Care Approach

To understand the use of a social care approach for older adults and their caregivers, one must learn how tailored practice models have evolved over time by incorporating new theoretical assumptions and interventions as they have become available and as societal demands have prompted social workers to begin using them (Greene, 2005c). Various stakeholders have responded to sociocultural and political influences and modified or created practice theories to address client needs (Klein & Jurich, 1993). The benefits of modifications to various models and the use of new concepts are discussed here.

Among the historical changes pertinent to this chapter are the growing size of the aging population, varying family constellations, and the increasing diversity of the older population over the past decades (Hudson, 1996). This chapter also describes the increased pressure on social services programs and health care delivery systems, which has a major impact on the constellation of social care.

Social Care Model for Older Adults and Their Families: Evolution and Development

One of the most important professional competencies a social worker needs to have is the ability to "distinguish, appraise, and integrate multiple sources of knowledge, including research-based knowledge, and practice wisdom" (CSWE, 2008, 2012, Educational Policy 2.1.3). One such source of knowledge is human behavior theory, which is used to assess and intervene in client functioning. According to Greene (2008a),

> No single theory to date has been able to provide the organizing principles to meet the challenge of understanding fully the person as well as the systems with which he or she interacts. The dual goals of improving societal institutions and assisting clients within their social and cultural milieu have led to the mining of concepts from different disciplines. Each concept or theory attempts to explain the complex interplay of physical, psychological, cognitive, social, and cultural variables that shape human behavior. (p. 29)

We will see how certain theories and concepts help shed light on specific caregiving situations.

Person-in-Environment: Theories and Models

Although the models, theories, and frameworks presented in this book can be considered separate entities, you will find that social work practice often necessitates linking theoretical concepts together to better address complex situations such as caregiving. In the case of family caregiving, using a *metatheory*, or a grand theory or series of theories, can help you approach your social care role. Combining concepts will allow you to better help your client system, learn about new activity in the field, and use revised models as a guide for future work (Klein & Jurich, 1993).

A *theory* is a set of rules, ideas, and assumptions about how a phenomenon functions. *Models* comprise theoretical assumptions taken from available theories and considered useful to practice. They are abstract ideas or a roadmap for combining practice elements to effectively serve clients.

Theories in social work provide concepts to use in assessment and suggest methods of intervention. Theories—which offer comprehensive, simple, and dependable principles for the explanation and prediction of observable phenomena—assist social care workers in identifying orderly relationships (B. Newman & Newman, 2005). Most important, social workers need to know how specific theories contribute to understanding and intervening in the person-in-environment construct (CSWE, 2008, 2012).

In this chapter, we are specifically interested in the goodness of fit between the older adult and his or her environment. In this context, *goodness of fit* refers to the quality of the match between the person and his or her environment over the person's life course. A social worker can create a better person–environment fit by addressing barriers so that an older adult's environment is more supportive. The following sections discuss concepts and theories that can facilitate this process and outcome.

Inception of FAM

FAM is itself composed of several theories. It was originally created in the 1970s by a clinical social worker at a family service agency to provide a means of assessing and intervening with older adults and their families in caregiving situations (Greene, 1986). Although researchers were developing a body of biopsychosocial information about older adults, few social work practice models specifically designed for work with older people were available. A review of the literature at the time also revealed a dearth of family-centered practice models available for use with families in their later years. Greene began to consider how she could devise a model in which the family could be appraised as a unit.

Biopsychosocial, Psychodynamic, and Systems Theory. During the 1970s, when FAM was originally constructed, psychodynamic theory was used as the basis for individual assessment and intervention. For example, Erikson's (1950) framework for the healthy personality, or eight life stages, provided the foundation for conducting life reviews with older clients—a method that taps naturally recurring reminiscences to resolve internal conflicts (Butler, 1963). Systems theory served as a foundation for family-focused interventions, offering a means of viewing the family as an emotional unit and settling old scores (Ackerman, 1970). These theories, together with extensive research on the biopsychosocial aspects of aging, helped bring about FAM.

Ecological Perspective. Another area of competence required for all social workers is conducting "dynamic and interactive processes of engagement, assessment, intervention, and evaluation at multiple levels" (CSWE, 2008, 2012, Educational Policy 2.1.10). Therefore, the FAM approach includes an ecological perspective that calls social workers' attention to both micro and macro level phenomena. During assessment and intervention with older adults, their families, and their support systems, social workers typically follow six steps to broaden their point of view:

1. Identify the client system to be assessed.
2. Identify the condition in the client system that the practitioner needs to understand.

3. Identify the factors in the client system itself that contribute to the condition.
4. Identify the factors in the social context of the client system that contribute to, or assist with, the condition.
5. Identify the resources available to the client system that exist within the system itself.
6. Identify the resources that exist within the environment of the particular system. (Longres, 1990, pp. 47–48)

With the passage of legislation that provided resources for older adults, such as the Older Americans Act, extensive case management systems were devised to allocate these resources. Social workers became responsible not only for helping older adults and their families talk about family issues, but also for assisting them in accessing programs and resources.

Spiritual Functioning. There has been a renewed interest in spiritual aspects of development and their contribution to adaptive functioning (Crowther, Parker, Achenbaum, Larimore, & Koenig, 2002; Greene, 2007). FAM was thus modified in early 2000 to include spiritual issues in mental health practice. This allowed for a better understanding of older adults' faith-based support systems.

Inception of REM

Frail and disabled older adults are usually the clients most in need of services. At the same time, social workers in the field of aging strive to promote a strengths-based approach to practice, one that recognizes the capacity of older adults to develop and even transform in old age (Chapin & Cox, 2001). Geriatric social workers are also interested in the application of evidence-based theory, such as how effective cognitive therapy might be with older adults (Cummings & Kropf, 2009b; Cummings, Kropf, Cassie, & Bride, 2004; Knight, 1999). Because risk and resilience theory addresses both of these concerns, its use led to an interest in resilience-enhancing practice (Greene & Cohen, 2005).

Risk and Resilience Theory. Risk and resilience theory is itself a multitheoretical framework, building on a systems-ecological-developmental approach to explain how people remain adaptive or overcome adversity (Fraser, 1997; Greene, 2007). When working with older adults, social workers examine their clients' adaptation or coping pattern over time to determine their relative risks, challenges, capacity for resilience, and strengths. Social care workers also explore which protective factors shield the older adult from negative aspects of his or her environment. The information gathered in this assessment contributes to a care plan.

Moreover, social workers interested in resilience-enhancing interventions focus on theories that "are more *contextualized*, that is, theories that emphasize multiple, individualized perspectives" (Greene, 2008a, p. 8). Consequently, REM emphasizes the idea that social workers need to create a partnership with their client. The goal is to develop new client meanings through a *narrative approach*, one that gathers and often reframes life stories (White & Epston, 1990). The reframing of their life stories is viewed as a key empowerment strategy. Using the steps outlined in Tables 3.1 and 3.2, we describe the implementation of the theory here, with Rachel as a therapeutic model.

Adoption of Models of Human Capital and Collective Efficacy

To "recognize, support, and build on the strengths and resiliency of all human beings," social workers need to understand collective well-being (CSWE, 2008, 2012, Educational Policy B2.2). Once practitioners focus their attention on the collective, additional practice models are required. One area is the physical and built environment of older adults—that is, the community level of practice. Unfortunately, a recent national survey of 10,000 local governments found that only 46 percent of communities have started to address the needs of an increasingly older population (National Association of Area Agencies on Aging, 2011). To address this issue, the World Health Organization (2007) has promulgated a series of recommendations to help cities become more aging friendly. Cities across the globe, including 15 within the United States, have signed on in support of these measures (Barusch, 2013). As the baby boom generation ages, planning for an older population is increasingly necessary. For individuals to remain engaged and involved in their communities, the physical and built environment must be able to accommodate their numerous physical and functional changes.

In addition to creating environments that foster interactions, community development models can harness the talents and experiences of the older population. Austin, DesCamp, Flux, McClelland, and Sippert (2005) reported on the Elder Friendly Communities Program, which uses a community development approach to increase the involvement of seniors in their local areas. These authors wrote, "The extent to which individuals are integrated into [the] larger society will influence the size, density, and nature of their neighborhood networks" (p. 403). The Elder Friendly Communities Program works with seniors to identify actions that can be taken in their local neighborhood to enhance community life. Examples of these actions include increasing intergenerational programs, creating senior columns in local newspapers, and enhancing infrastructure, such as through snow removal or more convenient placement of postal boxes. Through the Elder Friendly Communities Program and other similar programs, older adults become more involved in the lives and decision making of their communities.

Social Care Innovations

In the near future, the need for eldercare will outstrip the availability of formal services. Families will be challenged, and innovations in care will be vital. Some of these care-sharing innovations are already under way: For example, the Louisiana Chapter of AARP has sponsored a project to turn a senior center into a 21st-century wellness center, attending to preventive medicine and testing. AARP chapters are also establishing housing trust funds.

Because older adults generally prefer to live in their own homes rather than assisted living or nursing homes—a phenomenon known as "aging in place"—some organizations are creating innovations to support this effort. In the mid-1980s, the Federation of Jewish Philanthropies of New York established a new paradigm of healthy aging by creating a community-based social service program known as Naturally Occurring Retirement Communities (NORCs). These communities targeted older adults in a centralized area who were living in moderately priced apartment buildings. City and state programs provided case management and social work services; health care management and prevention programs; education, socialization, and recreational activities; and volunteer opportunities for program participants and the community.

Another example of an NORC is Beacon Hill Village, founded in 2001 in Boston. The village is a membership organization the nearby Cambridge, Massachusetts, designed to provide older "residents with an alternative to moving from their houses to retirement or assisted living communities by offering programs and services that support them to age in place." This nonprofit organization created by and for local residents is considered to be the pioneer of the increasingly popular "village" movement (Aged & Community Services Australia, n.d.).

Stigmatized and Politicized Caregiving Context

Caregiving for an older adult is performed in a context with many negative views about aging in general. *Ageism*, or discrimination and prejudice based on a person's age, is prevalent in U.S. society. At the same time, various positive social resources can benefit older adults and their caregivers. However, the current political climate makes some of these benefits (for example, Social Security and pension benefits) increasingly precarious.

Ageism

Just as in all fields, the ability to "practice personal reflection and self-correction to assure continual professional development" is a prerequisite to competency in geriatric social work practice (CSWE, 2008, 2012, Educational Policy 2.1.1). The presence of ageism in our society makes reflection and insight crucial in social work practice with older adults and their care providers. Ageism often involves both negative and positive systemic stereotypes about older adults and their abilities, such as whether older adults should remain employed after age 65. These stereotypes, which allow younger generations to see older people as very different from themselves, can affect service delivery and even a family's ideas about its older members' ability to thrive (Butler, 1975).

Furthermore, a long-standing problem in the helping professions has been the belief that older adults are less responsive than clients of other ages to mental health treatment (Butler, 1975; Greene, 2008c). Thus, *countertransference*, or a social worker's unintended and irrational feelings about a client, may interfere with the effectiveness of interventions. An honest self-examination of the social worker's views of older adults is therefore in order.

Benefits for Older Americans

Ironically, one of the best systems of care was designed for older adults and was initiated in the form of Social Security in 1935 by Franklin D. Roosevelt. Legislation conferring benefits to older adults, especially the regulations of the Older Americans Act, is extensive (see "Select Federal Aging Policies" on page 60). The Older Americans Act was passed by Congress in 1965 in response to concern about a lack of community social services for older people. The legislation gave authority for grants to states for community planning and social services, research and development projects, and personnel training in the field of aging. It also established the AOA, which administers grant programs and serves as the federal focal point for issues concerning older people. Today, the Older Americans Act is considered the major vehicle for the organization and delivery of social and nutrition services to older adults and their caregivers.

However, Social Security, Medicare, and Medicaid are currently up for debate in Congress. The debate centers on whether U.S. taxpayers can afford to continue paying for a range of aging programs and entitlements as well as escalating health care costs. This controversy has been intensified by the Affordable Care Act and its attention to health insurance coverage and the public's use of hospitals and other medical benefits. The rationing of health care in the United States and in other countries is also under scrutiny. This fast-changing landscape, a complete discussion of which is beyond the scope of this chapter, will affect caregiving well into the future (see chapter 12).

Demographics of Aging

The older population is growing, and projections indicate that the numbers will continue to increase over the coming decades. According to the AOA (2013),

> The older population—persons 65 years or older—numbered 39.6 million in 2009 (the latest year for which data is available). They represented 12.9% of the U.S. population, about one in every eight Americans. By 2030, there will be about 72.1 million

Select Federal Aging Policies

Social Security Act (enacted 1935)

- A sweeping federal policy passed to help ensure economic security for aged and, later, indigent populations; for surviving spouses and children; and for individuals with disabilities
- Originally included social insurance, unemployment insurance, old age assistance, and aid to dependent children; later additions included Medicare, Medicaid, Supplemental Security Income, and Supplemental Security Disability Income (Social Security Administration, n.d.)

Older Americans Act (enacted 1965)

- Provides access, in-home, senior center, nutrition, employment, and legal assistance services and additional services on the basis of local needs and resources to individuals age 60 and older
- Established the federal Administration on Aging and the aging network, comprising federal, state, and area agencies on aging (Greene, Cohen, Galambos, & Kropf, 2007)

Medicare (established 1965 under Social Security Act, Title XVIII)

- Makes those eligible for Old Age Insurance (commonly called Social Security) also eligible for the following health benefits:
  - coverage for hospital care
  - voluntary supplemental health insurance
  - subsidization of prescription medication purchases for seniors (Henry J. Kaiser Family Foundation, 2012b)

Medicaid (established 1965 under Social Security Act, Title XIX)

- A means-tested medical assistance program for categorically needy populations
- Pays a significant amount of long-term care expenses and other health-related expenses for the elderly population (see Henry J. Kaiser Family Foundation, n.d.)

Age Discrimination in Employment Act (enacted 1967)

- Promotes the hiring of workers based on ability, not age, and prohibits age discrimination in employment
- Later included government employers under these requirements

---

older persons, more than twice their number in 2000. People 65+ represented 12.4% of the population in the year 2000 but are expected to grow to be 19% of the population by 2030.

As mentioned previously, each older adult ages differently and has varied family and community supports.

The composition of the older population is also shifting in significant ways. The greatest increase is in the population older than 85, which will likely require some degree of assistance or support in activities of daily living. At this time in the life course, the gender distribution is also at its most extreme. In 2011, there were 23.4 million women 65 years of age and older and 17.9 million men 65 years of age and older: a sex ratio of 131 women for every 100 men. Among individuals 85 and older, this ratio increases to 203 women for every 100 men (AOA, 2012). As these numbers suggest, the typical pattern of caregiving involves a wife taking care of her husband. As this woman ages, her adult children assume care for her.

Because the majority of assistance for older adults is provided by informal sources of support, an important aspect of understanding aging is knowing who provides care:

> The "average" U.S. caregiver is a 49-year-old woman who works outside the home and spends nearly 20 hours per week providing unpaid care to her mother for nearly five years. Almost two-thirds of family caregivers are female (65 percent). More than eight in ten are caring for a relative or friend age 50 or older. (Feinberg, Reinhard, Houser, & Choula, 2011, p. 1)

As this summary indicates, care provision is the equivalent of a part-time job for many. These responsibilities are typically assumed in addition to other role responsibilities, such as being a parent, employee, spouse, or partner.

Caregiving is also associated with significant costs. About half of all individuals ages 55 to 64 spend an average of 580 hours per year caring for family members (R. W. Johnson & Schaner, 2005a). Although men assume some of the tasks of care, the majority of caregiving is provided by women, and this has consequences for women's economic security in later life (R. W. Johnson & Schaner, 2005b). It is estimated that the cost of unpaid caregiving supports provided to older family members is $450 billion per year (Family Caregiver Alliance, 2012).

One way in which older adults vary is in their health status, a key aspect of client assessment. According to the AOA (2012), 44 percent of older adults assess their health as excellent or good (compared with 64 percent of people 18 to 64 years of age). Most older people have at least one chronic condition, including arthritis, heart disease, cancer, diabetes, or hypertension, and 72 percent take medication for hypertension. Social workers in health care settings must become familiar with these and other health concerns.

Applying FAM in Assessment

The following case study is an example of caring for an older adult named Gerald. The example provides a way to use FAM in the assessment process and shows how a health crisis can affect a family. As Gerald's situation worsened, interventions were introduced to support him in the remaining weeks of his life and provide relief to the family care providers.

Case Study

Gerald was a member of the baby boom generation (individuals born between 1946 and 1964). Like most baby boomers, he had a small immediate caregiving family that consisted of his spouse and daughter. He was well educated and in the upper-middle class. He subscribed to a successful aging approach that included (1) freedom from disease and disability, (2) high cognitive and physical functioning, and (3) social and productive engagement (Rowe & Kahn, 1998). In everyday terms, this meant that Gerald had yearly checkups, exercised at the gym, did not smoke, and only drank socially. On retiring, he took classes to become a museum guide. He also took courses on world religions (the model of successful aging was later modified by Crowther et al., 2002, to include spirituality).

Unfortunately, Gerald developed atherosclerosis, or hardening of the arteries, which required bypass surgery. Over time, his condition worsened, leading to depression and a pulmonary embolism. He was on 10 medications daily, and these were managed by his wife, Rachel. Because Gerald had difficulty getting into and out of a chair, his daughter, Sarah, often had to help lift him. On the advice of the social worker, the family eventually bought a lift chair.

Gerald's case manager made finding ways to lessen the family's stress and burden a focus of her work. In the last six weeks of his life, Gerald became incontinent and more confused. He could no longer be cared for at home. The family decided that he should receive palliative care. (Although associated with the end of life, palliative care—care designed to relieve pain, stress, and symptoms—may be given at any time during an illness and is usually administered by an interdisciplinary team [NASW, 2013; Supiano & Berry, 2013].) Following Gerald's death, Rachel continued to see her social worker about bereavement transitions.

Biopsychosocial and Spiritual Assessment

The social worker conducted Gerald's biopsychosocial and spiritual assessment through interviews, observation, and the use of assessment instruments. Individuals from other disciplines, including physical therapists, nurses, and other medical specialists, were also involved. The family further provided information to the social work practitioner about Gerald's functioning in his home environment. The first interviews were critical for establishing trust. Shulman (1999) suggests the following steps for accomplishing this task:

- Clarify the social worker's purpose and role. Offer a simple statement of the reason for the encounter and the services of the social worker's agency.

- Reach for client feedback; that is, make an effort to understand the client's perceptions of his or her needs.
- Partilize or break down the client's concerns into manageable parts so that they are less overwhelming.
- Deal with issues of authority by striving to establish mutuality in the working relationship.

In addition, it is important not to patronize the older client. Some clients may require simple explanations of the social worker's role. Others who are hard of hearing may need to hear elevated speech patterns, whereas those with dementia may require a quiet location and several explanations of the ongoing process of care.

Biological Age. Biological age comprises physical status and limitations, such as hearing or vision loss; health, including medical regimes and chronic and acute illness; and activities of daily living, including bathing or grooming oneself. It is important to remember that some clients may be physically active well into old age.

When assessing a client's biological age, the social care worker is interested in how he or she traverses the environment. Among the questions that may be asked are the following:

- Is the client safe in his or her home? For example, can he or she reach items on higher shelves in the kitchen? Will rugs cause a fall?
- What is the client's energy level or stamina?
- Does he or she go out for leisure activity?
- What are the client's physical limitations or strengths? How have these changed over time?

In the case of Gerald, the biological age assessment was not static, as he had relatively good health that deteriorated over time. Eventually, he required more intensive interventions to remain in his environment, and the stress on Rachel and Sarah increased.

Psychological Age. Psychological age is the ability to adapt and cope in late life. It is influenced by lifelong adjustments or resilience and the capacity to meet environmental demands (Lawton, 1982). You will want to assess whether the client's behaviors enable him to her to deal effectively with reality, master his or her environment, resolve conflict, reduce stress, or feel personal satisfaction. In the case of Gerald, the social worker found that as time went by, he was less able to deal with reality and his environment. However, he still received personal satisfaction from going to concerts and playing video games.

Mental Health Issues. Because older adults may experience depression or dementia, as well as other mental illnesses, social workers need to become familiar with the major psychiatric disorders of late life (see Tables 4.1 and 4.2). Practitioners should also be conversant with mental status questionnaires, seek consultation

Caregiving and Care Sharing

TABLE 4.1
Differences between Grief and Depression

Characteristic	Grief	Depression
Onset of depressed feelings	Grief is triggered by one or more identifiable losses (loved one, independence, financial security, pet, and so on).	Depression may not relate to a particular life event or loss. The loss may be seen as punishment.
Expressions of anger	Anger is expressed openly and is often misdirected.	People who are depressed can be irritable and may complain; they do not express anger openly and often direct anger inwardly toward self.
Expressions of sadness	Feelings of sadness and emptiness are expressed; weeping.	People who are depressed have pervasive feelings of sadness and hopelessness; they experience a chronic sense of emptiness and may have difficulty controlling weeping.
Physical complaints	Grief may be expressed through temporary physical complaints.	Depression can lead to chronic physical complaints.
Sleep	Grief may sometimes cause difficulty getting to sleep and disturbing dreams.	Early morning waking, insomnia, or excessive sleeping (escape into sleep).
Insight	Grief may cause people to be preoccupied with the loss of a person, object, or ability; or they may have guilt over some aspect of the loss and temporary loss of self-esteem.	People who are depressed can be preoccupied with self, have generalized feelings of guilt, may have thoughts of suicide, and experience a longer-term loss of self-esteem.
Responsiveness and acceptance of support	Grief can respond to comfort and support; people may not want to impose grief on others.	A person who is depressed does not accept or seek support, but tends to isolate self and may be unresponsive.
Pleasure	The ability to feel pleasure varies with grief, but the person can still experience moments of enjoyment.	When depressed, people, often have a persistent inability to feel pleasure.
Others' reactions toward the person	There is a tendency for others to feel sympathy for a person in grief.	People who are depressed can find that others have a tendency to feel irritated with them.

Source: Adapted from *Mental Health, Mental Illness, Healthy Aging: A NH Guide for Older Adults and Caregivers* (p. 12), by National Alliance for the Mentally Ill, 2001, Arlington, VA: Author.

TABLE 4.2
Differences between Depression, Delirium, and Dementia

Characteristic	Depression	Delirium	Dementia	Normal Aging
Onset	Variable	Usually sudden, caused by acute medical disorders	Variable, often gradual or unnoticed	No specific chronological pattern for symptoms
Duration	Weeks to years	Days to weeks	Months to many years	Some changes begin in mid-30s
Progression	Variable	Symptoms suddenly severe in days	Varies with type of dementia	Small changes over long periods
Memory	Person usually complains of memory problems	Person often denies having problems	Person is often unaware; problems are noted by others	Person may complain of mild losses, forgetfulness
Attention	Often impaired	Impaired	Often intact	Normal
Judgment	Variable; person often believes it is impaired	Poor	Poor; person's behavior is frequently inappropriate	Normal
Insight	Cognitive distortion likely (self-doubt, negative thoughts, and so on)	Impairment likely, sometimes intermittent	Usually absent	Normal, consistent with personal history
Sleep	Early morning waking, insomnia, or excessive sleep are common	Typically disturbed	Often normal, day–night reversal possible	Increased likelihood of intermittent awakenings
Problems functioning	Mild to extensive	Mild to extensive	Mild to extensive	None or a few problems
Hallucinations and delusions	Unusual	Sometimes vivid	Sometimes present	Absent

Source: Reprinted from *Mental Health, Mental Illness, Healthy Aging: A NH Guide for Older Adults and Caregivers* (p. 24), by National Alliance for the Mentally Ill, 2001, Arlington, VA: Author.

from other health professionals, and help the family understand changes in the older adult's behavior.

Social Age. The sociocultural aspects of functional age explore how clients interact with family, friends, and support networks. What roles did the client once play, and what roles is he or she able to maintain? Does the client have friends he or she can depend on? Are outside formal services needed to supplement a low level of informal support? Gerald had a loving neighbor who took him out to lunch and maintained the music on his iPod. However, the social worker made a mutual agreement with Rachel and Sarah to get more respite services to help them in the home.

Spiritual Age. Spiritual age, like the other aspects of functional age, varies by individual. It may include a person's relationship with his or her faith, religious community, religious leader, or inner belief system. As we will see with Rachel in her bereavement, discovering meaning in older years is one aspect of spirituality and healing.

Environmental Press

Another way to view biopsychosocial and spiritual functioning among older adults is from the perspective of environmental press (see Figure 4.1 for a visual representation). Lawton (1982), who constructed the environmental press concept, was interested in the competence of older adults and their ability to function in their environment. He defined *competence* as "the theoretical upper limit of capacity of the individual to function in the areas of biological health, sensation-perception, motoric behavior, and cognition" (p. 38). When social workers examine the upper limit of an individual's capacity to function in the environment, they are exploring the least restrictive environment in which the person wants or is able to function. If clients prefer to stay in their home, or age in place, can they remain there? Do they need or want additional help?

Family Assessment

When assessing Gerald, the social worker explored the family as a unit, examining systems organization and communication as well as the family's roles and development across the life course.

System. FAM defines the family as a group of interdependent members. The family system has a set of rules, a power structure, and the ability to solve problems. The social worker learned through her assessment that Gerald's family was well organized and had good communication. This was demonstrated by joint decision making and consultation with two sons who lived in faraway states. The family was open to suggestions from professionals who provided guidance in Gerald's care.

Roles. FAM views the family as a set of reciprocal roles, involving the obligations and behavioral expectations members have to and for one another. Gerontologists have had a long-standing interest in how the nature of family relationships affects

FIGURE 4.1
Environmental Press

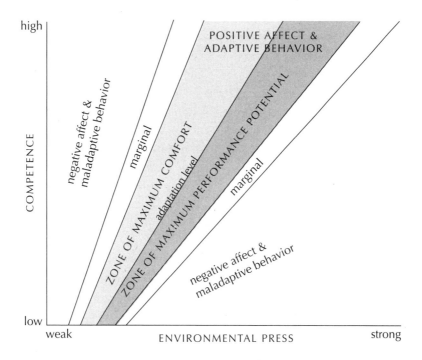

Source: Reprinted from "Ecology and the Aging Process" (p. 661), by M. P. Lawton and L. Nahemow, in *The Psychology of Adult Development and Aging,* edited by C. Eisdorf and M. P. Lawton, 1973, Washington, DC: American Psychological Association.

the aging process. For example, Boszormenyi-Nagy and Spark (1973) contended that the "major connecting tie between the generations is that of loyalty based on the integrity of reciprocal indebtedness" (p. 217). The relationship between older parents and adult children and the ways help is received and provided across generations was said to be maintained through emotional bonds, interdependence, and the exchange of goods and services.

Gerald's family comprised his wife, three children, their spouses, and his grandchildren. Because family members were able to delegate tasks to one another, the family was assessed as having clear, functional roles. Each member could be called on to carry out specific functions.

Development. Caring for a parent cannot be understood only as a part of the aging process. Rather, parent care involves a lifetime of interactions between parents and their children, often involving issues of independence versus dependence (Brody, 1985). FAM considers the family "a mutually dependent unit with interdependent pasts and futures" (Greene & Jones, 2006, pp. 12–13). Because the members of Gerald's family had a history of good communication and role assignment, they were better able to care for him in his old age. However, the bereavement phase was difficult (as described in a later section).

Caregiver Burden and Caregiver Resilience. A family assessment would not be complete if it did not explore caregiver stress, burden, and resilience. A 2004 report by the Family Caregiver Alliance acknowledged that the network of aging services now recognizes family caregivers as "valued consumer[s] in need of support services in their own right" (p. 21). Therefore, the term "client" has sometimes been expanded to include the caregiver, depending on the funding source. (Current data indicate that 30 percent of federal programs include the caregiver as a designated client [Family Caregiver Alliance, 2004].) The Family Caregiver Alliance report went on to state that strengthening families in their caregiving role is a necessary part of the long-term care system in today's aging society.

Caregiving tasks and responsibilities cover a wide range of activities, from helping with grocery shopping to changing the diapers of incontinent relatives. According to the National Alliance for Caregiving and AARP (2009; see also Redfoot, Feinberg, & Houser, 2013), the majority of caregivers (55 percent) in a Gallup study reported that they had cared for their relative for three years or more. The average number of days per month spent on shopping, food preparation, housekeeping, laundry, transportation, and giving medication was 13, and six days per month were spent on feeding, dressing, grooming, walking, bathing, and providing assistance with toileting. Gerald's spouse and daughter provided daily care in these activities. Like many members of the baby boom generation, they were able to afford occasional respite as recommended by their social worker.

As caregiving tasks may or may not lead to caregiver burden, social workers should give full consideration to the family caregiver in the assessment process. Caregiver burden, or difficulty maintaining care without negative effects on the caregiver, is related to how a person perceives stress. Does the caregiver see his or her caregiving tasks as manageable over time? The burden interview, written by Zarit et al. (1980), provides a list of statements to which the caregiver should respond yes or no:

- I feel that my spouse makes requests which I perceive as over and above what she/he needs.
- I feel resentful about my interactions with my spouse.
- I feel that my spouse does not appreciate what I do for him/her as much as I would like.
- I feel that I am contributing to the well-being of my spouse.
- I feel pleased with the interactions with my spouse. (p. 651)

In an interview exploring caregiver burden, Rachel was able to talk with the social worker about how her social life had declined as she continued to care for Gerald.

She also expressed feelings of embarrassment as Gerald exhibited inappropriate behaviors while friends were visiting.

Often caregivers feel both burden and resilience. They may enjoy being with their relative or recognize that they will miss their relative when he or she is gone (Farran et al., 1999). Walsh (1998) has proposed that to better help the client deal with mixed emotions, practitioners examine the belief system of the family, including how family members make meaning of adversity, take a positive outlook on life, and are able to transcend difficulties. Have they learned and grown from adversity in the past? Gerald's family displayed many signs of resilience as they pulled together to face adversity during the past.

Diversity

The older population is diverse in significant ways. First, later life spans several decades, and individuals in the younger range of this group are typically dissimilar from the very old. In addition, racial and ethnic differences exist. Finally, family constellations are changing in general, including in the older generations. Thus, practitioners need to use good assessment processes in their work with older adults and their care providers.

Age Variations

The population of older Americans is not homogenous. The U.S. Census Bureau (2010b) has projected that the population age 85 and older could grow from 5.5 million in 2010 to 19 million by 2050, while the number of people 85 and younger will remain relatively steady. This growth in the population known as the old-old may be of concern because frailty and the incidence of disease increase with age, requiring more caregiving.

Racial and Ethnic Diversity

According to data collected by the AOA in 2012, racial and ethnic minority older Americans made up 21 percent of the U.S. population 65 years of age or older: 9 percent were African American, 7 percent Hispanic, 4 percent Asian, and 1 percent Native American (AOA, 2012). The AOA (2012) also reported that older men were more likely than older women to be married. More than 3.6 million older adults (or 8.7 percent) live below the poverty line, with women and minority elders having higher levels of poverty (AOA, 2012). Poverty among this group must be attended to, as it may lead to disparities in health care.

Do ethnic differences result in differences in the caregiving experience or in caregiving configurations and practices? Pinquart and Sörensen (2005) conducted a meta-analysis of 116 articles related to ethnic differences involving objective stressors, beliefs about filial obligation, psychological and social resources, coping processes, and psychological and physical health. They found that compared with white caregivers, ethnic minority caregivers were of lower socioeconomic status, were younger, were less likely to be married, were more likely to receive informal support, and had worse physical health. In addition, ethnic minority caregivers provided more care and demonstrated stronger beliefs about filial obligation. Finally, African American caregivers experienced lower levels of caregiver burden and depression than white caregivers.

Janevic and Connell (2001) compared African American, Chinese, Chinese American, Korean, Korean American, Latino, and white caregivers as well as residents of 14 European Union countries. They found that white caregivers both in the United States and Europe were most likely to be spouses and reported greater depression than ethnic minorities. They also found caregiving more stressful than African American caregivers did. "Findings were mixed regarding differences in coping and social support, but suggested that minority groups may not have more available support than Whites" (p. 334).

The care-sharing context of older adults is shaped by their functional capacity, the family's cultural attitudes toward self-reliance and autonomy, and interrelationships among family members. For example, Cuban American families who migrated to the United States soon after the 1959 Cuban revolution may be somewhat assimilated and follow different caregiving patterns than their relatives who remained in Cuba.

> Mario, a 75-year-old great-grandfather, is invited to speak to a group of social work educators visiting Havana, Cuba. He relays that he decided to stay in Cuba when his brother left because he wanted to take advantage of the free education and health care systems. He attributes his positive functioning to the public health clinic in his neighborhood. He states that although his home is very crowded, he enjoys helping take care of his grandchildren and great-grandchildren. He has taken courses on grandparenting at the University of the Older Adult, sponsored by the University of Havana.

Patterns of Family Constellations

Most caregiving continues to be done by family. However, theorists and policy-makers are raising questions about the capacity for caregiving in the contemporary family (Greene, 2005b). For example, Popenoe (1993) characterized the family, particularly that of the baby boom generation, as stripped down to the bare essentials of childbearing and the provision of affection and companionship. This leads us to ask: If the modern-day family is already stressed, can intergenerational support among family members be maintained? Will the "fluidity of age-appropriate roles affect family structures and the norms of intergenerational family reciprocity"

(Bengtson, Giarrusso, Silverstein, & Wang, 2000, p. 5) remain feasible? Cultural attitudes and family forms and norms influence the answers to these questions.

At the beginning of the 20th century, the structure of most families was akin to a pyramid, usually with one older grandparent at the top. The 21st-century family, in contrast, is shaped more like a beanpole, with great-grandparents who are still living at the top, but with fewer branches, that is, members of their children's, grandchildren's, and great-grandchildren's generations (Hooyman & Kayak, 2005).

Baby Boomers. Baby boomers have experienced differences in the timing and tempo of human events (Corman & Kingson, 1996). They are the first generation raised in a postindustrial society, with its associated accelerated changes, the last generation raised by housewives. Baby boomers have higher rates of postponing marriage, a smaller family size, more dual-career marriages, and higher rates of preventing pregnancy and getting divorced than "general" society. In addition, this generation includes more single parents and blended households (Maugans, 1994). Furthermore, baby boomers will have a smaller pool of family members than previous generations because of falling birthrates.

Yet not all baby boomers meet this profile, particularly minority older adults. Those who have faced discrimination or poverty may experience double jeopardy from both frailty and social and economic issues. For example, older women of color who are unmarried are at risk for living in poverty during later life (Angel, Jiménez, & Angel, 2007; Kisor & Kendal-Wilson, 2002; Ozawa & Hong, 2006). These women may need to retain low-wage and physically demanding work to supplement insufficient Social Security and personal resources (such as pensions and savings).

Applying REM in Individual Intervention

In addition to experiencing biopsychosocial and spiritual concerns and frailty, older adults are at risk for losing friends and family, which often leads to sadness, depression, and prolonged bereavement. Among the most important protective factors for older adults are their families and support networks. Resilience among older adults is related to how they adapt to stress and continue to connect with others.

Triage

The burgeoning older adult population will test the capacity of families as well as health and social services systems. The longevity revolution will necessitate that social workers be prepared to conduct *client-centered assessments* "using the social work principle of basing the level of care (or intervention) on the individual's functional capacity—from those who are most independent to those who are least independent" (Vourlekis & Greene, 1992, p. 15). That is, care should be provided to those in the greatest need. To achieve the objective of *triage*, that is, providing the most services to the most frail or physically or mentally challenged people, practitioners must think of a far-reaching spectrum of services, ranging from preventive and supportive services to nursing home and hospice care (Greene, 2005b). A risk and resilience assessment is highly suited for this purpose.

REM

Following the death of Gerald, Rachel decided to avail herself of bereavement counseling. Believing that the helping process is facilitated by a client's natural healing process and the core conditions of treatment—empathy, nonpossessive warmth, and authenticity—her social care worker applied principles of REM. The goal was to examine both the positive aspects and challenges of caregiving (Farran et al., 1999) (see "Attitudes toward Caregiving Scale" on page 73).

Acknowledging Client Loss, Vulnerability, and Future. REM deals with the paradoxical effects of the client experiencing loss and simultaneously feeling hope for the future. Rachel told the practitioner that she could not imagine life without her husband of 40 years. Yet, at the same time, the practitioner encouraged Rachel to expand professional roles that she had relinquished to make room for caregiving.

Identifying the Source of and Reaction to Stress. The stress of caregiving, which may include hypervigilance, continues after the death of a care recipient. There also are new stressors, such as managing household affairs. Sorting through these is an important aspect of REM.

Stabilizing or Normalizing the Situation. Normalizing the situation helped Rachel understand her emotions: a combination of anger, sadness, and determination. How could she be angry that her husband died? The practitioner's nonjudgmental approach and reaffirmation provided support.

Helping Clients Take Control. Rachel expressed concern that she cried "at the drop of a hat!" The social worker explained that bereavement would diminish over time, especially as Rachel began to assume more of her customary roles.

Providing Resources for Change. Rachel was initially deeply troubled by Gerald's death. She gradually learned that she had her family as a resource for change. For example, her grandchildren often called for advice.

Promoting Self-efficacy. With the help of the social care worker, Rachel learned about volunteer opportunities in her community. She sought these out and gradually found that her sense of self-efficacy improved. This is an example of Rachel's collaborating in self-change.

Strengthening Problem-Solving Abilities. Many clients come to therapy with strong problem-solving capacities. Others may need to learn or be mentored in how to manage life events. Positive reinterpretation and acceptance of events leads to a lessening of the care burden that lingers after the care recipient's death (Dunkin & Anderson-Hanley, 1998).

Attitudes toward Caregiving Scale

Loss/Powerless Subscale (LP)

1. I miss the communication and companionship that my family member and I had in the past.
2. I miss my family member's ability to love me as he/she did in the past.
3. I am sad about the mental and physical changes I see in my relative.
4. I miss the little things my relative and I did together in the past.
5. I am sad about losing the person I once knew.
6. I miss not being able to be spontaneous in my life because of caring for my relative.
7. My situation feels endless.
12. I miss not having more time for other family members and/or friends.
13. I have no hope; I am clutching at straws.
18. I miss our previous social life.
19. I have no sense of joy.
24. I miss being able to travel.
25. I wish I were free to lead a life of my own.
30. I miss having given up my job or other personal interests to take care of my family member.
31. I feel trapped by my relative's illness.
34. We had goals for the future, but they just folded up because of my relative's dementia.
36. I miss my relative's sense of humor.
37. I wish I could run away.
41. I feel that the quality of my life has decreased.

Provisional Meaning Subscale (PM)

8. I enjoy having my relative with me; I would miss it if he/she were gone.
9. I count my blessings.
10. Caring for my relative gives my life a purpose and a sense of meaning.
14. I cherish the past memories and experiences that my relative and I have had.
15. I am a strong person.
16. Caregiving makes me feel good that I am helping.
20. The hugs and "I love you" from my relative make it worth it all.
21. I'm a fighter.
22. I am glad I am here to care for my relative.
26. Talking with others who are close to me restores my faith in my own abilities.
27. Even though there are difficult things in my life, I look forward to the future.
28. Caregiving has helped me learn new things about myself.
32. Each year, regardless of the quality, is a blessing.
33. I would not have chosen the situation I'm in, but I get satisfaction out of providing care.
38. Every day is a blessing.
39. This is my place; I have to make the best out of it.
40. I am much stronger than I think.
42. I start each day knowing we will have a beautiful day together.
43. Caregiving has made me a stronger and better person.

Ultimate Meaning Subscale (UM)

11. The Lord won't give you more than you can handle.
17. I believe in the power of prayer; without it I couldn't do this.
23. I believe that the Lord will provide.
29. I have faith that the good Lord has reasons for this.
35. God is good.

Note: Response options are strongly agree, agree, undecided, disagree, and strongly disagree.
Source: Reprinted with permission from "Finding Meaning through Caregiving: Development of an Instrument for Family Caregivers of Persons with Alzheimer's Disease," by C. Farran, B. Miller, J. Kaufman, D. Donner, and L. Fogg, 1999, *Journal of Clinical Psychology, 55*, pp. 1122–1124. Copyright 1999 by John Wiley & Sons, Inc.

Achieving Creative Expression. Finding activities that allow clients to reduce tension and to "escape from harsh realities" (Greene, 2007) contributes to positive emotions. Rachel joined the symphony league, telling her social worker that she was trying to arrange for pleasing activities.

Making Meaning of Events. Studies on resilience suggest that Rachel would better resolve Gerald's death if she were able to derive positive meaning from her caregiving experience (Farran et al., 1999; Thoits, 1995). As Rachel reviewed her accomplishments over her five-year caregiving experience, she was able to find benefit in this (seemingly) adverse event and transcend the immediate situation.

Updegraff and Taylor (2000) suggested three areas that practitioners can tap to help clients find benefits following traumatic events:

1. Improve clients' self-concept: strengthen the belief that they are stronger and better able to handle negative events
2. Increase clients' appreciation of relationships: enhance the sense that they have a stronger sense of belonging
3. Enhance personal growth: increase the conviction that goals can be accomplished

Caregiving as a Collective Action and Goodness of Fit

As the case studies in this chapter indicate, caregiving requires a goodness of fit between the care provider and care recipient. Social support from family and friends is critical for older adults as functional declines and health problems can overwhelm their ability to provide self-care. In a study that examined cases of abuse and neglect among older adults, individuals with the greatest risk for self-neglect were those who had low levels of social support (Choi & Mayer, 2000). Support that can meet the older individual's needs is important in maintaining functioning despite the challenges of later life.

Caregiving is a reciprocal relationship, however, and the experience affects the care provider as well. There is clear evidence that providing care to older adults can lead to increased problems with health and functioning for care providers. In a meta-analysis of care provision for older adults, Chappell and Funk (2011) highlighted the negative outcomes that caregivers can experience as a result of their role. These include emotional distress, such as depression and anxiety, as well as physical health problems that can lead to increased morbidity. To understand caregiving holistically, the social work practitioner needs to assess the experience of both members of the caregiving dyad.

In addition, social workers need to focus on the collective actions involved in care provision. Some cultures and ethnic groups have a more expanded orientation to care than the individualist model that tends to predominate in the United States.

In a study of care provision in Britain, for example, immigrant families reported a more collective approach to care provision than white British families (Willis, 2012). This was demonstrated by the use of more inclusive language to describe the experience of care (for example, the use of pronouns such as "we" and "our" to describe care provision) and a network orientation to task. In the United States, these findings are aligned with trends in African American culture, which has a collective orientation to care (Dilworth-Anderson, Williams, & Gibson, 2002).

Collective action is also needed to change the paradigm and policies regarding care provision in later life. As Hooyman, Browne, Ray, and Richardson (2002) asserted,

> Caregiving can be a labor of love, chosen by both the caregiver and the care receiver. More often, however, the choices of both are limited by public policy, in part because long-term community-based care, defined by our society largely as a private responsibility, is typically unpaid care by women. Such care, frequently motivated by cost-savings, is not "free" but has real costs and consequences for women, especially in old age. (pp. 10–11)

Thus, caregivers need to raise their collective voices to policymakers to change some of the current laws and practices that add challenge and stress to caregiving situations.

Collective Efficacy and Human Capital

The neighborhood context is important for health and functioning in later life. The environmental and social context for older adults can promote feelings of inclusion, engagement, and belonging. Conversely, older adults who live in neighborhoods with high levels of social disorganization are more likely than their younger cohorts to report negative emotional consequences (Payne, Monk-Turner, Kropf, & Turner, 2010).

From a care-sharing perspective, communities can provide support for families and older individuals who require care. The proximity of neighbors makes them potential sources of support for caregiving families in, for example, reporting risk situations (such as the wandering of older adults who were left unattended). In addition, training efforts to make natural gatekeepers within the community have been undertaken in some locations, with good success (Barrett, Secic, & Borowske, 2010). Individuals who naturally come into contact with older adults (for example, bank tellers and mail carriers) can be trained to spot risk situations that can compromise the health and well-being of the older adult.

For many older adults and families, however, the environment may not include the qualities important for promoting positive health and functioning. In a study on racial disparities in self-rated health, neighborhood affluence was a significant factor in positive health status, regardless of race (Cagney, Browning, & Wen, 2005). For those who lived in poorer neighborhoods, lower levels of residential stability (that is, living in the same house over time or owning one's home) had a negative effect on health status. This finding indicates that weak ties owing to transient and impermanent living situations are associated with poorer health and well-being and that lack of care sharing in the community can have a detrimental effect on the older adults who live there.

Social workers can be involved in interventions to strengthen social connections and cohesion in neighborhoods. The following is an example of a geriatric nurse practitioner who has taken the initiative to bring together a group of individuals who are interested in sharing their talents with one another as they grow older:

> Elaine is a nurse geriatric practitioner with more than 20 years of experience. She works in an office on a multidisciplinary team, and in this role, she participates in the evaluation of distressed older clients, many of whom reside in nursing homes. Having witnessed the struggles many families face as they try to locate resources for their loved ones, Elaine has decided to arrange a community similar to Beacon Hill (discussed previously) in her hometown. She has gathered together a group of close friends who will either buy or build homes within walking distance of one another so that they can be of assistance to members of the group. They have engaged a law-yer to incorporate their idea and work out funding and entitlements. When needed, each member of the community can use a concierge to pick up laundry, a driver to get to doctor's appointments, as well as a system for delivering groceries.

This arrangement is playing out in communities across the nation where older adults are constructing care-sharing situations. In some areas, home sharing is another option that provides mutual and economic aid. A 2013 National Public Radio story featured a group of women who had moved into a house together to share expenses, social experiences, and support (Rovner, 2013). Because the gender gap increases in later life and older women have fewer economic resources than older men (see Angel et al., 2007; Ozawa & Hong, 2006), creative ways to share resources can provide an important buffer against the social and economic stresses of later life.

In summary, caregiving for older adults is becoming a normative part of the life course. The role of the social worker is to assess how families handle the associated tasks and to assist care providers in preserving their own health and functioning. From a social care perspective, families need assistance from both formal and informal networks that can share the responsibilities of these roles. As the baby boom generation continues to age, even more creative ways of providing care and care sharing will be needed to support older adults and their families.

CHAPTER FIVE

Disability through the Life Course

This chapter explores caring for a family member with an early-onset disability, specifically, intellectual or developmental disability (IDD). Caregiving for people with IDD starts early in life, as these disabilities are diagnosed early in the child's development. IDD requires many families to provide care for a child significantly past the usual time frame for raising children. In fact, some parents remain in a caregiving role until their death or incapacitation. In many ways, this type of care provision is different from that for an older family member, as described in chapter 4.

Using a Social Care Approach

Using a social care approach begins with identifying the population with a disability. As previously stated, individuals with IDD have developmental delays that appear early in the life course. This section covers the effect of an early diagnosis on the person with IDD and the family as well as intragroup variation across diagnostic categories.

IDD Defined

An *intellectual disability* is "a condition of arrested or incomplete development of the mind, which is especially characterized by impairment of skills manifested during the developmental period, which contribute to the overall level of intelligence, i.e., cognitive, language, motor, and social abilities" (World Health Organization, 2001). The American Association on Intellectual and Developmental Disabilities (2013) further defines it as "a disability characterized by significant limitations both in intellectual functioning (reasoning, learning, problem solving) and in adaptive behavior, which covers a range of everyday social and practical skills. This disability originates before the age of 18."

A major piece of legislation relevant to IDD is the Developmental Disabilities Assistance and Bill of Rights Act of 2000 (P.L. 106-402). This legislation sets up a policy agenda for individuals with developmental disabilities and their families. Within this piece of federal legislation, a *developmental disability* is defined as a

Developmental Disabilities Assistance and Bill of Rights Act of 2000

DEVELOPMENTAL DISABILITY is defined:

(A) IN GENERAL.—The term "developmental disability" means a severe, chronic disability of an individual that—

    (i)   is attributable to a mental or physical impairment or combination of mental and physical impairments;

    (ii) is manifested before the individual attains age 22;

    (iii) is likely to continue indefinitely;

    (iv) results in substantial functional limitations in 3 or more of the following areas of major life activity:

        (I)   Self-care.

        (II)   Receptive and expressive language.

        (III) Learning.

        (IV) Mobility.

        (V)   Self-direction.

        (VI) Capacity for independent living.

        (VII) Economic self-sufficiency; and

    (v)   reflects the individual's need for a combination and sequence of special, interdisciplinary, or generic services, individualized supports, or other forms of assistance that are of lifelong or extended duration and are individually planned and coordinated.

Source: Reprinted from *Administration on Intellectual and Developmental Disabilities (AIDD): The Developmental Disabilities Assistance and Bill of Rights Act of 2000*, by the Administration for Community Living, 2013, retrieved from http://www.acl.gov/Programs/AIDD/DDA_BOR_ACT_2000/p2_tl_subtitleA.aspx

---

chronic disability that appears before age 22 and that leads to limitations in three or more areas of functioning. See "Developmental Disabilities Assistance and Bill of Rights Act of 2000" on page 78 for an excerpt of the definition used in this legislation.

According to this definition, numerous diagnostic categories make up IDD. "Intellectual and Developmental Disabilities Defined" on page 79 summarizes the most common categories of disabilities. These different conditions reveal the variation in behavior and in mental and physical ability within the population with IDD.

Incidence

The rate of developmental disabilities has increased over previous decades (see "Incidence of Developmental Disabilities" on page 80). One reason for this is the availability of sophisticated diagnostic measures that provide more accurate evaluations for disabilities. However, some unknown factors—such as environmental agents or physical conditions—may also partially account for these increases.

Intellectual and Developmental Disabilities Defined

Autism spectrum disorders are developmental disabilities that can cause significant social, communication, and behavioral challenges.

Cerebral palsy refers to a group of disorders that affect a person's ability to move and maintain balance and posture. Cerebral palsy is the most common motor disability in childhood. The CDC estimates that on average 1 in 303 children in the United States has cerebral palsy.

Developmental disabilities are impairments in physical functioning, learning, language, or behavior. About 1 in 6 children in the United States have one or more developmental disabilities or other developmental delay.

Intellectual disability, previously known as "mental retardation," refers to limits to a person's ability to learn at an expected level and function in daily life. Delays in developmental milestones may include

- sitting up, crawling, or walking later than other children
- learning to talk later or having trouble speaking
- finding it hard to remember things
- having trouble understanding social rules
- having trouble seeing the results of one's actions
- having trouble solving problems

Source: Adapted from Specific Conditions, by the Centers for Disease Control and Prevention, 2012, retrieved from http://www.cdc.gov/ncbddd/developmentaldisabilities/specificconditions.html

An examination of trends in developmental disabilities showed that diagnoses of these disabilities are not uncommon among children (Boyle et al., 2011). The estimate indicated that in 2006–2008, 15 percent of U.S. children ages three to 17 had some type of developmental disability. It also showed that the prevalence of parent-reported disabilities increased 17.1 percent between 1997 and 2008. This increase in the incidence of disability requires additional services and supports for these individuals and their families.

Diversity Issues

Because IDD includes multiple diagnostic categories, there is substantial diversity in the population with IDD. Some individuals have serious health challenges related to their disability. For example, a common difficulty for people with cerebral palsy is ambulation. In research describing the functional ability of adults with cerebral palsy, one-third of the study participants either had never been able to walk or had lost the ability to walk over time (Andersson & Mattsson, 2001). Although individuals with cerebral palsy may have extensive physical challenges, many do not

Incidence of Developmental Disabilities

- The prevalence of any developmental disabilities in 1997–2008 was 13.87 percent.
- The prevalence of autism was 0.47 percent.
- Over the last 12 years, the prevalence of developmental disabilities has increased 17.1 percent—that's about 1.8 million more children with developmental disabilities in 2006–2008 compared with a decade earlier—and the prevalence of autism increased 289.5 percent.
- Males had twice the prevalence of any developmental disability than females and more specifically had a higher prevalence of attention deficit/hyperactivity disorder, autism, learning disabilities, stuttering/stammering, and other developmental disabilities.
- Hispanic children had a lower prevalence of several disorders compared with non-Hispanic white and non-Hispanic black children.
- Children insured by Medicaid had a nearly twofold higher prevalence of any developmental disability compared with those with private insurance.
- Children from families with income below the federal poverty level had a higher prevalence of developmental disabilities.

Source: Adapted from *Key Findings: Trends in the Prevalence of Developmental Disabilities in U.S. Children, 1997–2008,* by the Centers for Disease Control and Prevention, 2012, retrieved from http://www.cdc.gov/ncbddd/features/birthdefects-dd-keyfindings.html

have impaired cognitive functioning. In one study, 44 percent of individuals with cerebral palsy had normal mental functioning (Hutton & Pharoah, 2002). Clearly, there are significant differences in the functional ability of people with IDD.

There are also differences in other sociodemographic factors. As is indicated in "Incidence of Developmental Disabilities," more male children than female children are diagnosed with IDD. In addition, children from lower socioeconomic backgrounds have higher rates of disabilities.

Cohort effects are important in understanding the lives and experiences of individuals with IDD and their families. The philosophy and paradigm of caregiving and care sharing has changed dramatically since the 1960s. Before that time, families had to choose between being the sole source of support for their family member or placing him or her in an institution. Today's services are founded on a care-sharing perspective in which various services (educational, behavioral, and medical) are provided in partnership with the family.

Service systems for people with IDD have changed dramatically, and cohorts within this population have different experiences that affect their level of trust and involvement with formal service providers. Just as the aging population is increasing (see chapter 4), adults with developmental disabilities are also living longer. It used to be that people with developmental disabilities had shorter life expectancies than their peers in the general population. On average, people with IDD still die earlier than their counterparts in the general population, yet some live as long (or outlive) their peers without disabilities (Janicki, Dalton, Henderson, & Davidson, 1999). Therefore, aging has become an important issue for the families of individuals with IDD.

Stigmatized and Politicized Caregiving Context

To understand the experience of caring for someone with IDD, the practitioner needs to be sensitive to and aware of the dramatic shift in services for this population. These major changes have taken place within the lifetimes of the current cohort of older individuals. Thus, the experiences of families with younger children are significantly different from those of people who have witnessed these shifts in care. Sadly, a historical perspective of the treatment of individuals with disabilities reveals inhumane treatment conditions until the mid-1900s. Legislation has shifted to focus on community integration and support for families of individuals with a disability. To help you understand these dramatic changes, we present some of the major milestones here.

Historical Perspective

As recently as the mid-20th century, people with IDD were treated poorly in U.S. society. The photographic essay *Christmas in Purgatory* vividly portrays the deplorable conditions in mental institutions for people with disabilities (Blatt & Kaplan, 1966). The pictures that make up the essay convey the inadequate and cruel standards of care that existed in such institutions during these years. They depict the mass warehousing of children and infants in environments without stimulation, impoverished living conditions, and the disengagement and hopelessness of institution residents. *Christmas in Purgatory* was a catalyst for efforts to change the conditions for and treatment of people with developmental disabilities.

In 1963, President John Kennedy authorized the Community Mental Health Act (P.L. 88-164, also known as the Mental Retardation and Community Mental Health Centers Construction Act of 1963). Besides being the impetus for change in service provision for people with mental illness and developmental disabilities, the act marked the first time that a president had sent a message to Congress about mental health issues (National Institutes of Health, 2013). This legislation created hope that people with disabilities (both developmental disabilities and mental illness) would be able to receive treatment in their own communities. In the act's wake, community mental health organizations were formed across the country. Yet in spite of these changes in policy and treatment, resources (including funding and staffing) continue to be insufficient to provide effective and comprehensive services to individuals and families.

Summary of Legislation Related to Individuals with Disabilities

Individuals with Disabilities Education Improvement Act of 2004 (P.L. 108-446)

- Amended the Education for All Handicapped Children Act of 1975 (P.L. 94-142)
- Guarantees free and appropriate public education in the least restrictive environment for every person with a disability
- Gives federal funding to people who meet minimum education standards
- Has six principles:
  - Free education
  - Appropriate education
  - Individual education programs
  - Least restrictive environment
  - Parent and student participation in decision making
  - Procedural safeguards

(See idea.ed.gov.)

Americans with Disabilities Act of 1990 (P.L. 101-336)

- Created to protect people with disabilities from discrimination within the community and the workplace
- Signed into law by President George H. W. Bush in 1990
- Provides civil rights protections to people with disabilities similar to those provided on the basis of race, gender, national origin, religion, and age

(See http://www.ADA.gov.)

Olmstead Act: *Olmstead v. L.C.* 527 U.S. 581 (1999)

- Maintains that community-based treatment programs must be provided for individuals with mental disabilities
- Based on a case in which the state of Georgia forced two women with intellectual disability to remain in a state hospital after their service providers had deemed them ready for discharge
- Ensures that under the Americans with Disabilities Act, a state will provide community-based services to qualified individuals and make "reasonable accommodations" to do so

Rehabilitation Act of 1973 (P.L. 93-112)

- Authorizes grant programs of vocational rehabilitation, supported employment, independent living, and assistance
- Includes sections that prohibit discrimination against individuals with disabilities by federal agencies, employers and businesses that contract with federal agencies, and programs receiving federal financial assistance

Since the 1960s, several other pieces of legislation vital in the lives of individuals with disabilities have been passed (see "Summary of Legislation Related to Individuals with Disabilities" on page 82). These policies have the goal of providing individuals with access to education, employment, and the community in general. In addition to the major legislation summarized in the box, other laws and statutes include language about people with disabilities as well.

Even after the passage of federal legislation, however, people with IDD were subjected to inhumane practices. Like treatment for psychiatric diagnoses (see chapter 6), treatment approaches for IDD could involve pain and suffering. For example, some people with disabilities were involuntarily sterilized to curb their sexuality (and reproduction). This issue continues to gain exposure as individuals who were involuntarily sterilized are now demanding legal recourse and compensation. In 2011 the *New York Times* told the stories of men and women who had been involuntarily sterilized in North Carolina, one of the states that practiced eugenics (Severson, 2011). Sadly, social workers were part of these movements and advised families that this practice was for the good of their family member. Remember that historically social work professionals did not always act in the best interest of people with IDD and their families. In particular, older adults and their families may have had negative experiences that color their perception of services today.

Creating Supportive Communities

At the community level, the availability and accessibility of resources is crucial in helping families who are caring for individuals with IDD. In 1981, the Home and Community-Based Service Waiver program was authorized by Congress to allow groups at risk for institutionalization (for example, people with IDD and older adults) to remain in their homes and communities (Gettings, 2012). As services have changed to reflect more of a community-based focus, this program has grown tremendously—to more than $25 billion in 2009 (Braddock et al., 2011). Because this program is administered at the state level, services authorized under it vary greatly. However, these support subsidies offer families resources to promote family functioning, for example, waivers to purchase a van that can accommodate a wheelchair or to engage respite services for after-school hours. An important aspect of the program is that families can decide how to use these funds to suit their particular needs.

Managing Stigma

In the past decades, policies regarding individuals with IDD have shifted dramatically, yet attitudes have been much slower to change. Research indicates that individuals with disabilities experience negative attitudes and stereotypes that make achieving full integration in the community challenging (Rao, 2004; Tervo, Azuma, Palmer, & Redinius, 2002). Some research suggests that attitudes toward individuals with IDD are improving (Goreczny, Bender, Caruso, & Feinstein, 2011). However, some areas remain less positive (for example, there is still often hesitation to establish close personal relationships with people who have disabilities).

Over time, the language used to describe people with IDD has changed to become less stigmatizing. Until the mid-1900s, terms such as "idiot," "feeble minded," "mongol," and "moron" were used to describe people with IDD. In addition to avoiding these condescending terms, people today use person-first language to emphasize the individual and deemphasize the disability (McCoy & DeCecco, 2011). For example, instead of talking about a "disabled person," we talk about a "person with a disability." This change emphasizes the personhood of the individual. In addition, terms have been changed to lessen some of the stigma. Rosa Marcellino, an 11-year-old girl with Down syndrome, and her family worked to have the term "mental retardation" changed because of its historical negative connotation. In October 2010, President Barack Obama signed Rosa's Law (P.L. 22-256), which changes references in federal statutes from "mental retardation" to "intellectual disability." The term "intellectual disability" is the one most commonly used in current legislative and academic documents.

Applying FAM

Case Study: Family Caregiving in Transition

The Grogan family lives in a large urban area in the Midwest. Parents Nathan and Penny were wed right after college graduation and have been married 14 years. They have three children: Kevin, age 11, who has cerebral palsy and an intellectual disability; Andy, age eight; and Mallory, age five. Nathan works as a middle school assistant principal, and Penny is a librarian at a local community college. Overall, the family is financially stable and lives in a three-bedroom home in a suburb of a large city.

Kevin was born with a disability as a result of complications during delivery. His parents have received support services from the community disability agency since he was born. In addition, both sets of grandparents live in the area and have been involved in helping care for Kevin from birth. Because Andy and Mallory are younger, they have always known Kevin as having a disability; they all get along well. Andy in particular is protective of his brother and spends a great deal of time interacting with him. The kids like to be outside together and enjoy playing with their family dog, Romper, who is well behaved and does well with the children.

Kevin is nonambulatory and uses a wheelchair. He is also nonverbal but uses a few idiosyncratic words that are understood by his family and teachers. He has limited use of his upper body but no fine motor skills. He requires assistance in all activities of daily living, including eating, maintaining hygiene, and using the bathroom.

The family is starting to experience some stress as the children age. Kevin and Andy currently share a bedroom on the ground floor of the home, and the master bedroom and Mallory's bedroom are on the second story of the home. Most of the boys' room is taken up by Kevin's wheelchair and adaptive equipment, and Andy has limited space to call his own. As Andy ages, this is becoming a bit of a problem; he is starting to ask for more space and privacy (for example, to have his friends over to play). Andy has also started to express jealousy that Mallory has her own room but there is no available room for him.

Also, there have been some changes in the supports for Kevin's care. Previously, his grandparents shared the responsibility for meeting Kevin's school bus and helping him in the house. Now they are aging (both sets of grandparents are in their early 70s) and are starting to experience some age-related health challenges. At the same time, Kevin is maturing physically, and it is more difficult to provide care. This situation is causing some stress in the family, as both Penny and Nathan have jobs that require them to be at work until 5 p.m.

Thus, Penny and Nathan are considering whether Penny can reduce her hours to half time. Although this will free up some time for her to be home, she loves her job and is reluctant to give up her time at the community college. Penny's work provides her with a group of friends as well as a meaningful career. In fact, her supervisor is close to retirement age and has made it clear that she would like Penny to assume her position when she leaves in another year or two. The drop to half-time employment will require that Penny relinquish this possibility, and the thought saddens her.

There are also financial considerations related to this change. Moving to a half-time position would mean a loss of more than 50 percent of the family's income because, as a full-time employee, Penny is on the payroll in the summer, when fewer students are on campus. Part-time employees are ineligible for summer employment, which means that the family will have only one income during the summer months.

These changes are creating tension in the family. Penny and Nathan have been fighting more frequently, and Nathan has been staying longer at work, sometimes coming home after 8 p.m. This infuriates Penny, who is absorbing the responsibility for the children and household most weekdays. Weekends are also chaotic, as Andy has joined a soccer league and has games most Saturdays. Mallory is taking dance lessons and also has practice and performances on weekends. Although Nathan thinks that the children should slow down, Penny is adamant that her two younger children "have a normal childhood." That is, she feels that they should be able to pursue activities that other children their age do and should not have to curtail their interests because they have a brother with a disability. Overall, the family is experiencing a number of changes that have consequences for the individual family members' functioning as well as the relationships within the family.

FAM Assessment

The experiences of the Grogan family are highlighted here to illustrate the various components of FAM. This family is experiencing stress as a result of the aging of a child with a disability as well as the life course changes the family is undergoing. Although the family has experienced challenges in the past, the current situation is putting stress on the family in new ways.

From a biological perspective, several issues are affecting the family at this point in time. First, Kevin is maturing into a young adolescent with a disability, and he is experiencing physical changes and growth. Second, his grandparents, who have been important sources of support, are also aging. These intersecting aging processes are creating difficulties for family functioning. Third, Kevin's physical health trajectory is unknown. Although he is fairly healthy currently, he does require specialized equipment and care. His parents are also in good health currently, but their ability to care for him in the future may place additional stress on the family.

In terms of the psychological assessment, Penny and Nathan's challenges relate to their parenting experience and their ability to cope with Kevin's needs. In addition, they both must find balance between being available for the family and respecting individual needs, such as Penny's gratification in her career. Kevin's siblings, Andy and Mallory, are also growing older and becoming more independent. They are exerting autonomy and beginning their own lives away from their family. As they develop, mature, and gain additional abilities, their parents may be sad that their younger children's skills are now eclipsing those of their oldest child.

With regard to social functioning, Nathan and Penny may find themselves in the role of providing care across Kevin's entire life course. Significant issues are involved in caring for individuals with IDD; as a result, mothers and fathers in these roles have been termed "perpetual parents" (Barrett, Hale, & Butler, 2014; Jennings, 1993; Kelly & Kropf, 1995). These experiences, and the related consequences for family choices and relationships across the life course, are significant.

One area of concern for the Grogan family is the career trajectory of the parents. Both Penny and Nathan are ascending in their careers. As an assistant principal, Nathan aspires to become a principal. Although rewarding, his current position has responsibilities that require he work weeknight and weekend hours. In addition, Penny's supervisor at work has been grooming her for a new position, which is appealing to her. However, it may be unrealistic for both parents to achieve increased responsibility in their careers. Clearly, Penny is feeling some disappointment about having to curtail her job opportunities.

In addition, the younger children are growing older and achieving more independence. As they begin to cultivate more relationships outside the family home, Kevin's companionship and friendship will come into question. He and Andy are close, and Andy's independence may cause Kevin to feel loneliness.

Although limited information about the Grogan family's spiritual functioning is available, other families that have children with disabilities experience spiritual crises. Parents might wonder why their child was born with such a condition. Conversely, they might think that their child was placed in the family for a reason and that the family should bear all the responsibility for the child's care. An assessment of spiritual functioning is important in working with families that include a child with IDD.

Family Assessment

Some family issues require assessment and possible intervention. Families are social systems. Because the primary relationships for many people with IDD are with their families, family therapy may be helpful in navigating the various transitions and junctures through the life course (Hill-Weld, 2011). Therapy can assist with making decisions, decreasing guilt, and promoting bonds between various family members that may shift because of care responsibilities.

When a family member has a lifelong disability, bonds between subsystems can decrease within the family. In the Grogan family, for example, Kevin and Andy have a strong bond. What characterizes the bonds between Kevin and Mallory or Andy and Mallory? How do the parents relate to the younger children? Do the younger children have a relationship with the grandparents, or are these relationships based primarily around Kevin's care needs? It is critical to know whether the care needs of the child with a disability are affecting relationships among all members of the family.

Although children with Kevin's type of disability have certain unique care needs, assessment also must consider the sources of joy and rewards that are present in caregiving for a child with IDD. Through their relationships with siblings with disabilities, brothers and sisters can find happiness and have character-building experiences (Dykens, 2005). The positive aspects of these relationships are important.

In addition, people with disabilities may play important roles within the family and household as their parents age. One of the authors once worked with an older mother who lived alone with her son, who had Down syndrome. As the mother aged, the son would go grocery shopping with her and push the cart, carry the bags, and help put the food in the cupboards. In addition, he ran the vacuum in the house. Without this assistance, the mother may not have been able to remain in her home alone. In this example of familial interdependence, the collective skills of all members are necessary in the successful functioning of the family.

Applying REM in Individual Intervention

Families need support in caring for family members with IDD, and a care-sharing perspective suggests that interventions would enhance families' abilities to perform in caregiving roles. As Chan, Merriman, Parmenter, and Stancliffe (2012) stated, "The social model of disability emphasizes the shared role of the family and the state in caring for individuals with disabilities" (p. 122). Two types of interventions—relieving stress and planning for future care needs—are presented here as ways to enhance family competence in care.

Stress Reduction: Reducing Risks

Because the care needs of individuals with IDD can be intense and complex, care-givers benefit from breaks in their responsibilities. Respite care services provide substitute care either in the care recipient's own home or at another site (such as a group or foster care home) so that primary caregivers can have time to themselves. The need for respite care is most acute when the care recipient exhibits behavioral challenges, has a severe disability, or is exceedingly dependent on the care provider (Chan, 2008; Chan & Sigafoos, 2000). In these situations, respite care may be the primary means for care providers to find relief from their caregiving tasks. This time away can be rejuvenating and can provide caregivers with an occasion to relax and distance themselves from their typical care experiences.

Respite care could provide Nathan and Penny Grogan with opportunities to spend time with their other children. In addition, it would allow them to spend time together as a couple, which is also important for their marriage and partnership. Respite care could also enable Kevin, who enjoys social interactions, to spend time with non–family members. Although respite care is often considered a support for the caregiver, it also provides social time for the person with the disability.

Families also benefit from receiving support as they consider their care responsibilities, plan for transitions in the life course of the person with the disability, and make decisions. Family therapy can assist families with these challenges and with any stress that occurs within the marriage or other subsystems of the family (for example, between siblings and between parents and their typically developing children). The additional family stress is evident in the Grogan family, as the transitions around Kevin's care, the impending situation with Penny's work, and the maturation of Andy and Mallory are destabilizing the family. Because many individuals with IDD have their family as their primary source of care and support, support and intervention with the family unit alone can address these issues (Hill-Weld, 2011).

Future Planning: Enhancing Resilience

A major concern for families with a son or daughter with IDD is future care. That is, what will happen if the parents can no longer provide care? In many families, future planning does not start until some type of crisis, such as the death or incapacitation of the care provider, arises. Care planning is complex, however, and becomes more difficult when superimposed onto another family crisis.

Future planning can enhance the resilience of the family. It provides a plan that allows for transitions in care. If the person with IDD will eventually move to a supported living arrangement as an adult, future planning should include short respite stays away from the family for him or her. These transitions help the person with IDD to learn coping and independent living skills and also allow caregivers opportunities to move out of the care provision role. Especially for those caregivers who have provided care for many years, this transition can be difficult.

Many individuals are involved in transition planning. The individual with IDD is an integral part of the process and should be involved in making choices about his or her own living and working arrangements. Families and formal service providers share the responsibility of assisting the individual with IDD with achieving his or her goals and desired outcomes. Research on the outcomes of person-centered future planning indicates that this process helps families make plans for future care, releases anxieties about care transitions, and enables individuals with IDD to make choices about their own lives (Heller & Caldwell, 2006).

Future planning needs to take place at various points along the life course, even now while Kevin is young. At this point, the Grogans should consider what plans to put in place as Kevin ages. If the family encountered an emergency or unplanned situation, would it have the necessary plans (financial, support, and so forth) in place to address it? Families may resist planning, as the process can be an emotional one. Yet navigating a crisis can be more complex if there are no plans for dealing with changes in health or financial emergencies.

Case Management: A Life Course Perspective

Families experience different issues in care provision at different points in the life course of the person with IDD. In the person's early life, the family adapts to having a child with a cognitive or physical disability. During adulthood, individuals with IDD integrate into adult roles, such as in employment or vocational settings. Physical health issues may become more prominent for both the aging parent and the individual with IDD. During the individual's later life, the source of caregiving may change as a result of declines in the primary caregiver's health or the caregiver's death. Families may also face end-of-life issues for the person with IDD.

Case managers help families and individuals with IDD access services within the community. These services can be especially helpful in times of transition, such as when the person with IDD develops a need that requires more involvement with formal services (Bigby, Ozanne, & Gordon, 2002). At these points, case managers can assess what has occurred in the family and create a care plan that incorporates one or multiple service sectors (for example, health, mental health, and disability). At point-of-care transitions, family needs are often complex and require coordination across networks.

Early Life

Environmental influences, including social interactions, are crucial in the development of all children in early life. The quality of early relationships, especially the relationship with the primary care provider, is significant in children's development

(Fenning & Baker, 2012). Children with parents who can evaluate the abilities of their children and structure interactions that increase competence and foster resilience achieve higher levels of development. Clearly, the quality of interaction between parents and a child with a disability is critical to the subsequent development of that child. Case management services can link parents with organizations that can help them develop effective parenting skills to match the needs of their child with IDD.

However, parents are not always able to adequately handle raising a child with a disability. Research on the maltreatment of children with disabilities has consistently indicated that these children are at greater risk for abuse, neglect, and out-of-home placement than children without disabilities (Lightfoot, Hill, & LaLiberte, 2011; Rosenberg & Robinson, 2004; Sullivan & Knutson, 2000). Moreover, older children with disabilities in the child welfare system experience a longer out-of-home placement time and greater rates of placement instability than their peers without disabilities (Hill, 2012). The early life experiences of significant numbers of children with disabilities can be difficult and traumatic indeed.

Early intervention programs provide support and education for young children with disabilities. The Individuals with Disabilities Education Improvement Act of 2004 (P.L. 108-446) is federal legislation that allows states to provide therapeutic and educational programs to infants and toddlers. Although these services are important in the development of all young children, their provision reflects a care-sharing approach, as families are provided with the support and skills they need to deal with their child's unique needs and situations (Tomasello, Manning, & Dulmus, 2010). The case manager evaluates the whole family system to determine congruence between the child's care needs and the available resources and to establish goals that are consistent with the family's abilities.

Midlife

As the child with IDD develops into an adult, new challenges emerge for the family and in care provision. One is a concern about how the individual with IDD will spend his or her time. Case managers can help families by providing information about employment and habilitation service options. Unfortunately, after the individual completes his or her education, job opportunities may be limited; unemployment rates for this population are well beyond the typical rate. In 2012, only 17.8 percent of people with disabilities were employed, and 33 percent of workers with disabilities worked part-time compared with 19 percent of those with no disability (Bureau of Labor Statistics, 2013). Clearly, these statistics indicate that adults with disabilities have more limited employment options than those without disabilities. As a result, their economic self-sufficiency is low, and they often depend on support from their families across the life course.

Physical health issues are also significant for many adults with IDD; this population is in worse health than the general population is. Some health conditions, such as the musculoskeletal issues of individuals with cerebral palsy, are related to the disability itself, whereas other conditions result from an unhealthy lifestyle or lack of access to quality health care. Across the life course, obesity rates are higher for people with IDD than for those in the general population (de Winter, Bastiaanse, Hilgenkamp, Evenhuis, & Echteld, 2012; Hinckson, Dickinson, Water, Sands, & Penman, 2013). In addition, adults with IDD face inequities in multiple areas, including access to care and the quality of care received (Ward, Nichols, & Freedman, 2010). Families may require assistance from case managers in accessing qualified care providers who understand the health issues of adults with disabilities.

Because the majority of adults with IDD are supported by their families, the aging of their parents can precipitate a crisis in care. Unfortunately, many families in this situation have limited or no plans for the future care of the individual with IDD. This can be because they do not understand their options, they believe future planning is unnecessary, or they want to avoid undergoing this potentially painful and emotional experience. If no alternative plans are in place, a health crisis for the care provider can mean a crisis for the family. In this situation, case managers can intervene by identifying a group or respite situation or working with other family members to coordinate an adequate care plan for the individual with IDD.

Late Life

The concept of late life for people with IDD is relatively new, thanks to medical and social transformations of the past few decades. For example, life expectancies for individuals with Down syndrome have increased dramatically; previously, individuals with this condition were not expected to live past adolescence (Janicki et al., 1999). Individuals with IDD are now typically living into their late 50s, 60s, and beyond. This trend signifies that family caregiving involves many transitions in late life, and case managers can assist by providing information and being involved in decision making with the family.

End-of-life issues become more prominent as adults with IDD age. This population faces the normative experiences of grief and loss when someone close to them dies, but they also face some unique challenges (Botsford, 2000). For people with limited cognitive abilities, death is a difficult concept to understand. In addition, family members may withhold medical information from the individual to protect him or her. Instead of helping, this strategy can create confusion or anger and exacerbate an already complex situation. Case managers can assist with these transitions as well.

Collective Efficacy and Human Capital

The diagnosis of a disability is a second-order change for families and alters the nature of interaction and care provision in the family. In addition, families must be ready to assume advocacy roles for their son or daughter. One of the greatest needs for families with children with IDD is to find social acceptance and to engage with others (Banach, Iudice, Conway, & Couse, 2010). Interventions that bring families together and promote interaction and advocacy skills will enhance parents' sense of efficacy.

Advocacy for Services

Interventions can enhance the collective efficacy of underrepresented groups within service systems. Families that are not used to being assertive or engaging in self-advocacy may have difficulties in programs that require these skills (Huang et al., 2004).

From a care-sharing perspective, the Grogan family will require community services and support as Kevin ages. Although Kevin is currently in school, his parents are already fearful about his future after he graduates. He will have few employment options because of his physical and cognitive abilities. In addition, vocational programs and services often have a waiting list. His parents have started to worry that there might be a gap between Kevin's leaving school and entering a day program. Because Kevin thrives on social interaction, his being home without any social involvement is a serious concern for the family.

Community access is also a big concern for the Grogan family. As Kevin matures, physical management of his needs is becoming more challenging. Even small family outings like going to dinner have become complex. Navigating his wheelchair across streets, through parking lots, and into buildings can be difficult. As he reaches adulthood, he will have limited options for getting around in the community, as public transportation is minimal. With greater numbers of individuals with disabilities remaining in their homes and communities, access issues must be addressed more comprehensively.

Policy and Program Initiatives

As previously stated, services and interventions for individuals with IDD and their families have changed dramatically over the life course of the older adults in this cohort. Institutional placements are fewer, and community-based and family-centered care is now the norm. Yet in spite of this progress, additional changes are needed to more adequately support families in their caregiving roles across the life course.

In some states, families receive support subsidies to help with care for their child with disabilities. Although this method of support has yielded positive outcomes, not all states offer this option. Agosta and Melda (1995) reported on states that provide cash subsidies that allow families to purchase resources tailored to their particular situation. This type of program provides families with choices and empowers them to determine the best way to meet their needs.

Consider this type of initiative for the Grogan family. With enough funds, the family might be able to pay a neighbor or community member to provide after-school respite care for Kevin. Without support to do this, the Grogans bear this additional expense, which may be too costly. This additional income could make a big difference in the life and experience of a family that is providing care to a child with a disability.

An additional issue is the allocation of funds across different initiatives in IDD services. In an analysis of funding for various developmental disability services, researchers concluded that family support remained a low priority according to budget allocation amounts:

> The majority of people with developmental disabilities are cared for in their family homes, yet state developmental disabilities resources are allocated disproportion-ately for the care of those who live in residential settings, not with their families. There have been calls from advocates around the nation to push states to remedy this fundamental inequity in the distribution of services and support. Even after 2 decades of recognition that family support services are vital to caregivers, the programs continue to comprise a tiny portion of state developmental disabilities resource allocations. (Parish, Pomeranz-Essley, & Braddock, 2003, p. 185)

Therefore, political changes that provide additional methods to support families in their caregiving roles are necessary.

A care-sharing approach for people with IDD involves a shift in the paradigm regarding who is the client for these services. Formal services must be available when family care is absent or no longer feasible, and programs must be available to help families in their care responsibilities across the life course. Chan et al. (2012) made this point as they discussed the need for professionals to share in the care of people with IDD through programs such as respite care: "There are social and eco-nomic gains to be achieved from [such] a shared understanding as family already contribute significantly to the care and support of the person with a disability in the family home" (p. 124).

As in the general population, additional attention needs to be paid to aging in the population with IDD. As these individuals live into later adulthood, later life services (for example, residential options and hospice care) need to be provided so families do not undergo crises when transitions happen within the family. In addi-tion to using direct practice skills with families, social workers need to undertake efforts in advocacy and coalition building (Parish & Lutwick, 2005). Social work-ers need to take more direct professional action to enhance family caregiving in later life.

In summary, families that care for someone with a disability often have extensive caregiving horizons. Many families are in these care roles across the life course of the person with IDD. The cumulative demands of care can be extensive, as they occur in multiple domains, including physical, financial, and emotional.

Through a care-sharing perspective, families benefit from assistance to enhance their caregiving roles and functions. As this chapter has highlighted, approaches to care (and family support needs in care provision) differ at various points in the life course. Social work assessment must continually address the changes in the individual with IDD, the needs and experiences of this individual, and the experience of the caregiver.

CHAPTER SIX

Care Provision and Severe Mental Illness

Mental illness includes numerous diagnoses that have differing presentations, manifestations, and care needs. Sadly, psychiatric conditions continue to carry a stigma that is experienced not only by the person who is diagnosed with the condition, but also by his or her caregiver. For this reason, caregivers for individuals with mental illness have been termed "stigmatized caregivers," and they often remain outside the service system (Kelly & Kropf, 1995). As you will discover as you read this chapter, providing care for a child, adult, or older adult with a psychiatric condition is often challenging and must be done without the care-sharing resources of many informal and formal support services.

The term "mental illness" refers to several diagnostic categories. In this chapter, care provision is discussed in relation to *severe mental illness* (SMI), which is defined as a mental illness that results in a "serious functional impairment that substantially interferes with one or more major life activities, such as work, school or interpersonal relationships" (National Survey on Drug Use and Health, 2012, p. 2). Examples of SMI include schizophrenia and schizophrenia-related disorders, bipolar disorder, major recurrent depressive disorder, and personality disorders. Other research has defined SMI similarly (see Cummings & Kropf, 2009a, 2011). In this chapter, we do not discuss some conditions that are termed "mental disorders" in other research (such as autism, eating disorders, and posttraumatic stress).

We use the life course perspective to explore the experience of caring for an individual with SMI during different life phases. Changes in behavior and experience at different points in the life course are highlighted in this chapter, and implications for assessment and intervention with families are explored. In addition, we present the experiences of caregivers at different times of life (for example, parents growing older and sibling involvement in later life) to emphasize differences in the support needs of families at different points in the life course.

Using a Social Care Approach

Incidence and Statistics

Childhood and Adolescence. As assessment and clinical procedures have become more sophisticated, they have become more sensitive to the existence of mental health conditions in childhood. In fact, some studies have identified mental health and behavioral disorders in children as young as one or two years of age (Carter, Briggs-Gowan, & Davis, 2004). As a result, day care and educational programs have begun to provide treatment and therapeutic interventions very early in life (Furniss et al., 2013).

The National Alliance on Mental Illness (NAMI) (2010) provides statistics on the prevalence of and risk factors for mental disorders among U.S. children and adolescents:

- Four million children and adolescents in the United States suffer from a *serious* mental disorder that causes significant functional impairment at home, at school, and with peers. Of children ages 9 to 17, 21 percent have a diagnosable mental or addictive disorder that causes at least minimal impairment.
- Half of all lifetime cases of mental disorders begin by age 14. Despite effective treatments, there are long delays, sometimes decades, between the onset of symptoms and when people seek and receive treatment. An untreated mental disorder can lead to an illness that is more severe and more difficult to treat and can lead to the development of co-occurring mental illnesses.
- In any given year, only 20% of children with mental disorders are identified and receive mental health services. . . .
- Suicide is the third leading cause of death among youths ages 15 to 24. More teenagers and young adults die from suicide than from cancer, heart disease, AIDS, birth defects, stroke, pneumonia, influenza, and chronic lung disease *combined.* More than 90% of children and adolescents who commit suicide have a mental disorder. In the United States in 2002, almost 4,300 young people ages 10 to 24 died by suicide. . . .
- Approximately 50% of students age 14 and older who are living with a mental illness drop out of high school. This is the highest dropout rate of any disability group.

Adulthood. In the United States, mental health disorders are part of many families' lives. Estimates indicate that about 26.2 percent of individuals age 18 or older suffer from a diagnosable mental health condition. Fewer individuals suffer from a more severe form of mental illness; however, 6 percent of Americans (or one in every 17 individuals) fall into this category (Kessler, Chiu, Demler, & Walters, 2005). With advancements in treatment, more people with severe forms of mental

Incidence of Severe Mental Illness in the United States

Major Depressive Disorder

- Major depressive disorder is the leading cause of disability for Americans ages 15 to 44.
- Major depressive disorder affects approximately 14.8 million American adults, or about 6.7 percent of the U.S. population age 18 and older.
- Although major depressive disorder can develop at any age, the median age of onset is 32 years.

Bipolar Disorder

- Bipolar disorder affects approximately 5.7 million American adults, or about 2.6 percent of the U.S. population age 18 and older.
- The median age of onset for bipolar disorder is 25 years.

Personality Disorders

- Approximately 1.0 percent of people age 18 or older have antisocial personality disorder.
- An estimated 5.2 percent of people age 18 or older have avoidant personality disorder.
- Approximately 1.6 percent of Americans age 18 or older have borderline personality disorder.

Schizophrenia

- Approximately 2.4 million American adults, or about 1.1 percent of the U.S. population age 18 and older, have schizophrenia.
- Schizophrenia often first appears in men in their late teens or early 20s. In contrast, women are generally affected in their 20s or early 30s.

Source: Adapted from *The Numbers Count: Mental Disorders in America,* by the U.S. Department of Health and Human Services, National Institutes of Health, National Institute of Mental Health, 2012, retrieved from http://www.namigc.org/documents/numberscount.pdf

illness are involved in community life and social organizations. In a survey of college counseling center directors, for example, 77 percent of participants indicated that the number of students on campus who have a severe psychological disorder, especially anxiety, has increased (Sieben, 2011).

Prevalence estimates vary across different diagnostic categories, as shown in "Incidence of Severe Mental Illness in the United States" on page 97. Overall, about 45 percent of those with an SMI have multiple psychiatric conditions (Kessler et al., 2005).

Late Life. About 2 percent of older adults, or 1 million individuals, have an SMI (Cohen, 2003). It is estimated that by 2050, the number of older people with an SMI will increase dramatically as baby boomers enter later life. In fact, it has been estimated that by 2030 as many as 15 million older adults might have an SMI (Bartels, 2003).

Years ago, institutionalization was common for individuals with SMI who lived apart from their families. However, now about 85 percent of older adults with SMI live in community-based settings, and up to 50 percent live with family members (Cohen & Ibrahim, 2012). Most of their care providers are spouses, adult children, or siblings (Lefley, 2003). Like other types of caregivers, the majority of these care providers are women (Tessler & Gamache, 2000), which suggests that they are juggling multiple roles. As a result, caregivers may feel significant stress and burden as they try to manage various responsibilities across social contexts.

Life Course Perspective

Because a mental illness can exist at multiple points in the life course, caregiving takes different forms and involves various responsibilities. Parents of a child with a mental illness must resolve grief about the future for their child, help negotiate the social issues and challenges of childhood and adolescence, and learn effective parenting skills for dealing with the child's conditions. Caring for an adult with mental illness may mean reassuming a caregiving role later in development; such is the case with Philip, whom we discuss later in the chapter. Finally, late-life issues include the challenges of dealing with aging issues as well as the cumulative stress of years of caring for a person with SMI.

Parenting a Child with a Mental Illness

In a study of parents of young children and adolescents with mental health conditions, a major theme was the grief and loss felt in accepting such a diagnosis for their child. In addition, parents expressed anxiety about what the future would hold and struggled with the loss of support from family and friends (Richardson, Cobham, McDermott, & Murray, 2013). With the onset of atypical behaviors, parents are initially frightened and confused about their child's development and often struggle to adjust to what a psychiatric diagnosis will mean for the child and the family. Clearly, having a child with a mental health condition charts a course for parents that involves emotional and behavioral ups and downs.

As stated earlier, rates of childhood mental illness have increased as better diagnostic assessments have been developed. Psychiatric assessments are now sophisticated enough to diagnose mental illness in toddlers and preschool children. Early intervention is critical, as there is rapid brain and behavioral development during this period (Dawson, Ashman, & Carver, 2000). One promising, family-oriented treatment is provided as part of the Preschool Family Day Hospital (Furniss et al., 2013). This treatment program works with children and their families separately at the infant, toddler, and preschool levels. In addition to treating the child, the program provides support, education, and skills building for parents to gain efficacy and confidence in their parenting.

Regardless of age or time in the family life course, stigma is a major issue for families of individuals with a mental illness. However, the stigma is especially acute for children and adolescents who have a psychiatric condition. The National Stigma Study of Children was conducted to investigate the experience of stigma for children with a psychiatric condition (Pescosolido, Perry, Martin, McLeod, & Jensen, 2007). The researchers reported several major issues related to stigma management and subsequent functioning. Among them was the child's experience of outsider status, which leads to problems in interpersonal relations and peer interactions. Another problem was the possibility of long-term drug use and the overmedication of children and subsequent fears about the negative effect of drug use on health. Parents' experiences were also reported to include feelings of grief, loss, and responsibility.

Children who behave in atypical or eccentric ways are targets for bullying and ostracizing by peers. Unfortunately, children who have psychiatric conditions or developmental disabilities are maltreated by peers at higher rates than children without disabilities (Cappadocia, Weiss, & Pepler, 2012). Thus, parents need to act in advocacy roles in school systems, neighborhood groups, or other social contexts in which these interactions occur.

Parents of children with mental disorders frequently need to provide care for health conditions as well. In research on children with mental illnesses, those with physical health conditions, and those without either of these conditions, children with mental illnesses fared worst on several dimensions of health functioning. Children with mental illnesses scored higher on perception of pain, higher on health-related interference in overall family functioning, and scored lower on quality of general health (Sawyer et al., 2002). Raising a child with a mental illness requires that parents oversee a number of physical health and social responsibilities in addition to dealing with the psychiatric condition itself.

Providing Care to an Adult with a Mental Illness

Dealing with physical health conditions is a part of caring for a person with SMI, as individuals with SMI are more likely than individuals without SMI to suffer from disabilities in health and functioning. The World Health Organization reported that individuals who suffer from major depression or schizophrenia have a 40 percent to 60 percent higher probability than the general population of dying prematurely from conditions that are left untreated, such as cancer, cardiovascular disease, diabetes, or HIV. Thus, caregiving involves paying attention to problems of physical as well as mental health and dealing with the higher health care costs associated with greater levels of disabilities (Scott et al., 2009).

Because of low levels of employment and tumultuous social relationships, many adults with SMI enter their later years with few financial and support resources.

They thus rely on formal and informal support for assistance with their care needs. Significant numbers of these older adults live with their care providers; it is estimated that up to half live in coresidential arrangements (Cummings & MacNeil, 2008; Dyck, Short, & Vitaliano, 1999). This type of living arrangement can be difficult for caregivers. For many women, the caregiving role competes with other responsibilities, including taking care of household tasks, caring for other family members, and working outside the home. In addition, many caregivers assume financial responsibility for the care recipient as part of the care arrangement. In one study, care providers who made more financial contributions reported feeling more burden (M. S. Thompson, 2007).

Notwithstanding the level of support that many families provide, older adults with SMI continue to have significant unmet care needs. In a study of older adults' reliance on formal and informal support, great need was reported in the areas of management of physical illness, psychological pain, social connections, and assistance with daily activities (Cummings & Kropf, 2009a). Formal services were more likely to provide assistance with managing psychiatric distress, managing physical health, providing information, and managing dangerous behavior (such as self-harm). Informal supports were more likely to assist with self-care, psychiatric distress, and money management. Despite receiving both informal and formal support, more than 70 percent of the older adults with SMI in this study continued to report needs that were not addressed by either support system.

Another aspect of care is the aging of both the person with SMI and his or her care providers. As people with SMI grow older, their psychiatric symptoms change, and new care demands, such as the need for managing health conditions, may emerge. As caregivers age, their ability to manage the demands of care may decrease at the same time additional age-related needs emerge in the care recipient. This combination creates substantial difficulties in care provision, a phenomenon that has been termed the "double demand for care" (Cummings & MacNeil, 2008). This situation is evident in the case study of Philip and his aging parents, presented later.

Although the caregiving role can cause significant stress, caregivers also report positive aspects of their relationship with the person with SMI. One factor that buffers against the stress is the caregiver's feeling of pride in his or her relationship with the person with SMI (Chen & Lukens, 2011). In Chen and Lukens's (2011) research, pride was operationalized as the ability to find enjoyment with the individual with SMI in spite of the challenges involved in care. Some caregivers also report experiencing a higher level of emotional intimacy with their family member because of the caregiving experience (J. S. Greenberg, Greenley, & Brown, 1997). In research specific to caregivers of older adults with SMI, caregivers reported enjoyable interactions (Cummings & MacNeil, 2008). More than half of the sample reported positive experiences with their family member. Specifically, the caregivers reported enjoying their relationship with the person, feeling good about providing care, and feeling appreciated as a result of their involvement.

Stigmatized and Politicized Caregiving Context

Historical Perspective and Trends

Since the 1960s and 1970s, major changes have taken place in the delivery of services to individuals with psychological disorders. These changes have had a dramatic effect on the experience of care and on the shared responsibility for care provision between families and formal service providers. Although the shift from a system based on institutionalization to a community-based system represents major progress, the sad fact is that individuals with SMI and their families still face challenges to receiving and providing effective and comprehensive care.

Before the passage of the Community Mental Health Act of 1963 (P.L. 88-164), people with impairments in cognitive and mental health were routinely institutionalized. Unfortunately, many residents suffered from poor-quality care, limited social interaction, and abuse from staff and other residents. Erving Goffman (1961, 1963), a prominent sociologist, researched the stigma associated with mental illness and the subsequent avoidance that society displayed toward individuals with psychiatric conditions. Residents were mostly disconnected from their families and had no interaction with or access to the community. For example, Central State Hospital in Milledgeville, Georgia, was once the largest institution in the world (Cranford, 2008), yet a visitor can easily drive through the town without ever seeing the campus or buildings. Like Central State Hospital, many institutions were hidden away from the rest of the community, and residents were not assimilated into or engaged in life beyond the institutional campus.

This level of disengagement was also evident on an individual basis. Goffman and Helmreich (1961) wrote about the patient as one who was disempowered. A patient who was ill had limited involvement in his or her own care and treatment. The authors argued that this apparent submissiveness fostered dependency and reduced patients' capacity to live in the community.

During the 1970s, the deinstitutionalization of people with mental illness and intellectual disability took place. In the ensuing years, institutions literally opened their doors, and residents left the hospital grounds. Without ties to families and communities, these individuals often ended up in precarious or dangerous living situations. Prison statistics indicate the magnitude of this issue. In the decade after the beginning of the deinstitutionalization movement, the prison population increased dramatically. Between 1985 and 1990, it increased by 91 percent. During the 1990s, the prison population grew at seven times the rate of the overall U.S. population (Diamond, Wang, Holzer, Thomas, & Cruser, 2001). A significant proportion of the new prison population had psychiatric conditions, leading some to conclude that SMI had been criminalized, that jails had become a substitute for mental health treatment (Ringhoff, Rapp, & Robst, 2012). Because people with SMI lacked resources, instead of receiving treatment, they often received no support or intervention. This led to a number of social problems, including incarceration and homelessness.

In addition to changes in the setting for treatment and intervention, the types of treatment available to people with SMI have changed dramatically since the mid-1900s. Previously, the dominant paradigm for understanding mental illness was intrapsychic and early life social conditions (Drake, Green, Mueser, & Goldman, 2003). For example, one theory about schizophrenia, published as *Interpretation of Schizophrenia* (Arieti, 1955), argued that the family constellation and dynamics associated with having a child who develops this disorder were of particular importance. The "typical" parental dyad for a child who developed schizophrenia was a dominant, controlling woman married to a weak, dependent man. A child emerging from this configuration would suffer from intense anxiety and have difficulty with individuation from the dominant parent; this would subsequently damage his or her internal development. This theory cast causation and blame for the condition on the parents, especially the mother.

Since those earlier years, various treatment approaches have dominated interventions in this area. Drake et al. (2003) outlined the evolution of treatment for individuals with SMI since the 1950s. During the 1960s and 1970s, the emphasis was on symptom control, with the overarching goal of keeping individuals out of psychiatric hospitals. In the 1980s, rehabilitation became the dominant theme, with intervention approaches that provided opportunities for individuals with SMI to learn the skills necessary to assume societal roles in social and employment situations. In the 1990s, programs shifted to a recovery framework, with a goal of helping people with SMI pursue individually meaningful activities and a higher quality of life. *Recovery* is broadly defined as an orientation within mental health services that stresses

> optimism, personal empowerment, and a deep commitment to accepting people for who they are. The recovery movement gathered momentum when evidence became available that the diagnosis of a chronic mental disorder was not a life sentence of ever-worsening functioning, but that for many people symptoms remitted, and work and social lives were restored in meaningful ways. (Greeno, 2013, "The Recovery Movement")

The use of psychopharmacological approaches has also increased dramatically, as a greater emphasis has been placed on the neurobiological causes of mental illnesses. Various drug therapies have been discovered that have reduced or alleviated symptoms enough to allow individuals with SMI to function in social and interpersonal roles (Mellman et al., 2001). Although negative side effects have been reduced overall, certain psychotropic medications still cause problems, such as weight gain and lethargy (Drake et al., 2003). As a result, individuals may stop taking prescribed medications because of negative side effects.

Mental Health Services: Care Sharing or Burden?

Although formal services should provide assistance and relief to care providers, interactions with the mental health system can be a source of stress. Families seek help in understanding and handling the symptoms and behaviors associated with the diagnosis of the SMI (Shankar & Muthuswamy, 2007). Studies of experiences with mental health professionals have indicated that satisfaction with services is significantly related to involvement with providers (Perreault, Rousseau, Provencher, Roberts, & Milton, 2012).

Unfortunately, numerous studies report that families feel left alone with their care responsibilities, unheard regarding their experience of care, and even blamed for having a mentally ill family member (Rowe, 2012; Weimand, Hedelin, Hall-Lord, & Sällström, 2011). In addition, caregivers who have had greater exposure to the mental health system through experiences such as admitting a family member to a psychiatric facility multiple times have reported higher levels of burden in their relationships with staff (Östman, 2004).

From a care-sharing perspective, mental health professionals and caregivers seem to hold different expectations about their roles and interactions. A review of studies of the relationships between professional and informal caregivers identified several expectations that differed between the two groups (Rowe, 2012). The informal caregivers, mostly family members, perceived an obligation to help provide support; they wanted assistance with managing disruptive behaviors and information about services and the psychiatric condition. In contrast, the professionals tended to limit the involvement of families and exclude them from receiving information that could help them carry out their caregiving role. Sadly, care-sharing interactions with mental health providers seem to increase the stress and burden on informal caregivers instead of provide support.

Applying FAM

Case Study: Philip

The following case study describes parents who care for an adult son with chronic mental illness. The case demonstrates the episodic nature of psychiatric disorders and the parents' attempts to reconcile the changed behaviors of their son after his first psychotic episode. The case also highlights how the stigma of mental illness is attached to the whole family, not just the client.

Philip is a 40-year-old, single, white male with a diagnosis of schizophrenia. He lives at home with his 75-year-old parents and has a 22 year history of mental illness. Philip experienced numerous psychiatric hospitalizations but has remained out of the hospital for the past two years. Currently he has a flat affect, depressed mood, and mild paranoid ideation concerning his parents. He reports bizarre hallucinations involving religious themes and sexual thoughts. He and his parents live in a small southern town where his father is a retired pastor from the local Baptist church. Although there are two other brothers in the family, neither assists the parents with caregiving responsibilities.

Despite the overprotective and strict nature of his parents, Philip was by most standards a "normal" child. In school, he usually received A and B grades and had plans for attending seminary. He was somewhat shy and withdrawn in his school years, but it was during his senior year that he began to exhibit strange behaviors. For example, he made bizarre sexual statements during his father's Sunday sermons. He also became reclusive and refused to bathe.

Since the family was prominent in the town, the community overlooked and ignored Philip's increasingly bizarre behavior. His parents were at a loss to understand the behavioral change and assumed it was part of an adolescent phase. Eventually he became violent, culminating in an incident when he shot out windows in the town square and held the police at bay for several hours. His explanation was that he attempted to kill the evil spirits that were "eating at his brain." Philip was sent away to the state hospital which was located more than 100 miles from the community. This was the first of many hospitalizations for him.

At the time of his first psychotic break, Philip's parents were in their mid-50s. They were looking forward to retirement, spending time with their grandchildren, and reaping the benefits of life in a small coastal area. His parents blamed themselves for Philip's illness and prayed fervently for him to be "cured and return to being normal."

Instead of regaining his emotional health, Philip's condition has worsened over time. After each hospitalization, he would return home over medicated but manageable. Eventually, he would resume bizarre and aggressive behaviors. His father retired prematurely, believing that if he devoted all his time to caring for his son, Philip would improve. However, the retirement caused the father to become isolated from his support system, and eventually family and friends stopped visiting.

The cumulative stress of caregiving have taken a toll on all areas of family functioning. Philip's parents are older now and have less energy to deal with his periods of decompensation. They continue to be isolated, fatigued, withdrawn, and depressed. They are financially ruined, and their glamorous old house is in a state of disrepair. Five years ago, Philip became psychotic and pushed his mother down, breaking her arm. She is developing osteoporosis and lives in fear of another violent attack.

Despite the numerous problems that accompany the caregiving for Philip, both parents have a strong desire to continue caring for him. Their determination, loyalty, and love are remarkable. A major worry that plagues the parents is the future of Philip's care when they die. Despite the long history of his illness, both parents continue to lament the "old Philip." (Kelly & Kropf, 1995, pp. 10–12)

FAM Assessment

FAM provides a method for assessing needs and resources in families that are caring for a person with SMI. Because of the extended and episodic nature of care, families in this situation need to be understood in terms of their current issues as well as their historical methods of coping.

From a biological perspective, assessment needs to consider the functioning of each of the family members. Philip's parents are both in their mid-70s and are experiencing some changes in health and functioning. These can potentially compromise their ability to provide care. Philip's mother experienced a broken arm after her son knocked her down. In addition, the stress and ongoing responsibility of caring for Philip have possibly taken a toll on the parents' health in other ways, including through hypertension and cardiovascular conditions.

Philip's health should also be assessed. As we have mentioned, the health of individuals with SMI is often worse than that of the general population. In addition, it is important to determine whether Philip is adhering to his medication regime.

Psychological assessment involves the evaluation of emotional health and coping. The parents feel a tremendous amount of guilt and sadness about Philip's disorder. They blame themselves for his condition, and Philip's father even took early retirement to be at home and provide his son a different type of family environment. In addition, the parents continue to deal with feelings of grief and loss over the "old Philip," who is no longer part of their lives. They also live in fear about what will happen to him when they are no longer able to provide care.

In addition, Philip's condition continues to be unstable. An evaluation of his medication regime, as well as his adherence to his prescribed medications, must be conducted. Also, little is known about Philip's own insight into his present situation and functioning. How much does he understand about his diagnosis and current life circumstances? Does it make sense for him to continue to live at home, or does he have any thoughts about alternative possibilities (for example, residential options)? These issues should be explored as part of the assessment process.

In the area of social-cultural functioning, the social worker should assess social relationships and support for the parents. The father's early retirement seemed to increase his sense of loneliness and isolation from this support. In addition, both parents have decreased their involvement in pleasurable and rewarding experiences (for example, church and community roles) to have more time and energy for caregiving.

Stigma management is also an issue, and this may be another factor in the parents' decreased social ties. This situation may be even more acute for them because of the small town in which they reside, where relationships are more dense and interconnected. Because part of Philip's past behavior involved public displays (including disruptions in church and damaging of community buildings), the meaning and experience of these episodes may continue for both the family and the community.

There is a lack of information about Philip's social functioning and relationship to peers. Does Philip have any relationships with others of similar age? How does he function in these relationships? What is his sexual history and ability to have an adult relationship? The answers to these questions are important in understanding Philip's social network and connection to people other than his parents.

The Family as a Social System

Part of assessing a family includes understanding how the various members of the family relate to one another. In this case study, there is virtually no information about Philip's brothers or their lack of involvement. The brothers might not want to be involved, or perhaps the parents are reluctant to have them assist with care. The dearth of information about these connections is significant and needs to be explored. These additional family members could potentially participate in a care-sharing arrangement and provide relief and support to the primary care providers.

The onset of Philip's mental illness altered the family's developmental history. That is, the family had previously operated under the assumption that Philip would develop as an independent adult. But in their 50s, the parents had to reassume the caregiving role for their adult child. This scenario involves two processes: letting go of expectations and hopes for the "old Philip" and accepting and understanding Philip as a person with SMI. The family has thus experienced role transitions and shifting expectations, such as the loss of the ability to retire and travel at leisure.

Future planning is important for this family. In one study of parents of adults with SMI, only 18 percent of caregivers had completed future care plans for the care recipient (Hatfield & Lefley, 2000). The most common reasons for not engaging in this planning were high levels of anxiety about the process on the part of the parents, resistance to change on the part of the person with SMI, lack of knowledge about how to plan, and the availability of few financial resources. In Philip's family, a combination of these factors seems to be present, and these need to be identified to help the family with this critical task.

Community-Level Factors

Sadly, many people with SMI do not receive the support they need to function adequately in the community. A national survey of mental health treatment rates in the United States, published in 2005, determined that less than half (41 percent) of individuals who had a mental health diagnosis had received some form of treatment in the past year. In addition, the majority of those who did receive treatment were likely to have had minimal contact with a mental health provider (Wang et al., 2005). The report further stipulated that the most underserved groups were most at risk in the community and included older adults, members of racial and ethnic minority groups, and people who lived in rural areas.

The small and conservative community in which Philip and his family live appears to have limited supports for individuals with SMI. For example, Philip was hospitalized numerous times in facilities several hours from the community where he and his family lived. There is limited information about the types of supports for dealing with mental illness in the area, including information and support groups for the parents and activity and employment opportunities for Philip. Also, it is unknown how connected the health and mental health service networks are in this community setting. Overall, the case study provides limited information about the capacity of the community to support families who are caring for someone with SMI.

Applying REM in Assessment and Intervention

According to a risk and resilience framework, Philip's case exemplifies how caregiving issues change across the life course and during periods of particular challenge. The parents' aging brings up issues to address now and in the future. In addition, coping strategies and social support resources should be assessed to understand family functioning.

Risk Assessment

Although Philip's parents continue to care for him, several aspects of this case are cause for concern. Philip's behavior has not appeared to stabilize, and he continues to act erratically and sometimes violently. For this reason, a thorough risk assessment should be completed with the family to determine whether there have been additional episodes and whether any elements in the home (for example, guns and weaponry) could potentially increase the family's risk.

Caregivers often prioritize the care of the other before their own health and well-being. In this situation, little is known about the health of Philip's parents except that his mother has osteoporosis. The conditions in which the parents have lived for years have been volatile, and such stress can have negative effects on physical and emotional health. Thus, the parents should have thorough physical examinations to determine their underlying health status.

Because Philip has spent time in extended care, the family is at risk for financial insolvency. Financial stresses that result from extended caregiving contribute to a sense of burden among care providers (M. S. Thompson, 2007). Because the parents have been responsible for Philip's needs for most of his adulthood, they have had limited opportunity to save money for their own retirement. Thus, they may be unable to meet their own later life needs.

In addition, it seems unlikely that Philip will be able to live independently once his parents can no longer provide care. Yet no plan or structure for transitioning care to another family member, such as one of Philip's brothers, is in place. Philip's only involvement with mental health services was when he was institutionalized. At this point, his parents have primary responsibility for his care, and their own health is at risk.

Resilience Assessment

In spite of numerous stresses, Philip's family shows commitment and resilience. The parents are devoted to Philip and demonstrate a desire for ongoing engagement and involvement with him. At every crisis situation, the family has tried to solve the problem and get Philip the help that he needs.

Although they have experienced some stress, Philip's family members have sustained ties to their family. The family's faith is important to its resilience and coping and has been a priority until recently. In addition, ties to the community are evident, although Philip's care has put a strain on the family's engagement in community life.

Using the assessment, the social worker will work with the family members to determine how to meet the challenges they are experiencing. Given the precariousness of Philip's uncontrolled symptoms and potential disruptive and violent behavior, his family is approaching a crisis situation. To mitigate the crisis and address the reality of his parents' advancing age, the social worker needs to work with the family to develop a future care plan.

Future Care

Part of the future care process is to determine the family's priorities and preferences for care. Although little information about the parents' health is available, part of this discussion needs to center on the parents' functional ability to remain in their caregiving roles. The osteoporosis of Philip's mother is concerning and should be assessed as part of the plan. In addition, the parents' emotional ability to continue providing care needs to be taken into account.

As part of the future care plan, Philip's functional level and ability should be assessed. If Philip were stabilized medically and socially, would he be able to participate in employment, education, or some other social role? The living arrangement should also be considered: Is it adequate for Philip to continue to live with his parents at this point? How do the parents (and Philip, if he is capable of making decisions) see the future unfolding? How would they want the future to take shape?

Other potential sources of support that are currently absent also need to be assessed. How do Philip's brothers play into his future? An important intervention in the future care planning process is a family conference to discuss this issue openly and as a group. To date, this type of full family meeting has not taken place in Philip's family.

Future planning needs to involve mental health service providers, as well as legal counsel in many cases. Discussions should focus on services that are available both within the local community and at the state and regional levels. Unfortunately, the grim reality is that people with SMI may not receive services that are appropriate for them in their own community. Is it feasible to look beyond the local level to other resources that might be helpful? Philip's ability to make independent decisions and provide consent may also need to be discussed. Finally, paying for future care costs and inheritance issues should be carefully planned.

Stress Reduction

Philip's parents are currently under a great deal of stress. Their isolation adds to their sense of aloneness in their role, and they appear to be unconnected to the mental health system in an ongoing way. NAMI (www.nami.org) provides information, advocacy, and support for caregivers of individuals with mental illness. In addition, *Today's Caregiver* (www.caregiver.com) has "channels" for different caregiving situations, including one for caregivers of individuals with schizophrenia and bipolar disorders. Families that are not aware of these resources might feel less alone in their caregiving role after learning more about them.

Besides information, Philip's family could use support from others in similar situations. Even if no support group exists locally, alternative methods of connection, such as online support groups, are available. This type of forum allows caregivers to tell their stories and exchange information and advice and provides an emotional outlet (Perron, 2002). This is a good alternative for families that live in communities with few resources, cannot physically attend meetings, or prefer to be involved in a less intense interpersonal experience. For Philip's family, this type of group might fill an unmet need for support.

Case Management: Enhancing Person-in-Environment Congruence

As part of the caregiving model of practice, the congruence between the family and the environment needs to be assessed. What must be in place to promote stable functioning in situations involving mental illness when conditions create unpredictable experiences for families? In addition, an intervention plan must address the intersection of aging and mental health.

Linking to Resources

Intensive case management can be helpful in reducing Philip's frequent hospital admissions. In a meta-analysis of case management research, assertive community treatment had positive effects on reducing readmission rates (Burns et al., 2007). In this approach, an interdisciplinary care team works with a small caseload of clients, is available around the clock, and has daily case consultations about the clients with whom they work (Bond, Drake, Mueser, & Latimer, 2001). Of course, the question is whether Philip would be eligible for this type of intensive service or whether it exists in his community at all.

A case manager could also be helpful in linking the family to available resources. Even if few formal services are available, it might be possible to develop some informal services to provide support for the family. Although the church has been an important part of the family's life during Philip's illness, the community has not been involved in assisting with the situation. The case manager might help the family develop ways to gain community support (such as an emergency plan if the parents require some help with the upkeep of their home). In addition, a case manager might be able to link the family to resources that could relieve stress (for example, programs that assist aging individuals with home remodeling).

Safety and the Physical Environment

The physical environment contains several risks that can compromise the safety of the family, and a case manager can complete an environmental risk analysis. Because of the costs of care, Philip's family has neglected caring for their home, which is an old, stately house. Especially given Philip's mother's osteoporosis, a home accident is a potential—even lethal—danger. A thorough evaluation of the home environment is needed, with possible modifications to enhance physical safety. AARP (2007) has published a checklist that can be used to assess safety risks and provides suggested modifications that can prevent a fall or accident within the home.

Because Philip has already exhibited violent behavior, taking steps to prevent future violent episodes is important. Any kind of weaponry (such as guns and sharp knives) should be locked up and kept safe. This precaution will keep the parents safer and prevent Philip from causing himself harm.

Increasing Social Support and Capital

Evidence suggests that strong ties within communities are protective factors in mental health functioning and development, especially for children and adolescents. The quality of relationships within a neighborhood is also important, as not all social connections have positive outcomes for children. In one study in neighborhoods of higher socioeconomic status, parents who knew few of their neighbors had children with higher rates of depression and anxiety than those who knew many neighbors. In poorer neighborhoods, however, the opposite was true: Children fared better emotionally when their parents knew fewer neighbors (Drukker, Kaplan, Feron, & van Os, 2003). In neighborhoods where there are significant deficits in social relationships between adults, children may feel unsafe, which has negative consequences for emotional development.

Other research has found that strong family bonds reduce the probability of adolescent suicide. In addition, a higher level of collective engagement within neighborhoods is a positive factor in promoting attachments within the family (Maimon, Browning, & Brooks-Gunn, 2010). Therefore, community-level interventions that promote strong, stable social bonds between families have a positive effect on the health and well-being of children raised in these environments.

In Philip's situation, the family has become disengaged from community life. Although some reintegration might be possible, the family might also need to develop new relationships that have functional outcomes. As already discussed, providing linkages for the parents can decrease their sense of isolation and aloneness in providing care. Philip would also benefit from making connections with others besides his parents. The Compeer Program matches trained community volunteers with individuals who have mental illness to provide social connection, positive role modeling, and general friendship experiences (Skirboll, Bennett, & Klemens, 2006). An evaluation of the program with adults with SMI indicated that Compeer was effective in enhancing social support and decreasing symptoms (McCorkle, Rogers, Dunn, Lyass, & Wan, 2008). If a Compeer chapter exists in Philip's community, this type of structured, intentional friendship program might provide him with some additional social connections outside his family relations.

Advocating for Social Policy

Because of the nature of mental illness, public policy in other areas has a direct impact on the lives and functioning of individuals with psychiatric conditions. One such area is housing policy, as individuals with SMI are at risk for living in substandard housing or being homeless. The U.S. Department of Housing and Urban Development produces the *Annual Homeless Assessment Report to Congress*, which provides national estimates on the number and circumstances of homeless individuals and families in the United States. According to the report, in 2011, more than half (54.6 percent) of homeless adults had either mental illness or combined substance abuse and mental illness (U.S. Department of Housing and Urban Development, 2012).

Philip could end up in a dangerous or substandard living arrangement. His current living situation is precarious at best, and the resources available in the community seem minimal. Even if he were to live in a supported or independent living situation, his unstable behavior could easily lead to life on the streets. This case clearly demonstrates the importance of a case manager's identifying alternative living arrangements for adults with SMI. A major policy initiative for mental health is adequate and safe housing for people with mental illness (S. Newman & Goldman, 2008).

Jails and prisons also house a disproportionate number of individuals with SMI (see "Mental Illness and Prisons: Issues and Suggested Policy Changes" on page 113). Various policy initiatives have been developed to address this issue, mostly with regard to treatment and reduction of symptoms of the psychiatric condition. As described by Ringhoff et al. (2012), current policy initiatives include the following:

- *Jail diversion programs* that divert individuals with an SMI or substance abuse from jail to a community-based treatment program (Substance Abuse and Mental Health Services Administration, n.d.)
- *Crisis intervention teams* comprising police officers trained to intervene in situations that involve a mental health condition
- *Mental health courts*, a specialized courtroom program in which (Steadman, Davidson, & Brown, 2001)
  - people with mental illness are referred to community-based services on initial booking and are handled on a single court docket
  - a courtroom team devises treatment and supervision plans
  - existing appropriate treatment slots are verified before the judge rules in the case
  - the individuals charged are appropriately monitored under court auspices, with possible criminal sanctions for noncompliance
- *Crime prevention programs* that coordinate with mental health services to target risk and are augmented with resources from criminal justice (such as specialized training and parole officers)

New or revised public policy is needed to help support Philip's family members, who have not received much assistance from formal service systems. Care providers can help Philip gain as much self-sufficiency and autonomy as possible (for example, through employment opportunities) by working with mental health professionals; this would have the overall benefit of decreasing the family's stress. Considering social policy in general, and the benefits to high-risk groups such as individuals with SMI in particular, is an important part of mental health policy overall.

In summary, SMI can first manifest during childhood, adolescence, or adulthood. When symptoms begin, a family has to change its behaviors, and caregivers often have to change their roles and their expectations for the development and trajectory of the affected family member. In some families, such as Philip's, parents extend their caregiving journey well past the expected time in a typical family life cycle. In these cases, the aging of the care providers intersects with the psychiatric condition and aging of the person with SMI.

Psychiatric conditions are associated with a host of difficult behavioral manifestations. Living with someone with a mental illness can be like "walking on eggshells" (Swan & Lavitt, 1988), as he or she will have episodes of difficult, erratic,

Mental Illness and Prisons: Issues and Suggested Policy Changes

As many as 400,000 inmates held in the nation's prisons and jails suffer from mental illnesses.

- Between 25% and 40% of all Americans with mental illness will at some point pass through the criminal justice system.
- In 2000, approximately 70,000 prisoners were actively psychotic.
- State prison inmates with a mental illness received sentences an average of 12 months longer than those of other offenders.

Treatment can benefit both the public and people with mental illness.

- Most jail inmates with mental illnesses are charged with nonviolent offenses. Treatment is the best way to prevent recidivism.
- A total of 53% of inmates with a mental illness were in prison for a violent offense, whereas only 46% of inmates without a mental illness were incarcerated for violence. Treatment is the best way to prevent violence.
- Inmates with mental illnesses cost more to incarcerate than other inmates. Treatment is the best way to prevent these costs.

Mentally ill prisoners need treatment to prevent reincarceration.

- More than half of all inmates with a mental illness report three or more prior sentences.
- Only 6 in 10 state inmates with a mental illness reported receiving treatment since their incarceration.
- Only 4 in 10 local inmates with a mental illness reported receiving treatment since their incarceration.

Source: Reprinted from *Spending Money in All the Wrong Places: Jails and Prisons,* by National Alliance on Mental Illness, n.d., retrieved from http://www.nami.org/Template.cfm?Section=Fact_Sheets& Template=/ContentManagement/ContentDisplay.cfm&ContentID=14593

eccentric, or violent behavior. The cumulative stress can affect the health and mental health of care providers (for example, leading to depression, guilt, and anger).

As a social worker, you will find that practice with these caregivers involves multiple levels of intervention. Families that care for a person with SMI can be assisted with understanding the nature of the mental illness, identifying resources to decrease caregiving demands and burden, and accessing resources in the community.

CHAPTER SEVEN

Returning Veterans

For tens of thousands of troops, returning from war is a difficult process filled with both physical and psychological challenges. A December 2012 *Huffington Post* report indicated that between October 2001 and June 2012, a total of 891,903 troops from the wars in Iraq (Operation Iraqi Freedom) and Afghanistan (Operation Enduring Freedom) had been hospitalized: 153,936 for physical injuries and 161,385 for mental health diagnoses (Wood, 2012). Many soldiers have lifelong physical needs. Traumatic brain injury (TBI), posttraumatic stress disorder (PTSD), and depression are among the many difficulties experienced. Marital stress, substance abuse, and suicide are far too common. These issues have a ripple effect throughout families, as the majority of service members are married, and approximately two in five have children (*Mental Health Treatment*, 2008).

In a fact sheet from the U.S. Department of Veterans Affairs (VA), Norris and colleagues (Norris, Stevens, Pfefferbaum, Wyche, & Pfefferbaum, 2008) discussed the importance of family-focused interventions. They encouraged families of returning service members to talk to each other, resume normal activities to the extent possible, and handle conflict appropriately. In addition, the National Center for PTSD (2006), in *A Guide for Families of Military Members*, cautioned that everyone in the family must work toward and acclimate to a new family pattern that fits all involved. Families should also be aware that problems in relationships that existed before deployment may return. Finally, returning service members need to relearn how to feel safe, comfortable, and trusting with family members.

Unfortunately, as the need for services increases, the accessibility and availability of mental health support is declining (Williamson & Mulhall, 2009). This chapter examines how social workers can be part of the solution, helping returning veterans to maintain or regain their resilience and reunite with their families.

Three case studies in this chapter will help you apply your caregiving models: (1) The case of John and his caregiver, Deborah, illustrates a caregiver's struggle to cope with the physical disabilities of war; (2) the case of Conner shows how REM can be used to explore struggles with the meaning of war; and (3) the case of the F. family, which works to reunite after the father's multiple deployments to Afghanistan, uses

115

FAM and the family resilience template (FRT) to examine the factors that contribute to family resilience.

Politicized and Stigmatized Caregiving Context

On March 20, 2003, the United States invaded Iraq. On December 15, 2011, the war officially ended. The war in Afghanistan began on October 7, 2001. In 2013, President Barack Obama announced that 34,000 of the 66,000 troops would come home and that the war in Afghanistan would end in 2014 (Tapper, 2013). How will returning veterans in need of services be served effectively?

Veterans Services

The adequacy of care for returning veterans has been under review since the Vietnam War era. In the mid-1990s, the VA called for a transformation of its fragmented health care system. Between 1995 and 1999, numerous systemic changes were made to VA hospitals to ensure the accountability of management and the quality of care (Ashish, Perlin, Kizer, & Dudley, 2003; Kizer & Dudley, 2009).

Nonetheless, the multiple deployments and injuries that have marked the wars in Iraq and Afghanistan have severely tested the VA system. In February 2007, the American Psychological Association Presidential Task Force on Military Deployment Services for Youth, Families, and Service Members issued a preliminary report on the psychological needs of U.S. military service members and their families. The report contended that bureaucracies such as the Department of Defense and the VA have been inexcusably slow to respond to the growing mental health crisis, often allowing veterans to fall through the cracks.

Moreover, a March 2013 Institute of Medicine report requested by Congress and funded by the Pentagon stated that when surveyed, almost half of the 2.2 million troops sent to Iraq and Afghanistan reported they had had difficulties on return to civilian life. Efforts to deal with this crisis are ongoing, and some are discussed in this chapter.

Stigma of Mental Illness

The inadequacy of veterans' services is compounded by a stigma in the military associated with seeking mental health services. Soldiers who seek mental or behavioral health counseling may face career difficulties or have trouble obtaining security clearances. In 2008, the Pentagon, under the leadership of Secretary of Defense Robert M. Gates, issued a directive against the stigmatization of mental illness in the military. Unfortunately, at a mental health summit the next year, Gates commented that "failure to take advantage of some of the programs we offer is, I believe, also related to my greatest concern: that, despite our best efforts, there is still a stigma associated with seeking help for psychological injuries" (R. M. Gates, 2009; Miles, 2008).

The stigmatization of mental illness in the military is a long-standing problem (M. Thompson, 2013; Tucker, 2012). The alarming rise in mental illness among returning service members is still talked about in hushed tones among military health professionals (M. Thompson, 2013; Tucker, 2012). Those returning from war zones say, "I told them he was not able to remain in battle. They waited until it was too late and he was so distressed he had to be sent home" (personal communication with returning veteran, March 14, 2013).

In August 2012, President Obama issued an executive order aimed at improving access to mental health services for veterans, service members, and military families. Section 1 of the policy states the following:

> Since September 11, 2001, more than two million service members have deployed to Iraq or Afghanistan. Long deployments and intense combat conditions require optimal support for the emotional and mental health needs of our service members and their families. The need for mental health services will only increase in the coming years as the Nation deals with the effects of more than a decade of conflict. . . . We have an obligation to evaluate our progress and continue to build an integrated network of support capable of providing effective mental health services for veterans, service members, and their families. (Obama, 2012)

NASW has joined in this campaign. On September 14, 2012, Dr. Jill Biden, wife of Vice President Joseph Biden, announced the association's commitment to advancing work with military families, including through free online courses.

Understanding the Nature of Return

Although most service personnel are resilient and gradually return to civilian life, some experience difficulties that can require the help of mental health professionals. One of the major concerns is PTSD. To be diagnosed with PTSD, a person must experience anxiety following a traumatic event. For example, a soldier may feel that he or she or a loved one is in danger. However, not everyone who experiences trauma will develop PTSD. Therefore, scientists are attempting to identify the critical risk components that contribute to this complex syndrome, including both genetic factors and epigenetic factors (environmental influences on the development of genes) (Yehuda & LeDoux, 2007).

According to the National Center for Biotechnology Information (2013), symptoms of PTSD include nightmares, flashbacks, difficulty sleeping, and emotional numbness. These symptoms may in turn lead to other difficulties, such as marital strife, occupational instability, and problems in parenting.

Another concern among returning veterans is TBI. TBIs are caused by a violent blow or jolt to the head. The blow can cause a mild concussion or major brain injury that leads to long-term health complications (National Institute of

Neurological Disorders and Stroke, 2014). It is thought that many mild concussions go undiagnosed.

Depression is still another cause for concern among veterans. Among the symptoms veterans may show are difficulty concentrating, remembering details, and making decisions. Service members may also experience insomnia, loss of interest in activities, or thoughts of suicide. Suicide is a particularly alarming problem among returning veterans. In 2012, there were an estimated 349 suicides among active personnel (RT, 2013). Social workers and members of the health care team need to diagnose and treat depression among veterans as early as possible so that progress toward stability may be made.

Physical Injuries of War: Context and Case Study

The physical injuries of war may include TBI, spinal cord injury, hearing or vision loss, amputation (as many as 1,500 have been recorded during the Iraq and Afghanistan Wars as of November 2012), burns, and chronic pain (Wood, 2012). Chronic pain is often underdiagnosed or underreported and can lead to self-medication, including alcohol use (personal communication with returning veteran, October 4, 2012).

Social workers often assist caregivers with identifying much-needed resources or coping with caregiver burden. A survey by the National Alliance for Caregiving and EmblemHealth (2010) showed that the overwhelming majority of military caregivers (96 percent) are women. Although similar to civilian caregivers in some respects, they differ in important ways. Civilian caregivers are often women caring for older parents with dementia. Military caregivers are younger women caring for their spouses; most live with both the person they are caring for and dependent children. In these families, children often share some caregiving responsibilities. Unmarried veterans often rely on their parents to provide this care.

Because of the stress associated with caregiving, caregivers themselves may experience PTSD or *secondary trauma*, which results from helping a person suffering from trauma. Therefore, when helping a returning veteran, the social care provider should consider the caregiver as part of the client system and work to mitigate the stresses of combat and promote resilience (Bride & Figley, 2009). This dynamic can be seen in the case of John and Deborah:

John was hit by an explosion in Afghanistan when his right leg was blown away by stepping on the pressure plate of a roadside bomb. He was in great pain but remembers thinking about his wife and [the] men under his command. He says to himself that he must keep breathing, keep breathing. "If you do that you'll make it back to your wife." John's life was saved, but he is now a quadruple amputee who must return to civilian life.

John remembers being at the hospital, Walter Reed Army Medical Center, where many soldiers faced their struggles together, forming a natural support group. The veterans learn about the Tunnels to Towers Foundation formed to assist with building of homes with smart technology, such as stoves and sinks that move up and down, elevators, wheelchair ramps, and other appliances controlled by computer voice commands.

The staff at Walter Reed witnessed John's resilience when he went into another wounded soldier's room to tell him there is "life after a hospital bed." "I now walk with prosthetic legs, and plan to go to college."

However, the social worker noted that John's wife, Deborah, was showing signs of depression, anger, and fatigue. Deborah was offered counseling for what appeared to be secondary trauma. She is now in touch with other spouses in similar situations helping them make transitions. John and Deborah have moved into their new home and must build community ties (Almasy, 2012).

Using a Social Care Approach:
Resilience as Survivorship

A social care philosophy of social work practice directs attention to survivorship among returning military. A survivorship approach recognizes that traumatic events cannot be undone, nor can they be erased. At the same time, a survivorship perspective emphasizes veterans' ability to overcome the damaging events of trauma, to rebuild their lives, and to maintain a coherent family narrative. Veterans will grieve their loss and the ways their lives have changed forever. However, a survivorship approach helps them to explore what is feasible and decide what opportunities and choices can be made today (Greene, 2002).

Survivorship is a complex phenomenon that describes how individuals, families, and communities return to the basic functioning of life after trauma. It "involves innate and learned abilities (traits/capacities) to take action (follow adaptive/coping strategies) to survive, and to deal with feelings of distress and anxiety" (Greene & Graham, 2009, p. S75). Helping professionals can assist veterans in

- prioritizing their concerns
- delineating what they want to achieve
- articulating past success
- identifying what is going well
- distinguishing small but important changes that can be made
- examining how roles are played out with the family
- promoting active survivor engagement in family and community
- examining whether they and their families are becoming more optimistic
- identifying helpful resources in the family and community
- accessing resources
- planning for continued availability and follow-up

Risk and Resilience Intervention

Survivorship is closely associated with risk and resilience. Veterans of the wars in Iraq and Afghanistan have faced risks similar to those faced by veterans in other combat situations, illustrating the association or relationship among stressors, coping, and health (Antonovsky, 1979, 1987). What makes the risks seemingly more powerful here are the multiple deployments and the danger of TBI, the "signature wound of the Iraq War" (Williamson & Mulhall, 2009, p. 1). Many veterans are going undiagnosed for TBI, PTSD, and depression because distinguishing among these difficulties can be problematic (Williamson & Mulhall, 2009).

Given these issues, the goal of the social worker is to help the veteran regain his or her resilience. Although resilience is a natural human capacity, social workers can actively teach their clients how to adapt to stress, trauma, and tragedy during therapeutic situations (Bonanno, 2004). That is, the social worker's task is to help a client regain *functioning*, or the ability to carry out daily life tasks, particularly those dealing with family and work situations (Greene, 2008b).

Family Resilience and the Military

Around 2005, the Department of Defense implemented a resilience approach to promote well-being among military personnel and their families (Meridith et al., 2011). The department shifted the emphasis of its health care for military personnel from illness to prevention and health. It also began to focus on a family's strengths and survival skills and the difficult transition to civilian life.

The resiliency of veterans who have experienced trauma might be difficult to accept, considering that many service members have experienced two, three, or even as many as five extremely stressful combat deployments as well as physical injury. During combat, stress reactions are not uncommon. These reactions usually fade over time, but changes in behavior may be brought home and triggered by seemingly innocuous events (see Table 7.1). Coming home to family might not include the excitement and relief the returning veteran imagined it would. The families that soldiers left on deployment may not be the families to which they return home: Children will have grown, and spouses will have taken on new responsibilities (see the case of the F. family later in this chapter).

Therefore, family-centered social work interventions are important at this time. One such intervention suggested by Hollingsworth (2011) is *community family therapy*, a "modality designed to promote resilience both within and beyond the four walls of the therapy room, to facilitate family connections in the community, and empower them [veterans] for local leadership" (p. 215). This type of therapy allows families to be treated through outreach within larger systems.

TABLE 7.1
Battle Mind

	During Combat	*Returning Home*
B	Buddies (cohesion)	Withdrawal
A	Accountability	Controlling
T	Targeted	Inappropriate aggression
T	Tactical awareness	Hypervigilance
L	Lethally armed	Locked and loaded
E	Emotional control	Detachment
M	Mission operational security	Secretiveness
I	Individual responsibility	Guilt
N	Nondefensive driving	Aggressive driving
D	Discipline/ordering	Conflict

Source: Adapted from *After the war zone: A practical guide for returning troops and their families* (p. 57), by L. B. Slone and M. J. Friedman, 2008, Philadelphia: Da Capo Press.

Evidence-Based Resilience Programs

A Rand Corporation study by Meridith et al. (2011), commissioned by the Defense Centers of Excellence (DCoE) for Psychological Health and Traumatic Brain Injury, identified an initial set of factors that promote psychological resilience. The research team reviewed 270 publications and obtained the views of experts, yielding 20 evidence-based resilience factors at the individual, family, unit, and community levels (see "Evidence-Based and Evidence-Informed Factors That Promote Resilience" on p. 122). The study concluded with recommendations for the Department of Defense, including creating a department-wide definition of resilience, strengthening existing programs, standardizing resilience measures, developing a resource guide, ensuring scientifically proven resilience factors, and engaging senior military leaders in program evaluation.

Applying FAM

Many soldiers returning from armed conflict come back with multiple areas of trauma. FAM reviews their current level of functioning in multiple domains and determines how physical and psychological wounds affect their social relationships and spiritual selves. In addition, the model helps practitioners determine how social relations and spirituality help with trauma experiences.

Evidence-Based and Evidence-Informed Factors That Promote Resilience

Individual-Level Factors

- *Positive coping.* Manage taxing circumstances and seek to reduce stress.
- *Positive affect.* Have positive emotions and feel enthusiastic, active, and alert.
- *Positive thinking.* Process information, apply knowledge, reframe, have positive expectations.
- *Realism.* Accept what is in one's control, master what is possible.
- *Behavioral control.* Use self-management, monitor and modify emotional reactions.
- *Physical fitness.* Function effectively and efficiently.
- *Altruism.* Be motivated to help without reward, have concern for others.

Family-Level Factors

- *Emotional ties.* Bond with family members, take leisure time together.
- *Communication.* Exchange thoughts, opinions, information.
- Support. Give and receive emotional, tangible, instrumental, informational, and spiritual support.
- *Closeness.* Give and receive love, intimacy, and attachment.
- *Nurturing.* Use effective and loving parenting skills.
- *Adaptability.* Make changes or transitions within the military, including role flexibility.

Unit-Level Factors

- *Positive command climate.* Facilitate and foster intraunit interaction.
- *Teamwork.* Coordinate team members, be flexible.
- *Cohesion.* Perform combined actions, bond to sustain commitment.

Community-Level Factors

- *Belongingness.* Form friendships, protocols, participation opportunities.
- *Cohesion.* Develop bonds and shared values and interpersonal ties.
- Connectedness. Make a sense of community, commitment, roles, responsibility, and communication.
- Collective efficacy. Perceive the group as working together.

Source: Adapted from Promoting Psychological Resilience in the U.S. Military (pp. xiv–xv), by L. Meridith, C. D. Sherbourne, S. Gaillot, L. Hansell, H. V. Ritschard, A. M. Parker, and G. Wrenn, 2011, Santa Monica, CA: Rand Center for Military Health Policy Research. Retrieved from http://www.rand.org/pubs/monographs/MG996.html

Biological Factors

The wars in Iraq and Afghanistan introduced new sophisticated weaponry, and soldiers have sustained more severe and unique wounds in these theaters than have the personnel in other conflicts. Yet because of advances in body armor, helmets, and battlefield medical care, about 90 percent of soldiers have survived serious injury. The weapon most widely used by Iraqi and Afghan troops is the improvised explosive device, which produces terrible wounds and burns. Other major biological complications that affect returning veterans are PTSD, TBI, and amputation.

The U.S. Department of Veterans Affairs has established polytrauma centers that offer treatment through multidisciplinary medical teams that include cardiologists, internists, physical therapists, nurses, transition patient case managers, and social workers. The goal of these teams is to optimize wounded soldiers' independence and functionality. In addition, the VA (2014) offers spinal cord centers as well as rehabilitation for blindness. Of course, these biological concerns have psychosocial and spiritual components that the social worker may tap to contribute to resilience and healing.

Psychological Factors

Many returning veterans are able to reintegrate into civilian life without difficulty. Others find that they are returning to a very different world. All who return face some psychological aspects of what is termed "a return from Battle Mind" (see Table 7.1). For example, during battle, soldiers must be tactically aware, but when they return home, they find they are unnecessarily hypervigilant. Or, in combat they have emotional control, but at home they appear withdrawn.

One of the primary roles of boot camp is to socialize recruits into military life. The values of "duty, honor, loyalty, and commitment to comrades, unit, and nation" must be instilled (Demers, 2011, p. 162). When soldiers return home, they experience the difference in values between military and civilian life known as the "civil-military cultural gap" (J. Collins, 1998). By using a narrative approach, the social care worker can help a client become conscious of these bicultural personal identity factors that can sometimes interfere with reintegration into civilian life.

One soldier recalls,

> I felt indoctrination . . . like a cult in the sense of the single minded focus and allegiance but different in that the military develops traditionally socially accepted values and behaviors within individuals, such as honor, selfless service, and duty to country and the men in your unit. Indoctrination in that you are being called upon to protect your unit brothers and to KILL another person (personal communication with returning veteran, October 2011).

An injured contractor who served in Iraq recalled his "mind racing from the never-ending deluge of headlines and information, trying to decipher the future of the world" (Fair, Williams, & Janis, 2013). Studies have shown that when deploying to war, veterans felt that they were warriors, had little or no fear, and had a general feeling of being high. On their return, they often feel that they are time travelers, that no one understands them, and that they have a crisis of identity (Demers, 2011). By helping a soldier to reframe these negative narratives, a practitioner can have a healing effect.

Social Factors

The military unit in which a soldier has served plays a powerful role in his or her ability to share information and feelings with mental health professionals. Often a group of "therapy buddies" is needed to provide group support:

> The cohesion of the unit lets members grieve and share fears in particular ways that are acceptable within the group. If a soldier talks about something being "all fucked up" (the old FUBR—fucked up beyond all repair), he or she is expressing the anxiety and stress of the situation in an acceptable way, and others will usually confirm the statement. Men and women will at times actually cry, and this is most often accepted by the members of the unit given their experiences and losses. The question is how to make this support possible once a soldier has returned home. (Blundo, Greene, & Riley, 2012, p. 312)

One of the most powerful factors contributing to resilience and healing among returning veterans is the extent and involvement of their support networks. Practitioners should explore whom a veteran feels he or she may turn to and how often he or she may turn to that particular person or group.

Spiritual Factors

Veterans who survive trauma have the potential to find new meaning in negative events and to experience posttraumatic growth. *Posttraumatic growth* involves living with loss and distress in a new way (Calhoun & Tedeschi, 2006). Not only can a veteran reframe his or her feelings of stress and pain, but he or she may also come to have a greater appreciation of life, family, and friends.

Applying REM in Individual Intervention

The following case study involves an army reservist who returned from active military duty to his wife in a rural area. Suffering from PTSD, he had difficulty reintegrating into his family and community. This example highlights the various issues of trauma and the veteran's effect on other members of his family.

Context and Case Study

Social workers should apply REM with an eye toward the context in which practice will occur. They can use critical thinking to synthesize some of the following concerns:

- In what geographical locale does the client live?
- What is the client's cultural milieu?
- What is the design of the social service delivery systems?

The Western Interstate Commission for Higher Education, which attempts to recruit returning veterans to college in professional health fields, reported in 2012 that 44 percent of U.S. military recruits are from rural areas (McFaul, n.d.). Because individuals from rural areas serve in the military at higher rates than those from urban and suburban areas, rural areas have a higher proportion of returning veterans (McFaul, n.d.). Social workers who work in sparsely populated areas may have clients who do not have easy access to public transportation, health care, or government agencies, but these clients are likely to have strong ties or close connections with local friends and family (National Center for Veterans Analysis and Statistics, 2011). These factors shape help-seeking behavior at the local level, where rural campus colleges, criminal justice personnel, and postsecondary educators may become community stakeholders with whom social workers can partner (Kirchner, Farmer, Shue, Blevins, & Sullivan, 2011).

Conner is a 28-year-old from rural Kentucky. He is in the Army Reserve and has had four deployments to Afghanistan. He has his general equivalency diploma and works in a local hardware store. He went to war because he believed it was his duty to his father and two of his uncles, who had served in the military. Conner returned from war depressed, doubting his own ability to "get back to normal."

Acknowledging Client Loss, Vulnerability, and Future

Social workers working in rural areas may see clients who they know through social networks. The social worker Diane went to high school with Conner. A supervisor will need to monitor Diane's work, and she will need to be careful that her dual relationship does not interfere with treatment (NASW, 2008).

> Dual or multiple relationships occur when professionals engage with clients or colleagues in more than one relationship. A professional enters into a dual relationship whenever he or she assumes a second role with a client, becoming social worker and friend, employer, teacher, business associate, family member, or sex partner. A practitioner can engage in a dual relationship whether the second relationship begins before, during, or after the social worker relationship. (Reamer, 2001, p. 188)

Diane's supervisor confirms that is it is alright for Diane to acknowledge in conversation with Conner that the small town they live in has suffered more than its share of causalities in the Iraq War. It is "normal" for the veteran to grieve and wonder about his future. Later in his healing, he might reach out to families who have experienced loss.

Identifying the Source of and Reaction to Stress

Conner is experiencing nightmares and general sleeplessness. After working for weeks to establish trust with Diane, he is able to share that he witnessed military personnel shooting civilians. Diane is nonjudgmental and recognizes that this is a difficult burden for her client to bear. Her acceptance appears to lessen Conner's anxiety.

Helping Clients Take Control

Diane and Conner reevaluate his anxiety level before he goes to see a psychiatrist at the VA (an hour away) for his six-month checkup. Having identified the source of his stress, Conner is better able to stabilize, or normalize, his situation. Diane encourages Conner to make his own decision about sharing his "secret" about the civilians' murder with the psychiatrist. This gives Conner control and promotes self-efficacy.

Providing Resources for Change

Diane wants to introduce Conner to activities that will encourage his work toward self-change and strengthen his problem-solving abilities. He agrees to take advantage of online resources not available in his local community. Such resources are disseminated through extension services such as Project Youth Extension Service (Y.E.S!), a care-sharing program jointly sponsored by the U.S. Departments of Defense and Agriculture (Bush, Bosmajian, Fairall, McCann, & Ciulla, 2011; see also U.S. Department of Defense & U.S. Department of Agriculture, 2014). These services provide a means of reaching other REM goals, including addressing positive emotions and achieving creative expression.

Making Meaning of Events

Conner is experiencing great difficulty making meaning of his military deployment. Diane, who has kept up on the literature, knows that this feeling is not uncommon (Diacosavvas & Specjal, 2012). Diane learns that Conner's family is proud of his service and does not know that he witnessed civilian casualties. By talking through the various events of war with Diane, Conner is able to see the benefits of his service, such as helping to depose a totalitarian dictator and saving the lives of both soldiers and local civilians (see Tables 7.2 and 7.3). Having begun to appreciate these benefits, Conner decides to have a one-to-one conversation with his pastor. Months after treatment ends, Diane sees Conner attending church. She simply nods.

Diversity

Returning veterans' condition and experiences cause changes in family functioning. In addition, the diversity of the veteran cohort, which now includes more women and openly LGBT soldiers, has also changed how veterans' families are assessed. As veterans' families change, support and services to family members and caregivers must evolve to meet new demographics.

Military Culture

The military has a culture and language all its own that reflects the organization and hierarchy of the various branches of service. Military family culture is affected by

TABLE 7.2
Meaning Matrix

	Before War	During War	After War
Purpose	Having a sense of pride and patriotism Defending freedom and keeping the country safe Sharing in a family history of military service Having a "John Wayne" syndrome	Staying alive Keeping fellow soldiers alive Providing the people of Iraq or Afghanistan with a safer and better standard of living	Having saved lives Having been part of an effort to depose a totalitarian dictator Having kept comrades safe in the face of danger
Sacrifice	Knowing that hopes, dreams, and future plans need to be postponed Knowing that there is a risk of being killed	Giving up one's own morality Challenging one's physical integrity Forgetting individualism Missing interpersonal relationships	Losing time Leaving camaraderie behind Living with a changing self-image and shattered assumptions of the world or shattered sense of innocence Diminishing religious faith
Outcome	Hoping to perform the job well Making family and military leaders proud	Saving lives Reshaping or altering one's life perspective Having a greater appreciation for life, family, and things	Having deposed a totalitarian dictator Having assassinated the head of Al-Qaida Having saved the lives of soldiers and local civilians Having sustained physical or psychological wounds

whether a family lives on base or is being reassigned or whether a family member is being deployed. Service members develop their culture through basic training, rituals, and discipline that prepare them to act as a team in combat situations (Demers, 2011). In military culture, controlling one's stress and carrying out assigned duties is paramount. Yet these feelings and behaviors may not be conducive to reintegration into civilian family life.

Demographics

The military does not have the same demographics as the mainstream U.S. population. In "Who Joins the Military? A Look at Race, Class, and Immigration Status,"

TABLE 7.3
Sample Questions to Illicit Meaning

	Before War	During War	After War
Purpose	Do you remember what you were told when you were preparing to go to war? What sense of purpose did you have before you reached the combat zone?	Can you remember what it felt like while you were on missions? What was your sense of purpose while performing your job?	Looking back, what do you perceive your overall purpose was? How does this compare with your original sense of purpose? Can you think of other purposes you served? What would your comrades, spouse, children, parents, friends, and family say about your purpose?
Sacrifice	What did you think you would be sacrificing by going to war?	What types of sacrifices did you feel yourself making while you were deployed?	What did it ultimately cost you to be deployed in a war zone, considering spiritual and psychological costs? What would your comrades, spouse, children, parents, friends, and family say you've sacrificed?
Outcome	What did you hope to achieve during your deployment?	What personal or unit accomplishments were you aware of during your deployment? Is there anything you patted yourself on the back for while in combat?	Looking back, what do you think your greatest accomplishments were during the war? What do you believe your unit accomplished? What do you think are positive outcomes of the military action in which you served?

Lutz (2008) found that those with a lower family income are more likely than those with a higher family income to join the military and that a large percentage of Latinos who have served in the armed forces are children of immigrants.

According to data from the 2009 American Community Survey, an ongoing survey of the U.S. population, male veterans are older, more likely to be white non-Hispanic, more likely to be married, less likely to be uninsured, less likely to live below the poverty level, and likely to have higher personal incomes than male non-veterans (U.S. Census Bureau, 2009). Female veterans are more likely to be white non-Hispanic, more likely to be divorced, less likely to be uninsured, less likely to live below the poverty level, and likely to have higher personal incomes than female nonveterans (see National Center for Veterans Analysis and Statistics, 2011).

Diverse Family Forms

The military includes all the family forms that exist in civilian life. Therefore, social care providers must be prepared to learn about both the culture of the military and the specific culture of the military family.

Families of service personnel are eligible for Family and Medical Leave Act provisions. All soldiers who have dependents and who are either single or part of a dual-military couple must have a family care plan to ensure that their family is cared for during their absence. These plans reflect the culture of the family, the reach of the extended family, and other social supports.

LGBT Personnel

On September 11, 2012, the almost 18-year-old "Don't Ask, Don't Tell" policy was officially repealed by the Department of Defense. Today's policy states that "statements about sexual orientation or lawful acts of homosexual conduct will not be considered as a bar to military service" (Memoli, 2011). The "Don't Ask, Don't Tell" policy allowed gays to serve in the military as long as they kept their sexual orientation secret. Since "Don't Ask, Don't Tell" was repealed, partners of gays have been extended benefits, and support groups for LGBT service members have begun to meet in the Pentagon's main food court (Bumiller, 2012; Shanker, 2013).

Female Veterans

Of the 2 million people who have served in the military, women make up 15 percent of active-duty and 18 percent of National Guard and Reserve troops (National Center for Veterans Analysis and Statistics, 2011). On the basis of current trends, the number of female veterans and female VA users in all branches of service is expected to double again by 2020.

VA hospitals primarily serve women for PTSD, hypertension, and depression. Because female veterans underutilize VA care, on April 23, 2013, the VA launched a hotline to respond to questions from female veterans, their families, and caregivers about available services and resources. "The Women Veterans Call Center is aimed at increasing women veterans' knowledge of all VA services and benefits that they deserve," said Krista Stephenson, army veteran and Women Veterans Call Center director (VA, Office of Public and Intergovernmental Affairs, 2011)

Older Veterans

Older veterans in caregiving situations often experience the natural processes of aging, including physiological changes in the auditory system; frailty and the disease processes of old age, consisting of changes in skeletal and cognitive function;

and special issues related to the effects of their service in the military on themselves, their family, and their community.

Like returning veterans, older veterans may experience recurrences of PTSD, depression, and suicidal thoughts. For example, according to the VA's National Registry for Depression, "11% of Veterans aged 65 years and older have a diagnosis of major depressive disorder, a rate more than twice that found in the general population of adults aged 65 and older" (VA, 2011, p. 1). Older veterans thus require evidence-based treatment, including intensive case management approaches for those coping with SMI (Mohamed, Neale, & Rosenheck, 2009).

Family Resilience

The study of resilience has evolved from an examination of individuals to an understanding of the dynamic relational basis of resilience (Greene, 2002, 2012). The literature on family resilience is based on a multifaceted theory addressing the specific mechanisms that might undermine or support family functioning (Bowen & Martin, 2011; Bowen, Martin, & Mancini, 2013; Palmer, 2008; Riggs & Riggs, 2011). A review of the literature on the concepts of family dynamics produces the following:

- Risk and resilience theory deals with a the risks, protective factors, worldviews, and self-healing or transcendence of a family on reunification (Walsh, 1998).
- Attachment theory explores how parent–child relationships or bonds are challenged by military separations and reunions (Isserman, Greene, Bowen, Hollander-Goldfein, & Cohen, 2014).
- System theory examines organization and communication in families in order to improve reintegration (Buckley, 1968, Greene, 2008a).
- Role theory details the ways in which family tasks are assigned once a family has come together again (K. Thompson, 2008).
- Family stress theory discusses how a family perceives and reacts to the challenges of separation and war (Patterson & Garwick, 1998).
- Life course theory examines how a family unit (as well as its individuals) develops or varies over a lifetime, particularly in response to military service (MacLean & Elder, 2007).
- Ecological theory addresses how the family is supported by other social systems, including informal supports and groups, as it tries to reintegrate into society (Greene, 2008a).

FRT

The FRT, which can augment FAM in assessment, was first developed to study the reunification or re-creation of Holocaust survivor families (Greene, 2010). It poses questions based on the theories that the social worker may use in assessment listed previously (see "Family Resilience Template" on page 131).

Family Resilience Template

Section 1. Ecological-Systems Concepts

1. Family had positive interrelationships.
2. Family functioned as an effective structure.
3. Family members assumed viable roles.
4. Family had explicit rules, norms, and expectations.
5. Effective problem solving was based on effective communication.
6. Family engaged in successful decision making.
7. Family showed positive patterns of communication.
8. Successful parenting resulted in the success of the children.
9. Parents were caregivers to the children.
10. Family took on challenges in a direct manner.
11. Family had assets and strengths.
12. Family identified and responded to risks.
13. Family used its resources effectively.
14. Family members took time together.
15. Family was cohesive and worked together in its efforts.
16. Children functioned well in their environment.
17. Family was optimistic.
18. Family established connections with extended family and friends.
19. Family made affiliations in the community.
20. Family took the initiative to keep functioning well.
21. Family accepted what cannot be changed.
22. Family felt in control of life situations.
23. Family envisioned new possibilities.
24. Family learned and grew from adversity.
25. Family adhered to a faith system.
26. Family kept traditional practices.

Section 2. Attachment Theory from the Quality of Family Dynamics Paradigm

27. Closeness: There are frequent and positive contacts and ties with family members.
28. Empathy: The child experiences the parent as a caring and understanding adult.
29. Validation: The parent supports the child's feelings, thoughts, needs, and behaviors.
30. Expressions of positive emotions: Positive emotions, love, and affection are expressed.
31. Open communication: Thoughts about the war and about problems are expressed.
32. Distance: Contacts among family members are cold, infrequent, and negative.
33. Self-centeredness: The parent is focused on his or her own needs and desires.
34. Criticism: The parent's interactions with the child are negative, dismissive, and unsupportive.
35. Expressions of negative emotions: Predominantly negative emotions are expressed.
36. Closed communication: Sensitive topics are taboo or secret; problems are not discussed.

Source: Adapted from *Promoting Psychological Resilience in the U.S. Military* (pp. xiv–xv), by L. Meridith, C. D. Sherbourne, S. Gaillot, L. Hansell, H. V. Ritschard, A. M. Parker, and G. Wrenn, 2011, Santa Monica, CA: Rand Center for Military Health Policy Research. Retrieved from http://www.rand.org/pubs/monographs/MG996.html

Assessment and FAM

Case Study

This case study is based on the May 10, 2012, episode of National Public Radio's *Talk of the Nation*. The couple, Chris and Lisa F., shared their story, called "A Cycle of Deployment Strains Military Marriages." They said that their marriage appeared "to have it all together." Chris had risen through the ranks, and Lisa had taken care of family business. Yet they were growing more and more distant.

One of the most difficult aspects of their marriage was maintaining a "prepared state of mind"; both always needed to be ready for the next mission. The next deployment—and separation—loomed around the corner. But when they were together, they avoided this issue and instead talked about the kids' soccer games. The growing distance between Chris and Lisa became the elephant in the room. Their two daughters did not understand Chris's lack of participation in their lives. Why did he want to separate himself? Lisa found her husband putting up a wall, separating, or protecting, him from the family. A daughter remembers that "normal was when Dad was away."

Chris had an epiphany when his 18-year-old daughter asked why he had missed so many of her birthdays. He realized that he had not been at one of her birthdays since she was 10 years old. Chris realized he had put his "family into a compartment, and it was a very small compartment in my head." Chris said to himself, "We had to learn how to be part of a team/family again."

Family as a Caregiving System

A family's ability to care for its members depends on its organization, structure, communication, and belief system. The practitioner uses the questions on the FRT to elicit the family members' present understanding of their functioning as well as the challenges they think they are facing. The social worker can ask direct questions about finances ("Who is in charge?") or family rules. Questions should also address the family's narrative of success and the meaning it has assigned to events.

Roles Family Members Play in Caregiving

Families of service members are caregiving units when a member goes abroad and when he or she returns. The returning veteran needs more care at some points than at others, especially when he or she is experiencing a TBI or PTSD. Therefore, roles are allocated differently according to the caregiving context. It is important for the practitioner to learn from the family members what stresses they are experiencing. Does the family include a child with developmental difficulties? How do family members identify and respond to caregiving tasks? Research shows that a service member's increased time away from home on active duty is inherently stressful to military families and may contribute to detached parent–child and spousal relationships (Basham, 2008; Lowe, Adams, Browne, & Hinkle, 2012). The social worker's assessment of the family's expression of closeness, positive emotions, and validation can be essential in helping the family use its assets successfully (see Section 2 in "Family Resilience Template" on page 131).

Development of Family over Time

The life course of the family as a unit is influenced by the development of the unit itself as well as the development of each family member. As can be seen in the case of the F. family, military service may influence life transitions. A study by Elder, Gimbel, and Ivie (1991) supported this idea, finding that "military service creates discontinuity in men's lives by removing them from age-graded careers and subjecting them to the dictates of a world in which one's past or [particular] life history has no importance" (p. 215).

In addition, children of different ages react to stress in their own way and according to their developmental stage. In an American Red Cross workshop for returning veterans with young children, parents are taught to identify and respond to age-related differences in children's reactions to reunions with their returning family service member. For example, infants and preschoolers may act confused or clingy. They may exhibit changes in toileting, eating, and sleeping. Elementary-age children (ages six to 12) may show anger or jealousy. Finally, teenagers (ages 13 to 18) may appear apathetic or exhibit risky behavior. They may spend less time with family.

Caregiving Stress and Secondary Trauma

Caregiving stress or secondary trauma may affect the practitioner or members of the returning veterans' family (Figley, 1995). This phenomenon is related to "extreme" empathy or sympathy or to "over"-identification with traumatized persons. *Burnout* is another term used to describe the extreme exhaustion practitioners who work with many clients who have undergone trauma may feel (Maslach, Jackson, & Leiter, 1996). Supervisors should be mindful of this possibility, as should practitioners who work with families of returning veterans.

Resilience-Enhancing Family Intervention

REM and the FRT can be used to create an intervention plan for the F. family. The practitioner would begin by synthesizing what he or she already knows about the family and then decide what additional information needs to be gathered. The practitioner knows that the family has begun identifying some of the difficulties resulting from Chris's multiple deployments and separations and has thus begun the process of self-change. Therefore, the practitioner should first acknowledge this success and then ask further questions about how family organization (rules) and communication have changed in Chris's absence. The family members should speak to one another rather than through the social worker. When one member directs remarks to the social worker, the social worker should redirect the comments to the group.

Next, the practitioner could address the comment "Normal was when Dad was away." What roles did each family member play when Chris was on active duty? Was he locked out of the family on his return? Soccer seems to be an important activity for the daughters. Can Chris be more engaged as the family goes out into the community for soccer games and practice? How else will the family spend time together? Will there be better communication and recreational activity for Chris and Lisa, who once again must form a spousal and parental dyad?

Another area of family-centered work might focus on the daughter's comment that Chris had missed seven of her birthdays. How did this affect the closeness of their relationship? How can Chris make up for lost time? How can the daughters' needs be validated? Finally, what does each family member envision for the future? What growth will occur?

Care Sharing and Outreach Innovations

The social worker may want to work with programs sponsored by the military. Two programs established to help individuals and families with resilience include Comprehensive Soldier and Family Fitness and Seven Tools That Reinforce Psychological Strength. The Comprehensive Soldier and Family Fitness program, initially created by the U.S. Army to address physical strength, now addresses five dimensions of strength: (1) physical, maintaining healthy bodies through exercise, nutrition, and training; (2) emotional, approaching life's challenges with a positive and optimistic outlook and demonstrating self-control; (3) social, developing trusting relationships, communicating effectively, and exchanging ideas; (4) spiritual, finding strength in a set of belief and values; and (5) family, being an active member of a safe, supportive, and loving family (see U.S. Army, 2014).

The Seven Tools That Reinforce Psychological Strength program outlines seven actions service members can take to foster resilience: (1) call DCoE to reach out for help; (2) log on to Real Warriors live chats to connect instantly, anywhere in the world, 24 hours a day, with a resource consultant at DCoE; (3) watch videos of service members who have reintegrated with their families; (4) share stories about coping with change on message boards; (5) read others' stories; (6) find support during transitions, such as a change of status or new orders; and (7) send a Real Warrior an e-card showing support (see Real Warriors, n.d.).

Interactive tools for assessment and psychoeducational treatment are also available online. This multimedia outreach initiative was launched in 2006. It influenced the creators of *Sesame Street* to create and distribute a DVD for military families with young children (see http://www.sesamestreet.org/parents/tlc). The purpose of the DVD is to help young children cope with deployments and reintegrate with a returning parent. Two PBS television shows have presented these materials in prime-time specials. Another initiative, called Strong Bond, is sponsored by the U.S. Army Chaplain Corps. It provides retreats for families during which they can explore the effects of stress.

Saltzman et al. (2011) identified five major factors that can destabilize military family functions: (1) incomplete understanding of the effect of deployment and combat operational stress as well as inaccurate developmental expectations, (2) impaired family communication, (3) impaired parenting, (4) impaired organization, and (5) a lack of a guiding belief system. The researchers, along with the University of California, Los Angeles, and Harvard Medical School, developed a program called Families OverComing Under Stress (FOCUS) to teach practical communication skills and to create shared family stories. This program is available at designated installations and is supported by the Department of Defense.

Military Social Work: Micro- to Macropractice

Military social work requires an ecological mind-set to allow the practitioner to implement micro and macro level practice strategies. For example, a practitioner may have to become a vocal advocate for policy solutions that increase community support for returning veterans (Blow et al., 2012). Thus, military social work encompasses

> direct practice; policy and administrative activities; and advocacy including providing prevention, treatment, and rehabilitative services to service members, veterans, their families, and their communities. In addition, military social workers develop and advance programs, policies, and procedures to improve the quality of life for clients and their families in diverse communities. (CSWE, 2010)

Community Resilience

National health security depends on understanding and building community resilience in response to human-made and natural disasters. According to Chandra et al. (2010), "*National health security* is achieved when the Nation and its people are prepared for, protected from, respond effectively to, and able to recover from incidents with potential negative health consequences" (p. 2). Although more evidence is needed, it is thought that community cohesion and the ability to marshal resources quickly play an important role in building community resilience. Particular attention needs to be given to resource-poor neighborhoods.

Community Capacity

In his seminal book on social capital in current society, Robert Putnam (2000) suggests that we are all "bowling alone"—his metaphor for the erosion of social ties. This metaphor has also been applied to the military. Units such as the Air Force Family Advocacy Division attempt to establish a sense of community life both during and after service (Bowen, Martin, Mancini, & Nelson, 2001). Social care workers can contribute to building community capacity by "discovering the broad power of the community" (Huebner, Mancini, Bowen, & Orthner, 2009, p. 216). Briefly, *community capacity* consists of two elements: (1) *shared responsibility*, or caring for the general welfare of all or a general concern, and (2) *collective competence*, or taking action to meet community needs. If the social care worker effectively reaches out to formal and informal networks to assist veterans and their families, community capacity has the potential to grow.

Several model programs, such as the 4-H Army Youth Development Program and Operation: Military Kids, have been developed to enhance community capacity for military families. One such program, the Coming Home Project, provides community retreats during which family members cultivate psychoeducational life skills (Bobrow, Cook, Knowles, & Vieten, 2013). Where such programs are not available, social care workers may initiate programs of their own, as Diane did in her work with Conner.

Part of enhancing community capacity is increasing the sense of efficacy and human resources within the community (Huebner et al., 2009). This relationship and linkage between efficacy and human resources within a community is important, as many military families prefer to receive support through informal systems (Orthner & Rose, 2007). To enhance the bonds between families and professional services, a "'web of support' envelopes military families, which involves the reciprocal and synergetic effects from the combination of formal and informal sources of support" (Huebner et al., 2009, p. 220). In this way, veterans and their families feel connected to and supported by communities that have clear methods and articulated goals for engaging them in community life.

As communities receive male and female veterans, it is important that a policy and resource allocation philosophy founded on a care-sharing perspective be in place to assist with postservice transitions. In a study of the National Guard, researchers found a high level of commitment to providing resources and assistance to returning service members (Blow et al., 2012). Findings indicated that communities were seeking ways to better support these veterans, and citizens were willing to pay higher taxes for this purpose.

Rural communities may be especially challenged, as they have limited resources to assist returning service members. Kirchner et al. (2011) described a model program in one rural area that demonstrates a high level of involvement by key stakeholders in assisting veterans with mental health challenges. A training and outreach program was developed to help veterans reintegrate into community life and to help community members and stakeholders be more effective in working and interacting with this population.

Thoughts on Social and Economic Justice

In addition to the rights of freedom, justice, and an adequate standard of living (Rawls, 1971), people expect that their society will provide them with safety. How a society provides for its citizens is often linked to the relative benefits and costs of a social policy (Van Soest & Garcia, 2003). In 1970, the Gates Commission studied U.S. policy regarding a draft army. Its members recommended that the United States implement an all-volunteer army, arguing that sufficient military strength could be achieved without conscription. According to the *New York Times* (Tavernise, 2011), a smaller share of Americans currently serve in the armed forces than at any time since the period between World War I and World War II. Some segments of our population are more likely to have a service member in their family; as social care workers, we must explore what we think about this fact.

According to Diacosavvas and Specjal (2012), licensed clinical social workers who provide treatment to returning veterans at the VA, the debate about whether the United States has successfully met the foreign policy goals of the wars in Iraq and Afghanistan has led to a crisis of meaning among service personnel. The debate leaves to the service member the burden of deciding whether he or she has achieved the intended purpose of participating in the war. Were the intended outcomes achieved? Were the sacrifices worth the cost? Did his or her unit make a difference? These concerns can be incorporated into your social work practice at the individual, family, and community levels.

CHAPTER EIGHT

Caregiving Model
for People with HIV/AIDS

This book is intended to guide you through a social care approach to identifying the needs of various client caregiving systems. This chapter outlines the components of an integrated caregiving model for assessing and intervening with individuals, families, and communities who provide care for people with HIV/AIDS. Two of the major issues addressed are combating the stigma of HIV/AIDS and ensuring continuity and retention of care. We begin the discussion with a description of the early years of struggle to humanize the disease. To help you better understand how to synthesize your caregiving model, we then present case studies that focus on certain geographic locales and sociocultural contexts. This approach allows you to envision working with caregivers in multiple contexts in various communities in the United States and internationally.

The first case study involves Marvin, a gay white man in San Francisco. In this case study, FAM and REM are used to assess and intervene at the micro level. The case of a grandmother raising her grandson is presented next. The care in this family dyad is fragmented because of a poor case management system in the rural South. The next case introduces Leonard and Carolyn, who live in Washington, DC, and who have not yet been diagnosed as HIV positive. The final case study explores the care needs of Abeba, who lives in Ethiopia. The concepts of stigma, collective efficacy, and human capital will help you understand Abeba's situation. Methods for strengthening collective efficacy and human capital are explored. Caregiving strategies and medical advances are outlined to complement the model.

Using a Social Care Approach

A social care approach to social work practice involves walking alongside the client in order to provide quality, client-centered care. Social workers using this approach listen to the client's story, assess care needs, select interventions to maintain the stability of care, and promote resilience among individuals, families, and communities. When using a social care approach, the social worker may select from among many assessment concepts and intervention strategies at multiple system levels. No one family or caregiving situation necessitates the use of all assessment and intervention stratagems. Rather, the day-to-day practice of social work requires critical thinking about concepts and a synthesis of the most appropriate techniques. Research and master practitioners also inform action. Most important, client feedback is always necessary.

Incidence

The *incidence* of HIV is the number of new HIV infections that occur in a given year. The CDC estimates that approximately 50,000 people in the United States are newly infected with HIV each year. According to the CDC (2011b), 1.2 million Americans now live with HIV. In 2010 (the most recent year for which data are available), there were an estimated 47,500 new HIV infections. A total of 63 percent of new infections occurred in gay and bisexual men. African American men and women were also heavily affected, having an HIV incidence rate that was almost eight times as high as the incidence rate among whites (CDC, 2010).

Understanding HIV/AIDS

HIV is the human immunodeficiency virus, a virus that destroys CD4 cells, which help the body fight disease. The progression of the virus can be slowed dramatically through the use of medication, but if left untreated, HIV can lead to AIDS, or acquired immune deficiency syndrome. HIV can be transmitted through having unprotected sex, sharing needles, and being born to an infected mother. When a person has multiple sex partners who do not know their HIV status, his or her risk of contracting HIV increases (Mayo Clinic, 2014).

Stigmatized and Politicized Caregiving Context

The context of HIV/AIDS caregiving in the United States includes an early turbulent history involving attempts to find funding for medical research and to destigmatize and properly treat the disease. In 1981, the United States was the first country to officially identify AIDS as a new disease thought to be connected solely to gay men. At that time, the majority of Americans viewed HIV/AIDS as the most urgent health problem facing the nation (Henry J. Kaiser Family Foundation, 2012a).

Confronting AIDS: Directions for Public Health, Health Care, and Research, a seminal publication from the Institute of Medicine (1986), broke what appeared to be a logjam surrounding the proper treatment of the disease. So much tension arose around committing proper resources to conquering the disease that activists coined the term "AIDSgate" to characterize what was perceived as President Ronald Reagan's inaction surrounding the AIDS pandemic (Bronski, 2003).

Social work activists did not just address the policy context of HIV/AIDS. They also engaged in care sharing; educated people about the spread of the virus;

provided such basic information as how to wash sheets; delivered meals to the homebound; offered companionship and compassion; and when all else failed, attended funerals. Advocacy and the publication of the Institute of Medicine report finally convinced government officials to increase funding for research and treatment. In addition, a report by U.S. surgeon general C. Everett Koop (1986) urged the public to view HIV/AIDS as a public health emergency.

Since the mid-1980s, people have learned that all segments of U.S. society are at risk for contracting HIV/AIDS. Preventive methods are also better understood. Owing to the discovery of powerful antiretroviral medications, the diagnosis is no longer terminal, and interventions are no longer centered on death and dying. Rather, social workers help people who are HIV positive negotiate intimate relationships, notify their partners, and avoid mother-to-child transmission of the virus. In addition, attention is paid to people living with HIV, whose problems are often compounded by poverty (Bowen, 2013). In short, prompt identification and proper treatment of HIV/AIDS usually means that a person can live with it as a chronic disease. However, HIV/AIDS is still one of the most politicized, feared, and controversial diseases in the history of modern medicine, and stigma and prejudice associated with HIV/AIDS are prevalent today (NASW, 2012).

In this chapter, we show how *HIV prejudice*—or having an irrational fear of people with HIV—in society can lead to social isolation and loss of jobs among people with HIV/AIDS and to obstacles to getting tested for the virus for the general population (NASW, 2002). In addition, there are concerns that the number of HIV professionals—doctors, nurses, social workers—is not keeping up with the demand (Institute of Medicine, 2011). In the early years of the HIV/AIDS epidemic, research suggested that some professionals in health care avoided patients with HIV/AIDS (Riley & Greene, 1993). Does this fear still prevail? How comfortable will you be engaging clients with HIV?

Risk and Resilience Preventive Intervention

Concepts from risk and resilience theory can help social workers understand the role of prevention in combating HIV/AIDS. *Prevention science*, a relatively new discipline that focuses on risk reduction (Coie et al., 1993), is a research and intervention design that encourages the planned promotion of resilience and that fosters the development of competencies (Sandler, 2001). A person's *risk* of contracting HIV/AIDS, a factor that influences or increases the (statistical) probability that the person will experience the onset of the condition, is not evenly distributed across population groups in the United States; gay men, ethnic minorities, women, and drug users have historically been more likely to become infected with HIV.

Although prevention is at the core of HIV/AIDS treatment, experts generally recommend that those at "apparent risk" (Valdiserri, 2011) undergo HIV testing rather than promoting routine testing (Korthuis et al., 2011). According to the CDC (2012a), the population groups most at risk for contracting HIV/AIDS are youths between 13 and 24 years of age. In fact, one in four new HIV infections (26 percent) occur in this age group. In 2010, about 12,000 young people were infected, or about 1,000 per month (CDC, 2012a).

Making HIV testing a routine medical procedure would allow for population-specific prevention packages including education and outreach (Kurth, Celum, Baeten, Vermund, & Wasserheit, 2011; National Institutes of Health, 2010). For example, the CDC supports HIV risk education for parents, families, schools, community-based organizations, and Web-based prevention programs. With community support, social workers can be at the forefront of such psychoeducational programs (Hobson, 2007).

Social workers can promote or institute protective factors (that is, situations and conditions that help individuals to reduce risk and enhance adaptation). These may involve enhancing youths' internal personal characteristics, such as their problem-solving skills, or building external environmental support networks that modify risks (Rutter, 1987). For example, social work students in the Family Acceptance Project (http://familyproject.sfsu.edu) provide health and mental health care for lesbian and gay youths that aims to increase family involvement in the children's lives. Another model for external support is NASW's Spectrum Project (http://www.naswdc.org/practice/hiv_aids/spectrum.asp), which provides skill-building workshops for practitioners who work with people with HIV/AIDS. The goal is to promote sensitive and evidence-informed practice approaches for working with this client population, and to date, these workshops have reached over 18,000 providers in the United States and worldwide. Social workers can use these models to help clients maintain the continuity of their personal narrative or life story (Borden, 1992), a developmental process linked to demonstrated competence (Masten, 1994).

HIV/AIDS Service Organizations: Community-Level Action

Part of working with clients is understanding the service system that provides support and resources to enhance the functioning of individuals and their families. The early days of HIV/AIDS included significant turbulence and a reluctance to respond to individuals who were HIV positive. Given the slow or inappropriate responses of traditional health care services, AIDS service organizations (ASOs) were formed to specifically address the needs of those who were affected by HIV (Bielefeld, Scotch, & Thielmann, 2000). ASOs are alternative social service agencies that are designed to assist at-risk and marginalized populations. These organizations have strong missions that focus on issues of social justice, advocacy, human rights, and equitable services (Poindexter, 2002, 2007; B. Smith, 2004).

Care-Sharing Philosophy

ASOs were founded on a care-sharing philosophy. These organizations were started and staffed by mostly gay male volunteers whose communities and relationships were strongly affected by HIV. The early pioneers in these services served in all caregiving roles provided by these organizations (for example, as volunteer buddies, crisis workers, advocates, and educators). In a historical analysis of one ASO in a southern state, Poindexter (2002) shared a rallying cry from the organization's executive director. This gay man with AIDS stood on the steps of the state capitol and admonished the community to take action:

> I want to know how many of your friends have to die of AIDS before you folks get angry? I'm not suggesting that we not mourn our dead. But there is no victory in death, no pride in human misery and suffering. What I want is for you to put the anger in your grief to work. . . . Be generous of spirit, the AIDS horizon is still dark. (p. 59)

This director thus served as a community organizer, mobilizing continued action and commitment to overcome this disease.

Legislation

One of the major successes in the AIDS service expansion was the passage of the Ryan White Comprehensive AIDS Resources Emergency Act of 1990 (see Health Resources and Services Administration, n.d.). This federal legislation was the first comprehensive social and medical service package for individuals with HIV in the United States. Ryan White, the namesake of the legislation, was a teenager from Indiana who was critically ill with AIDS when the legislation was passed. White was a hemophiliac who had been infected as a result of a blood transfusion. This legislation was successful in part because it linked the disease to people like White, a young, innocent child who could not be faulted for contracting HIV; White stood in stark contrast to the conservative factions' depiction of gay men who were HIV positive.

The legislation was also successful because it was backed by a strong coalition. The National Organizations Respond to AIDS (NORA) network, a group of 125 national organizations, was formed to work on a legislative response to the HIV pandemic (Poindexter, 1999). On the surface, the groups that were part of NORA seemed to have few common goals; however, this diversity lent legitimacy to the coalition. Poindexter (1999) identified four categories of organizations that were involved: (1) traditional service providers and professional organizations (such as NASW and the American Red Cross), (2) specialized advocates (such as the National Parent-Teachers Association and National Gay and Lesbian Task Force),

(3) AIDS organizations (such as the National Association of People with AIDS and AIDS Action Council), and (4) a broad range of other religious and secular organizations (such as AIDS Education Care and Development).

In her analysis, Poindexter (1999) concluded that the NORA's effectiveness stemmed from three factors: (1) the large number of groups involved, (2) the presence of respected and long-term groups that gave legitimacy to the cause, and (3) the passion and urgency that the activist organizations lent to the cause. This method of organizing provided a means of creating a federal response to HIV/AIDS. As a social change agent practicing in the field of HIV/AIDS, you should understand the social welfare service climate, including grassroots service organizations. The history of organizations can also provide you with a context and purpose for being.

Demographic Shifts

Community-level practice continues to be an important approach for addressing HIV. Over time, the profile of those who are HIV positive has changed to include more people from diverse racial and ethnic groups (CDC, 2010). As the population of people with HIV has shifted from predominantly gay white men to predominantly people from diverse backgrounds, ASOs and other services for people with HIV/AIDS have changed. ASOs have been challenged to provide more culturally congruent services as well as tangible resources for people with HIV and their families.

Both domestically and internationally, HIV/AIDS has had wider transmission among heterosexual and ethnically diverse populations. Different types of service agencies emerged to provide complementary services, but potential clients sometimes struggled with issues of access. Urban centers were once the focal point of the epidemic, leaving rural communities and Native American reservations without service models that fit their needs (Duran et al. 2010; Poindexter, 2002). Like individuals, communities have unique characteristics and require assessment and intervention approaches that fit their culture, values, and behaviors. For example, treatment for HIV for someone who lives in a rural community typically involves a 50-mile trip (Sutton, Anthony, Vila, McLellan-Lemal, & Weidle, 2010). This commute alone can add stress to the caregiving aspects of this disease for both the individual and the care provider.

Faith-based communities are becoming more involved in HIV/AIDS service systems. For African Americans, the church provides information and education about HIV and thus is an important component of a prevention campaign (McNeal & Perkins, 2007). Religious organizations can partner with traditional service systems to offer a more comprehensive array of services to people with HIV/AIDS and their families (Derose, Dominguez, Plimpton, & Kanouse, 2010; Lentz, 2010; Weiss, Dwonch-Schoen, Howard-Barr, & Panella, 2010). This illustrates how partnerships outside of traditional service systems can be effective, extending and complementing existing services.

Applying FAM in Assessment

In 1982, at the beginning of the HIV/ADS epidemic in San Francisco, community leaders and physicians banded together to develop a collective response. They formed the San Francisco AIDS Foundation, providing a hotline with medical information, referrals, and resources. Their early work also involved education to combat the stigma associated with HIV/AIDS. In addition, they took on policy initiatives and public health campaigns, collaborating with community partners and legislators in what may be seen as an early care-sharing approach (San Francisco AIDS Foundation, 2012).

Case Study

Data from the San Francisco AIDS Foundation suggest that foundation clients are most likely to be gay white men. A large majority (71 percent to 90 percent) are receiving medical treatment. We can assume that most of these clients are also receiving some form of counseling, as in the case of Marvin. Marvin is a 45-year-old gay man who has been estranged from his parents since coming out as gay and divorcing his wife of 15 years. His parents are a middle-class religious couple and are embarrassed by Marvin's diagnosis as HIV positive. Marvin's attempts to reunite with his parents have been rebuffed. Marvin has two teenage sons and currently lives with his partner, John. His sons often visit Marvin and John on the weekend. Marvin works for a publishing company in a highly demanding job.

Biopsychosocial and Spiritual Assessment

As indicated in both FAM and REM, the care that Marvin needs depends on his biopsychosocial and spiritual age. To evaluate his biological age, the social care worker will want to know how HIV is affecting Marvin's immune system. Is he fatigued? Does he suffer from sleeplessness? What medications is he taking?

Physical routines vary from client to client depending on each client's antiviral therapy, its side effects, the client's nutrition, and the client's activity level. Among other medical complications, social care workers should become familiar with Kaposi's sarcoma (tumors that line the blood vessels) and *Pneumocystis carinii* pneumonia (a fungal infection of the lungs).

Medical advances have dramatically decreased the number of deaths caused by AIDS. For example, highly active antiviral therapy helped to decrease the number of AIDS deaths by 63 percent between 1995 and 1998 (CDC, 2011a). Routine screening of pregnant women in the United States and timely antiretroviral treatment for those found to be infected have resulted in a 92 percent decline in perinatal transmission of HIV (Fowler, Gable, Lampe, Etima, & Owor, 2010).

In assessing Marvin's psychological age, the social care worker should be aware that psychological adaptations are related to physical effects. When Marvin first tested positive, he denied that the diagnosis could be true. He then cycled through feelings of anger, sadness, and anxiety, which contributed to his stress (Taylor, 1995). The social worker gradually helped him accept the diagnosis and share it with his partner, addressing issues of intimacy and trust.

Another aspect of functional capacity for people diagnosed with HIV is their social-cultural age, which is related to their friends and social networks. Social supports have a profound positive influence on health (Farris, 2007), and HIV-affected health is no exception (Surface, 2007). How will the health care team and mutual aid groups at Marvin's clinic become involved in his care?

Finally, spiritual age is tied to biopsychosocial functioning and is known to relate to a client's quality of life. Will Marvin be able to overcome his estrangement from his parents and members of the church he attended as a child?

Applying REM in Individual Intervention

A verbal person who wanted to tell his story, Marvin sought out the clinic social worker. The social care worker decided to use REM to foster Marvin's resilience. The following steps for gathering the client narrative can be useful in arriving at the goal of resilience-enhancing therapy: transcending the immediate situation (Greene, 2007).

Acknowledge Client Loss, Vulnerability, and Future

When people first learn that they have contracted HIV, they often deal with a sense of loss, a sense of vulnerability, and the notion they have little future. For Marvin to make meaning of his HIV diagnosis, he must begin to come to terms with his sense of loss. What can his future hold? How can something positive come of this adverse event?

Identify the Source of and Reaction to Stress

Each individual with HIV/AIDS and his or her caregiver describe different sources of stress that accompany the disease. A person's reaction depends on personal factors, such as self-efficacy and problem-solving abilities, as well as on environmental support resources. Marvin indicates that he is most worried about his ability to continue carrying out his work and family responsibilities. He decides that he wants to brief his employers and have a family meeting with his partner and his teenage sons. He is not yet ready to include his parents in his care planning, as he is uncomfortable and disappointed with their homophobia.

Stabilize or Normalize the Situation

To normalize the situation, Marvin will eventually need to realize that he is experiencing emotions that many in his situation feel—a combination of anger, sadness, and determination. Affirming these emotions and framing them as positive should help Marvin move forward.

Help Clients Take Control

Moving forward begins with Marvin gaining a sense of control. As Marvin begins to make decisions regarding his medical treatment and family responsibilities, he will be initiating his own growth and transformation.

Provide Resources for Change

An important role of the social worker is to provide resources for change. Marvin's social worker informs him about a clinic-based program called LIFE—a multiweek workshop developed in San Francisco that provides people living with HIV with the motivation, skills, and emotional and practical support necessary to deal with life issues and improve their psychological, social, and physical health (Urban Coalition for HIV/AIDS Prevention Services, 2011). Marvin gains insight and support from this care-sharing group and decides to attend the program in conjunction with his personal counseling.

Promote Self-efficacy

Clients are often able to competently manage their own affairs before they experience a major life stressor. To the extent that his social worker can bolster his achievements, such as talking to his employers, Marvin will gain further self-efficacy.

Collaborate in Self-change

When dealing with what could at first be disastrous news for a client, the social worker can be helpful by tapping the client's potential for self-change. Does Marvin believe that he can make life-changing decisions? Are there people in his life, such as his partner, John, who will be supportive?

Strengthen Problem-Solving Abilities

A client's problem-solving capacity becomes stronger during the therapeutic relationship when the practitioner asks reflective questions intended to place the client in a reflexive position or trigger the consideration of new options (White & Epston, 1990). In his work, Marvin must make many decisions that affect his fellow employees. He is working on strategies to keep himself up-to-date with their assignments so that he does not fall behind. He will also eventually decide what information to disclose, as he knows people with HIV who have lost their jobs.

Address Positive Emotions

As social workers strengthen their relationships with clients over time, it is more likely that positive emotions, such as humor and hope, will emerge. Over the course of their therapeutic relationship, Marvin's social worker learns that her client's sense of humor is helpful in reducing tension and helping him to accept his limitations.

Achieve Creative Expressions

Letting one's imagination soar can put a client on a path to healing. Marvin, who has always loved opera, decides that he will make time to serve on the San Francisco Opera Board.

Make Meaning of Events

When Marvin was diagnosed with HIV, he perceived the event as a major life stressor (a *life stressor* is something that triggers a person's perception that harm or loss may take place). Through treatment, he can move to a secondary appraisal and consider the coping mechanisms and resources available to help him deal with his situation. By listening to and responding to his story, the social care worker can help him decide what is at stake and what can be done. Namely, Marvin will work to find meaning in the HIV diagnosis and to shape his emotional and behavioral response to it (see Lazarus & Folkman, 1984).

Find the Benefit in an Adverse Event

Finding a benefit in an adverse life event is closely linked to growth and transcendence. In some cases, clients may make a new start. The process of finding a benefit in an adverse event and growing as a result had been called "posttraumatic growth" (see Tedeschi & Calhoun, 1996). Marvin decides that he will try and revisit his relationship with his parents.

Attend to a Client's Spirituality

As Marvin reviews his narrative with the social care worker, she learns that one factor contributing to his depression is his rejection by members of his parents' church. He may benefit from the faith-based services available to the LGBT community in San Francisco (http://www.eastbaypride.com).

Transcend the Immediate Situation

As Marvin progresses through therapy, he realizes that life is more than survival and that he need not focus solely on his illness. He volunteers to work for Larkin Street (http://www.larkinstreetyouth.org), an outreach agency that provides HIV services for at-risk and vulnerable youths living on San Francisco's streets. He has become more resilient, looking for new opportunities and discovering new potential.

Assessment of Family Functioning

People with HIV/AIDS are part of various family configurations, including biological and chosen family systems. FAM and REM provide practitioners with an assessment and intervention framework to provide support and resources to individuals and their care providers. Marvin's health and social needs and those of his family are highlighted using these two models.

FAM

When using FAM to assess Marvin's case, the social worker will want to emphasize the development of relationships and roles in Marvin's diverse family form. This will include his *family of origin*, that is, the nuclear or extended family of birth (Marvin's parents), and his *family of choice*, which includes his partner. Marvin also has two sons and an ex-wife. The social worker will want to learn whom he considers part of his family. How do members interact? What will their roles be in care sharing? If Marvin becomes frail, who will assist him and his partner in performing basic caregiving tasks?

To understand the various roles in Marvin's family, the practitioner needs to determine what issues are disrupting or enhancing family functioning. Marvin says that he has long been estranged from his parents but is not happy with this situation. He acknowledges that he "always" had poor communication with them, and he would like to see whether they would attend a family session with the social worker. If successful, the attempt to resolve old family business could be beneficial. One method of family therapy that could be used is externalizing the problem. According to White and Epston (1990), the social worker would begin by coaching Marvin and his parents so that they could begin to understand that Marvin is not the problem. Questions would revolve around how all three could "take action to retrieve their lives and relationships and . . . cooperate in the struggle with [HIV]" (p. 39). Through this therapy, Marvin's parents come to understand that Marvin's sexual orientation does not mean that they failed as parents. They also are able to express their love through taking on care sharing with their teenage grandsons.

REM

Family resilience focuses on "the adaptive qualities of families as they encounter stress" (Hawley & DeHaan, 1996, p. 284) and involves natural resources, patterns of functioning, and capabilities that help family members overcome crisis situations. To manage these elements, the social care worker must first determine who belongs to a client's care-sharing system. To arrive at a care-sharing arrangement, the self-designated care-sharing group reframes and reinterprets the caregiving issues. The members of the group set mutual goals and mobilize the family system by drawing on strengths and past and present accomplishments.

An important goal of the family in enhancing resilience is providing emotional support. This support involves care sharing with the HIV-positive family member, that is, keeping him or her involved in his or her own care, including by helping out around the house. "Listening, trying to understand, showing you care, and helping them work through their emotions is a big part of home care" (CDC, 2007).

Macropractice roles are also important, as environmental change helps to decrease the incidence and prevalence of HIV. As the population with HIV/AIDS diversifies, different forms of education and outreach are needed. And as faith communities become more involved, clergy and church leaders can become important parts of a prevention and intervention plan (McNeal & Perkins, 2007). Social workers who are involved in HIV/AIDS work need to have the skills to develop coalitions and work across diverse segments of the community to bring together those organizations that will have the greatest impact in this area.

Partnerships can also be effective in tackling political or sensitive aspects of the disease. For example, one community-based participatory action project addressed HIV/AIDS and teenage pregnancy in a conservative, southern location (Weiss et al., 2010). In an educational campaign aimed at teens, a survey was performed to determine whether the community was amenable to social action that would address its higher than average rate of pregnancy and sexually transmitted diseases. This research led to a community-wide coalition that involved public schools, parents, and a committee of health providers. Educating the youths in this community became a shared responsibility, and the project's success was a result of the effective community partnership that was established. This type of coalition development is an important component of macropractice skills.

Caregiving as a Collective Action and Goodness of Fit

The year 2011 marked the 30th anniversary of the HIV/AIDS epidemic having a "broad and profound impact . . . on families, communities, systems of care, social norms, and collective scientific enterprise" (Valdiserri, 2011, p. 479). Although on the surface there appears to be a number of care services for people with HIV/AIDS—involving both government and nongovernment programs—it cannot be said that there is one delivery system. Nor is there always an organized care team. Care is often spread out among agencies that assist with issues of substance use, mental health, and homelessness. Furthermore, data systems that are usually not interoperable maintain separate program-planning processes that are often not well coordinated. Thus, care differs greatly depending on the program's size, financial resources, and the design of the organizational structure (Valdiserri, 2011).

Effective caregiving necessitates goodness of fit (that is, a nurturing or positive match) between the individual's adaptive needs and the qualities of the medical and psychosocial environment. Two of the most important factors in the medical environment that determine the effectiveness of personal treatment of HIV/AIDS are continuity of care and systems integration. *Continuity of care*, which is central to a social care model, involves the quality of care over time. High-quality care necessitates a "continuous caring relationship with an identified [health care professional]" (Guilford, Naithani, & Morgan, 2006, p. 248). This means more than patient satisfaction and positive health outcomes; as the Country Doctor (2010) suggested, "Continuity of care starts with caring."

Because the treatment of HIV/AIDS is complex, patient care is shared across vertical and horizontal systems, often leading to system disintegration and patient dropout.

> Like the multiple factors that influence, pro and con, the uptake of HIV diagnostic services, there is no single circumstance or variable that can account for all variations of retention in HIV care. Predictors of delayed linkage to HIV care and poor retention in care include demographic, socioeconomic, and psychosocial variables as well as measures of disease severity. (Giordano et al., 2007, p. 1494)

Even in systems with minimal financial barriers to HIV care, retention may be suboptimal. One means of improving linkages to and retention in HIV care is strengthening the integration of the various prevention, medical, and psychosocial components required to deliver high-quality HIV care (Torian & Wiewel, 2011). Through case management, social workers can perhaps do just that.

Integrated Multidisciplinary Care and Case Management

Because approximately half of all HIV-infected individuals are not engaged in regular medical care (E. M. Gardner, McLees, Steiner, del Rio, & Burman, 2011; Marks, Gardner, Craw, & Crepaz, 2010) and services are fragmented, social workers can play a major role in caregiving by acting as case managers, sometimes on multidisciplinary teams. Intervention approaches for people with HIV/AIDS often cut across multiple service networks, including health care, mental health care, substance abuse treatment, and financial aid and resource planning. Research evidence and practice skills for care management are presented and applied to individuals with HIV/AIDs and their care providers.

Research Evidence

Research indicates that health care for individuals with HIV/AIDs is effective when a case management approach is used to link individuals with resources. For example, the Antiretroviral Treatment Access Study assessed a case management intervention to improve linkages to care for people who had recently received a diagnosis of HIV (L. I. Gardner et al., 2005). Participants who lived in Atlanta, Baltimore, Los Angeles, and Miami were assigned to randomized trials that involved either a standard passive referral group or an intensive case management group that connected them to nearby HIV clinics.

The passive referral group provided information about HIV and local care resources; the intensive case management intervention included up to five contacts with a case manager over a 90-day period. Intensive case management is usually delivered by someone with a master's in social work with a small caseload. In this trial, case managers emphasized building a relationship with clients, identifying barriers to health care, and encouraging contact with a clinic. The outcome measure was a self-report of attendance at an HIV care clinic at least twice over a 12-month period. In another study, a nurse, a social work associate, and a nurse practitioner were able to connect to more than 90 percent of newly diagnosed, out-of-care HIV-infected patients who were tested in an emergency room setting in San Francisco (Christopoulos et al., 2011). These brief interventions are associated with a significantly higher rate of successful linkage to HIV care, demonstrating that case management is an affordable and effective resource that can be offered to HIV-infected clients soon after a diagnosis is made.

Practice Skills

Case management is a social work method carried out to ensure the delivery of comprehensive coordinated care to an individual with multiple care needs. The method is used in various fields of practice, including mental health services, HIV/AIDS services, and services for older adults. The case manager is responsible for ensuring the timely and adequate delivery of suitable community-based services (Rose & Moore, 1995). The client usually has decreased functional capacity and may need assistance with activities of daily living, such as keeping house, managing finances, using public transportation, preparing meals, and administering medication.

Social workers and public health nurses have engaged in case management since the 1880s, when charity organization societies were faced with scarce resources and many families in need of assistance (Vourlekis & Greene, 1992). A charity organization society friendly visitor was trained in "investigation, diagnosis, preparations of case records, and treatment, all of which required guidance, counsel, supervision, and the knowledge of scientific philanthropy"—a hands-on social care approach that ensured the delivery of care (Trattner, 1994, p. 238).

Many of these elements still characterize today's case management systems, which are designed to coordinate multiple care needs. However, some of these activities have been taken on by business entities interested in a streamlined, automated, and accelerated approach to decision making. Technology is increasingly used to find solutions for clients and resolve cases. Better process productivity and more effective internal collaboration are centralized and in some situations managed by information specialists. Thus, performing both the caregiving and the business aspects of case management is the challenge, and it requires a particular set of practice skills.

Case management involves several basic functions in which a social worker

1.   engages or identifies the client, often through outreach
2.   assesses client needs
3.   plans for service or treatment
4.   links or refers clients to appropriate resources
5.   monitors cases to ensure that services are delivered and used
6.   evaluates the treatment plan (and sometimes the service design system) (Rose & Moore, 1995; Weil & Karls, 1985)

Practitioners begin the case management process by working to establish a mutual relationship with the client. Once clients are identified, the setting of mutual goals for the service plan is at the core of the helping process. For example, Marvin decides which family members he is willing to include in family therapy sessions. By allowing the client to make decisions about his or her care, the social worker focuses on the client's strengths, blending therapeutic help with any needed resource allocation or referral. The goal is to help Marvin attain the highest level of functionality and competence.

While using REM with Marvin, the social worker wants to individualize service plans to improve her client's quality of life. She is also performing what is sometimes called a *broker role* to enhance her client's pattern of service usage, ensuring "the patient is not lost" (Ozarin, 1978, p. 168). This can be a challenge to the social worker who wants to ensure client self-determination and the use of the least restrictive but most supportive services. To find this balance between support and independence, social workers may use a social care approach of reaching out to natural support systems; informal support—ranging from emotional support to hands-on nursing care received from a family member, friend, or neighbor— constitutes the vast majority of help provided to vulnerable populations (Greene & Ubel, 2007). Family-focused case management requires that the individuals involved agree that the family should be the unit of the case manager's attention and have developed an agreed-on family care plan. The case manager will coordinate services within the scope of the family care plan and intervene clinically to ameliorate emotional problems in the family and any stress accompanying illness or loss of functioning (Vourlekis & Greene, 1992). The team of formal and informal caregivers will mutually evaluate service implementation and outcomes.

Intervention: Cultural Sensitivity

Disparities in HIV/AIDS data have been a problem since the mid-1980s (Institute of Medicine, 1986) and remain so today (CDC, 2011a). The White House Office of National AIDS Policy (2010) suggested that those of us concerned with eliminating

HIV/AIDS should strive to make the United States "a place where HIV infections are rare, and when they do occur, every person, regardless of age, gender, race/ethnicity, sexual orientation, gender identity, life-extending care, [should be] free from stigma and discrimination" (p. 2). Furthermore, we should work to "1) reduce HIV-related mortality in communities at high risk for infection; 2) adopt community-level approaches to reduce HIV infection in high-risk communities; and 3) reduce stigma and discrimination against people living with HIV" (p. 2).

In addition to reducing inequity, social workers need to promote collective action to reduce the stigma and discrimination related to HIV/AIDS. In 2002, NASW was part of a World AIDS Day campaign in the United States and Great Britain to end the discrimination and stigma associated with HIV/AIDS. The association is concerned with stigma at both the individual level (access to health care and status of family, friends, and caregivers) and the societal level (actions manifested in laws, policies, and popular discourse).

Poindexter (2009) argued that a human rights approach acknowledges that HIV and oppression or discrimination are linked in several ways. Furthermore, she argued that HIV is more than a public health, economic, and social crisis—it is a human rights crisis. She detailed four ways in which HIV and human rights are connected. First, groups of people who are susceptible to acquiring HIV are already challenged by oppression and marginalization both socially and economically. Second, acquiring HIV creates additional challenges and discriminations and may result in losses (for example, of family, relationships, jobs, physical safety) that add to the vulnerability of these individuals. Third, HIV stigma creates barriers that prevent people from seeking medical and mental health resources that are available. Fourth, when society takes a punitive approach instead of a human rights approach, overall health is compromised, as voluntary testing and access to medications are limited, affecting everyone. "Conversely, when human rights are respected in the battle against the HIV pandemic, including protecting dignity and privacy, it leads to better prevention, social and emotional care, and treatment" (p. 131).

Systemic Issues: Grandparents Raising Grandchildren

In some ways, caregiving in the era of HIV/AIDS involves unique arrangements for care provision. As discussed previously, HIV/AIDS has different consequences in different families. Sadly, this disease can affect multiple family members, including spouses or partners and children. When a parent is incapacitated by the disease, grandparents commonly assume care of the grandchildren. The number of grandparents who are raising grandchildren has increased as a result of several factors, including addiction and incarceration of parents (especially women) and HIV/AIDS. About 7.8 million children younger than age 18 (10.5 percent) live in homes in which the householders are grandparents or other relatives (U.S. Census

Bureau, 2010a). Almost 20 percent of these care providers live below the poverty level (AARP, n.d.).

Although there are no firm numbers, one estimate is that more than 125,000 U.S. children have lost parents as a result of HIV/AIDS (Joslin, 2002). When grandparents assume care because of HIV/AIDS, they face some unique challenges. For example, they may be experiencing the grief and loss of losing their own child, or they may be seeing their child's health decline while simultaneously assuming care for their grandchildren. Sadly, these grandparents face the off-time experience of losing their own child while once again assuming the role of caregiver (Levine-Perkell & Hayslip, 2002).

Case Study

This case study illustrates how uncoordinated care, lack of goodness of fit, and lack of case management can negatively influence kinship care. "Kinship care is the full time care, nurturing and protection of children by relatives, members of their tribes or clans, godparents, stepparents, or any adult who has a kinship bond with a child" (Child Welfare League of America, n.d.). Anita is an 89-year-old African American grandmother struggling to raise her troubled nine-year-old grandson, Albert, in the rural South. Albert was placed in kinship care by the child welfare system. Anita had promised her dying son that she would care for Albert, who was four years old when his father died of AIDS. Albert's mother was a drug addict and had disappeared from his life. Anita remembers, "Albert was very disturbed when he came to me." Yet the strength and warmth of Anita and Albert's bond is palpable when they are together. Under his grandmother's steadying influence, Albert has begun to flourish. But one morning, Anita suffers severe chest pains and is rushed to the hospital. Albert is visibly upset, continually shaking his head. Alone in his room, Albert sets a magazine on fire and subsequently burns down the house. Legal processes are undertaken. Albert is admitted to a psychiatric hospital. (This case study is based on a PBS documentary now online, *Big Mama*, an Oscar-winning film by Tracy Seretean, 2000. Names and locations have been changed.)

Intervention Issues

Social work practitioners must understand several critical issues in cases of grandparents' assuming care of grandchildren. In general, custodial grandparents report health-related and mental health issues that are result from, or are compounded by, responsibility for raising grandchildren (Hayslip & Kaminski, 2005a). In addition, the economics of care can be overwhelming, as the majority of families are not part of a formal child welfare system and do not receive financial support.

Although grandparents report that their caregiving role has its rewards, including keeping their grandchildren in the family and out of foster care, the stresses of care can have a detrimental effect on their health and functioning (Kropf &

Robinson, 2004). In addition, cultural assumptions and expectations affect decisions to assume care for grandchildren, even in situations in which the grandparent has limited resources (Yancura, 2013).

Poindexter (2008) highlighted several issues that grandparents in HIV-affected families face when they raise grandchildren:

- Children's health status and loss or trauma experienced as a result of losing a parent
- Social issues, such as low income, substance abuse, sporadic employment or unemployment, and other marginalizing conditions
- The emotional dynamic of losing one's own child combined with the possibility of losing a grandchild to AIDS
- The necessity of balancing their grandchildren's health care needs with their own health and aging issues

Another major challenge for custodial grandparents is managing the stigma of HIV/AIDS in the context of care provision. HIV continues to cast a stigma on the entire family of a person with the disease. For grandparents, the tasks of child rearing are compounded by the need to manage the associated stigma, and as a result, custodial grandparents often experience isolation, avoid social situations, and underutilize available resources (Poindexter, 2008; Poindexter & Linsk, 1999). To shield themselves and their family from negative experiences related to HIV stigma, grandparents may choose to keep the HIV a secret from others, even those with whom they have a close relationship.

Applying Models to Enhance Collective Efficacy and Human Capital

We have seen that the diagnosis of HIV/AIDS has different meanings depending on an individual's geographic location, gender, sexual orientation, family form, place in the life course or age, and so forth. This section describes issues of collective efficacy and human capital in the District of Columbia and in international locations.

District of Columbia: Center City Issues

Despite being home to clinics specializing in HIV/AIDS care, such as the Whitman-Walker Clinic, Washington, DC, has a greater proportion of HIV-infected individuals per population than any other U.S. city, and in its efforts to combat the disease, it faces issues similar to those faced in some developing nations. As of December 2010, an estimated 14,465 DC residents, or 2.7 percent of adults and adolescents in the city, were living with HIV. Unfortunately, the majority of these people were racial and ethnic minorities. Nearly seven in 10 (68 percent) DC residents between the ages of 18 and 64 (68 percent) have not been tested for HIV (Henry J. Kaiser Family Foundation, 2012a).

The issues are both personal and systemic. For example, many DC residents have difficulty accurately assessing the risk of HIV in their relationships (A. E. Greenberg et al., 2009). Moreover, DC Appleseed (2006), a center for law and justice in the district, found that the HIV/AIDS surveillance system in the city was ineffective at collecting and disseminating data in a timely fashion, that there was frequent turnover among personnel who support residents with HIV/AIDS, and that the city faced challenges to testing and condom distribution.

Leonard, an as-yet-undiagnosed 21-year-old black man, is an example of the DC Appleseed profile of a potential social work client. Leonard has received a flyer announcing National Black HIV/AIDS Awareness Day, but he is reluctant to go to the Whitman-Walker Clinic, a nonprofit community health center, which will be testing people in its mobile units at the Anacostia Metro Station in February.

Another person at risk might be an African American expectant mother. A 2012 study by the DC Department of Health (Sun, 2012) found that the HIV infection rate among heterosexual black women in DC's poorest neighborhoods nearly doubled in two years, from 6.3 percent to 12.1 percent. One of these women is Carolyn, who is three months pregnant. She does not yet know that there are effective treatments for preventing HIV in her newborn. Women like Carolyn could benefit from outreach and community-based mutual aid programs.

International Concerns

Worldwide HIV/AIDS statistics published by the United Nations indicate that 34 million people were living with the disease in 2010 (AVERT, 2013). Of these, around 68 percent reside in sub-Saharan Africa. Because of political debates and scarce treatment and resources, HIV continues to decimate the African population. Yet despite the bleak situation, programs funded by the United Nations Children's Fund (UNICEF) are having a positive effect.

UNICEF is assisting in the formation of mothers' support groups in the United Republic of Tanzania. These groups use home visits and drama to teach about mother-to-child transmission of HIV/AIDS. UNICEF is also supporting the Ethiopian government in a program to help more HIV-positive mothers deliver HIV-free babies. The program encourages women to use a birthing facility, which is not a cultural norm in Ethiopia, where less than 10 percent of women give birth in a health facility (Getachew, 2012), and is attracting mothers who need testing, prophylactic medicine, counseling, and mentor mother support groups.

HIV/AIDS Epidemic in Africa. Many countries experience great challenges because of HIV/AIDS, especially those in sub-Saharan Africa. In that region, Cameroon, Côte d'Ivoire, Kenya, Lesotho, Malawi, Tanzania, Uganda, and Zimbabwe have particularly high rates of the virus. More than four-fifths of children worldwide who have been orphaned by HIV/AIDS live in this region (U.S. Agency for International Development, 2008). Furthermore, resources for prevention and treatment are extremely limited, so the virus continues to be transmitted (Shetty & Powell, 2003). As in the United States, families (and especially grandparents) are taking on the responsibility of raising the children of those who have died of AIDS when possible (Karimli, Ssewamala, & Ismayilova, 2012). However, because the disease is so pervasive, some families are caring for several orphaned children. Although global initiatives are critical in addressing transmission of HIV/AIDS, they must also support families in this region who are shouldering extensive care responsibilities (Karimli et al., 2012).

Case Study. Abeba, who is expecting her first child, lives in a rural community in Ethiopia. Her husband drives a truck through more urban areas of Africa and frequents prostitutes, many of whom are likely to have HIV, along his delivery routes. Abeba learns that a group of Ethiopian mothers is going to visit her village to put on a play. She has been given permission to attend the play by the tribal elders. After attending the play, she decides to take an HIV test. On testing positive, she attends a UNICEF clinic and is able to deliver an HIV-free baby. Her virus is also now under control. She is in the process of persuading her husband to attend the clinic, especially to learn about safe sex practices.

In all the case studies presented in this chapter, the toll on human capacity is evident. HIV can affect multiple family members, and when this is the case, caregiving can become a complex task. Although medical breakthroughs allow HIV-positive individuals to manage the disease, treatment comes at a steep cost—between $2,000 and $5,000 a month, according to one estimate (Aguirre, 2012). Sadly, about half of the individuals with HIV who do not receive regular and ongoing care have Medicaid or are uninsured (CDC, 2011d). This number is staggering; treatment may be beyond reach if more than one individual requires care.

As HIV strikes globally, social workers need to continue to fight the spread of the disease. Models of community action that provide education and risk management, especially for women and children, are needed. In her powerful book on sexual violence and HIV/AIDS in Africa, Françoise Nduwimana (2004) narrated a story about a Rwandan woman:

> For 60 days, my body was used as a thoroughfare by all the hoodlums, militia men and soldiers in the district. . . . Those men completely destroyed me, they caused me so much pain. They raped me in front of my six children. . . . Three years ago, I discovered I had HIV/AIDS. There is no doubt in my mind that I was infected during these rapes. (p. 11)

These women certainly need health and trauma care, but they also need to have their stories told beyond the oppressive and torturous environments of their homeland.

Stories about the plight and resilience of women globally have been told in a powerful book by Nicholas Kristof and Sheryl WuDunn. This husband-and-wife team of reporters wrote *Half the Sky* (2010), about the adversities overcome by women around the world. Their accounts include ones similar to that of the Rwandan woman and tell about how women and girls have overcome these hardships and are making a positive impact on their communities and society. *Half the Sky* has been made into a movie and is also the name of a foundation dedicated to assisting women globally. The book shows how women's potential is critical in creating positive change in societies.

CHAPTER NINE

Grandparents Raising Grandchildren

Grandparents play a vital role within families and carry out various functions that support the well-being of their grandchildren. In particular, grandparents share a bond with grandchildren that serves different functions at various points in the life course. For many grandparents, this role brings a tremendous amount of joy and reward. They can enjoy significant involvement with their grandchildren without the responsibilities that accompany parenting. In addition, the involvement of grandparents is functional for the family as a whole because, for example, it provides bonding and couple time for parents (Lumby, 2010).

The following quote from a grandmother at a senior outing describes the experience of being a noncustodial grandparent:

> On Sunday afternoons, my grandchildren come to visit. Before they arrive, I sit in my chair and wait to see the car coming down my long driveway. I am just delighted! After four or five hours, they leave. I return to my chair and watch the car driving out my long driveway. I am just delighted! (Kropf, 2013)

This story captures the joy of having grandchildren visit but also returning to a life that does not include the energy and attention that grandchildren require.

Although grandparenting can be a positive and enjoyable role, significant numbers of grandparents experience challenges of being the primary care provider for their grandchildren. This chapter explores the reasons for grandparent caregiving. We present several cases of grandparents who have health concerns, who are dealing with the behavioral challenges of grandchildren, or who are dealing with grief and trauma. In addition, family diversity is highlighted, as custodial grandparents are represented in various racial, ethnic, and geographic populations. Interventions to support grandparents and grandchildren are provided, as are social policies that support or hinder these caregivers in their roles.

Using a Social Care Approach

Although grandparents have always been involved in raising grandchildren, the prevalence of this family form started to increase in the mid-1990s as a result of increased addiction and incarceration rates among women of childbearing age (Fuller-Thomson, Minkler, & Driver, 1997). Currently, about 2.5 million grandparents are responsible for raising one or more children within the same household (U.S. Census Bureau, 2010b). Often these family configurations are termed "custodial grandparenting" or "skipped-generation families."

These *grandfamilies*, or families in which a grandparent is raising one or more grandchildren, face significant challenges in health, mental health, child safety, and aging. For grandparents reporting responsibility for grandchildren, 33 percent are over age 60, which implies that these individuals are experiencing age-related changes that may affect their ability to care for their grandchildren (Goyer, 2010). Raising children is costly, but most of these informal caregivers are unable to receive assistance from child welfare programs. Financial and economic stresses are also present in many of these families. Finally, these caregivers are in child-rearing roles past the usual time frame for raising children. Therefore, they report feeling isolation and stigma that negatively affect their mental health status (Hayslip & Kaminski, 2005a).

Grandparent support is not a new phenomenon within families, as extended kin have historically been a form of help for parents. However, the prevalence of and reasons for this type of caregiving have changed dramatically since the early 1990s. Previously, grandparents and other family members were involved in raising children for the betterment of the family; for example, when others were available to care for the children, parents could relocate to another geographical area where they were able to secure jobs. Isabel Wilkerson, Pulitzer Prize–winning author of the book *Warmth of Other Suns* (2010), described the great migration of African Americans from the South to other parts of the United States. Between World War I and the mid-1970s, more than 6 million individuals and families left the South in search of work and better lives in urban centers such as Chicago, Cleveland, Oakland, Detroit, and New York City. During this time, grandparents and other kin enabled families to make these relocations by helping to raise the children. Often children were sent back home in the South to stay with extended family during the summer months. Family members thus held the role of surrogate parents when children were out of school, and children formed relationships with their extended family, which reinforced familial and cultural ties. Migration decisions frequently involved the entire family system, and well-defined plans were constructed to maintain connections between family members (Stewart, 2007). This is a good example of a care-sharing tradition within families.

During the mid-1980s, however, social changes precipitated different pathways into grandparent care. Grandparents increasingly became involved in raising grandchildren whose parents were affected by addiction, incarceration, or HIV infection. Concomitant changes also took place in the family experience and narrative about care. Whereas in years past families made a strategic and inclusive decision about sharing the care of children, more contemporary experiences resulted from problems or deficits in parenting. These changes presented challenges for grandparents and other family caregivers, as relationships between the caregivers and the children's parents often involved strain, stress, and the management of stigma (Poindexter, 2008).

Research on custodial grandparents of various races and ethnicities has found that when grandparents raise grandchildren of addicted parents, disruptions in the experience of care inhibit the transmission of customs and traditions within families (Yancura, 2013). In many ways, the care-sharing aspect of raising grandchildren, a shared role between parents and extended family, has eroded into a stressful care arrangement.

Diverse Family Forms

Custodial grandparents can be found among all racial and ethnic groups and community types. However, African American and Latino grandparents are overrepresented in this caregiving population, and both groups experience specific risks to their well-being (Kropf & Kolomer, 2004). Like other care provision roles, this role is gender based, as most custodial grandparents are women (Burnette, 1997; Kolomer & McCallion, 2005).

Race and Ethnicity

The concept of kinship has historical significance in African American families, and grandparents have traditionally held important roles within families. Since the days of slavery, grandparents have been called "kin keepers" and have provided support during times of economic and social stress within the family (Burton & Dilworth-Anderson, 1991). Compared with white grandparents, African American grandparents are less likely to "embrace norms of noninterference," and as a result, they are more likely to be involved in supporting and providing resources to family members (Pruchno, 1999). When grandparents raise grandchildren, it is not unusual to have the children's parent enter and exit the family with some regularity (Baird, John, & Hayslip, 2000).

Many grandparents assume responsibility for caring for their grandchildren despite having limited resources. African American grandparents have lower income levels than white grandparents (Harper, Hardesty, & Woody, 2001). Moreover, compared with their noncaregiving peers, African American custodial grandparents are more likely to be female, to lack a high school degree, and to live in poverty (Minkler & Fuller-Thomson, 2005). In addition, Minkler and Fuller-Thomson (2005) reported that that four-fifths of grandmothers who lived below the poverty line did not receive public assistance. These statistics underscore the level of economic vulnerability in this population and the degree to which any fluctuation in standard costs of living (for example, costs of food, rent, and transportation) will affect these families.

Like African Americans, Latinos are disproportionately represented in the population of custodial grandparents. A study that compared Latino, African American, and white custodial grandparents found that Latino families had the highest rate of poverty and lowest educational attainment in the sample (Goodman & Silverstein, 2002). For some Latino grandparents, being undocumented and having few language skills add to the difficulty of their caregiving role (Burnette, 1997). In addition, there is a cultural norm that women should be self-sufficient and refrain from disclosing family issues to non–family members (Cox, Brooks, & Valcarcel, 2000). This can lead to feelings of isolation, alienation, and shame for caregivers.

Another group of custodial grandparents who face significant challenges are Native American caregivers. Because large numbers of Native American children were being placed in homes outside their tribes and culture when their parents could no longer care for them, the Indian Welfare Act of 1978 (P.L. 95-608) mandated the placement of children within extended family settings when feasible. As a result, more children were placed in the care of extended family, especially grandparents (Matheson, 1996). In a study of Native American custodial grandparents, Fuller-Thomson and Minkler (2005) highlighted the reasons for and consequences of this caregiving arrangement. Reasons for this care included high adult morbidity and mortality, substance abuse, and the increase in female incarceration in native communities. Although committed to their role as surrogate parents, one-third of grandparents lived below the poverty line; this group had higher rates of health problems, overcrowded living arrangements, and functional impairments. Finally, compared with Euro-American custodial grandparents, Native American custodial grandparents have higher levels of depressive symptoms (Letiecq, Bailey, & Kurtz, 2008).

Gender

Like those in other caregiving roles, the majority of custodial grandparents are female (Burnette, 1997; Hayslip, Shore, Henderson, & Lambert, 1998). In fact, it is estimated that only about 6 percent of grandfamilies are headed by a grandfather (J. H. Patrick & Tomczewsk, 2008).

Those grandfathers who do assume the primary role in raising grandchildren have different experiences from grandmothers. One of the few studies that specifically analyzed the role of custodial grandfathers found some important differences between grandmothers and grandfathers (Kolomer & McCallion, 2005). Compared with grandmothers, custodial grandfathers were more likely to voice concerns about their own health conditions and the future of the care arrangement. In addition, a higher percentage of men in this study were employed (45 percent versus 21 percent of grandmothers) and reported a feeling of loss for their retirement years. Custodial grandparents clearly have concerns about the future of care and its impact on the caregiving arrangement.

Rural Families

Differences in custodial grandparenting also exist by geographic location. The earliest research on grandparents raising grandchildren was conducted in large cities (Burnette, 1997; Robinson-Brown & Brandon-Monye, 1995). Whether providing formal or informal care, grandmother caregivers most frequently live in inner cities, have less than a high school education, and are poor (Minkler, Roe, & Price, 1992; Woodworth, 1996). In contrast, factors that are especially challenging for rural grandparents raising grandchildren are feelings of isolation and the absence of caregiving supports in these areas (King et al., 2009; Robinson, Kropf, & Myers, 2000).

Some of the challenging behaviors that children may exhibit are incompatible with the culture and mores of rural settings. Grandparents, especially those who are older or transitioning into a custodial caregiving role, may be ill equipped to handle these challenges. In a discussion of case management with grandparents in rural areas, Myers et al. (2002) described an adolescent who became interested in witchcraft and defied her devoutly religious grandmother and her "old-fashioned" ideas. Without intervention from the case manager, this situation could potentially have created a rupture within the family and close-knit rural community.

Because many rural communities lack resources, social workers in these areas need to find creative and innovative ways to support these care providers. Myers et al. (2002) provided a framework for assessment that outlines factors relevant to understanding caregiving families in rural communities. For example, a comprehensive assessment includes understanding, among other things, the safety of the home living environment (for example, whether it is a mobile home, whether rodents or other vermin are present), financial issues (such as equity in home and worth of land), social issues (such as isolation of family and distance to neighbors), and health factors (such as proximity to groceries and health care services). Although these issues are important for any caregiving family, they are especially important for families living in smaller and more isolated areas.

Reasons for Care

Although grandchildren reside with grandparents for many reasons, several social issues play primary roles in the increase in the number of families with this care arrangement. One is addiction among women of childbearing age, often to crack cocaine. Another is the increased incarceration rate among women. In addition, the increase in HIV/AIDS among heterosexual families has created families in which one or both parents are incapacitated with or have died from the disease. Finally, compared with their urban counterparts, rural grandparents face some unique pathways to care.

Substance Abuse and Addiction

The prevalence of custodial grandparenting has increased with the increase in addiction to crack cocaine among women of childbearing age. The complexity of this addiction has had a dramatic and negative impact on families and children born to addicted mothers (Burton, 1992). One of the earliest comprehensive analyses of this phenomenon was *Grandmothers as Caregivers: Raising Children of the Crack Cocaine Epidemic* by Minkler and Roe (1993). This research followed 71 African American grandmother caregivers in Oakland, California, and their experience raising children with health, behavioral, and social challenges resulting from their mothers' addiction. This early study was one of the first to look comprehensively at the outcomes of the caregiving experience on the family.

Substance abuse creates specific challenges for grandparents and grandchildren. Because of the nature of addiction, there are periods when the parent is sober and wants to reenter the family. During these sober periods, parents may attempt to gain their children's favor by being permissive or more lenient than the grandparents; they may, for example, allow their children to stay up past their usual bedtime. When the parent inevitably departs, however, the children again experience the associated losses. This pattern erodes the structure of the household and can create confusion around boundaries and authority (Goldberg-Glen, Sands, Cole, & Cristofalo, 1998).

Incarceration

In a phenomenon related to substance abuse and addiction issues, the incarceration of women skyrocketed in the 1990s (Mumola, 2000). E. I. Johnson and Waldfogel (2002), in a study documenting increased incarceration rates among parents, reported that from 1986 to 1997 the number of mothers in prison increased 210 percent, more than the corresponding increase in incarceration among fathers (115 percent). Furthermore,

> about 10 in every 1,000 U.S. children had a parent in state or federal prison in 1986, while nearly 20 in every 1,000 children had a parent in prison during 1997. The number of women in prison more than tripled during this period. (E. I. Johnson & Waldfogel, 2002, p. 464)

One of every three women in prison have committed their crime for money or drugs. When either parent is incarcerated, the children most likely end up in the care of grandparents (E. I. Johnson & Waldfogel, 2002).

The effect of parental incarceration on children is profound. Children of incarcerated parents are five times more likely than those without a parent who is imprisoned to go to prison themselves (U.S. Department of Justice, 2002). In addition, adolescents of incarcerated parents are at risk for mental health problems. One study reported that 43 percent of those in a youth treatment program had an incarcerated parent (Phillips, Burns, Wagner, Kramer, & Robbins, 2002). Associated conditions of the criminal justice process, such as waiting, appealing, or in the extreme, dealing with capital punishment, have severe consequences for all family members but are especially deleterious for children (Beck, Britto, & Andrews, 2007). Interaction and interfacing with the criminal justice system, although intimately connected to substance abuse and addiction, can create additional challenges for custodial grandparents.

HIV/AIDS

As discussed in greater depth in chapter 8, some grandparents take responsibility for caring for their grandchildren when a parent is ill, incapacitated, or deceased from HIV/AIDS. Raising children in the shadow of HIV presents some unique issues for grandparents. These grandparents face the experience of losing their own child while simultaneously assuming the role of caregiver (Levine-Perkell & Hayslip, 2002). In addition, the grandchildren may be infected with the virus, and the grandparent may end up raising one or more grandchildren who are also HIV positive.

Although people are more educated about HIV/AIDS today than they were in the early days of the epidemic, this condition continues to carry a stigma that affects the entire family. Custodial grandparents may be reluctant to access services because they wish to avoid confronting the stigma (Poindexter, 2008). Therefore, these caregivers may be isolated from both informal and formal sources of support that could assist with their caregiving responsibilities.

Reasons for Rural Caregiving

In a study of reasons for custodial caregiving, the most common reason reported by rural grandparents was a shift from a multigenerational household to a skipped-generation household. Reasons for the parent generation leaving included the pursuit of better opportunities in another community and rifts between the two adult generations (Kropf & Robinson, 2004).

Risk and Resilience Framework

Custodial grandparents are often in this role because of challenges or problems experienced within the family. They experience risks related to the child's behavior, developmental factors, and their own health and well-being as care providers. Three case studies are provided to illustrate the risk situations encountered by custodial grandparents. Additionally, supports that can assist families experiencing risk situations are presented.

Risk

To assess and intervene with grandparent-headed families, social care providers must assess risks, resilience, and supports within the family system. Several issues related to risks need to be evaluated in a caregiving situation. Although one can be a grandparent at any age (that is, a grandparent can be 35 or 85), assessment processes should analyze the biopsychosocial functioning of both the grandparent and the grandchildren. In addition, it is important to observe the fit between the grandparent's ability to provide care and the grandchild's needs.

Phelps Case Study. Ms. Phelps is a 76-year-old grandmother raising her two granddaughters, who are 16 years old and 12 years old. The girls' mother, who is addicted to numerous substances, including crack cocaine, left them at Ms. Phelps's house one Saturday about five years ago and never returned. They have not heard from their mother since and are uncertain whether she is alive or dead. Ms. Phelps is raising her granddaughters informally and does not receive any support from the foster care system. She secretly holds out hope that her daughter is alive and will eventually return to the family and raise the girls.

Ms. Phelps has several health concerns, including diabetes, hypertension, and arthritis. She worked on the housekeeping staff of a major hotel chain until her health failed about eight years ago. Her main source of support is Social Security. Recently, 16-year-old Tiffany got a part-time job at a fast food restaurant. Her job has marginally increased the family income. However, it has also exposed her to a string of "boyfriends." A few times, Ms. Phelps has found a young man in the bedroom with Tiffany and has become very upset. This has set Tiffany off, and she has left home for a few days. This situation worries Ms. Phelps, who cares about Tiffany's health and safety. Tiffany's mother started her drug addiction during similar periods away from home.

This case example describes some serious risks to an adolescent's development. Grandparents may not be able to discriminate between a risk and normal teenage boundary testing. They may be hypervigilant about the circumstances that led to the parents' (their children's) problem behaviors, such as substance abuse and sexual risk taking. As a result, they may be extremely strict with their grandchildren in an attempt to prevent such behavior. Although rebelling and experimenting are normal parts of adolescence, grandparents may be too restrictive, and this may create additional challenges and problems for the family. The following case study illustrates this situation.

Bolton Case Study. Mr. and Mrs. Bolton (age 58 and 57, respectively) are raising their 10-year-old grandson, Kyle. They live in a mobile home in a rural area and have an immense amount of land. One of Kyle's only friends, Tim, age 12, lives on a parcel of land adjacent to the Boltons' property. One day while walking around the property, Mr. Bolton found Kyle and Tim smoking cigarettes behind a grove of trees. The Boltons were furious, grounded Kyle, and forbade him from having any additional contact with Tim.

Kyle is now isolated, as he has no other friends in the area. He has not gotten into trouble previously and is doing well in school. Although he loves his time in the Boy Scouts, he only sees the boys in his troop a few times each month. Kyle's mother, the Boltons' daughter, started smoking cigarettes as a teen and eventually developed a drug addiction. Although many adolescents experiment with tobacco and alcohol, the Boltons are terrified that smoking will be the first step in Kyle's pathway into addiction and a lifetime of substance abuse.

Thomas Case Study. Many grandparents raise one or more children in later life, when the incidence of chronic health concerns increases. Because of the emotional and physical burdens of caregiving, grandparents who provide care have more health concerns than noncaregivers of similar ages (Musil et al., 2011). Social care providers must therefore assess the goodness of fit of the caregiving situation in terms of the grandparent's ability to care for the children.

Mrs. Thomas is a 67-year-old grandmother who is raising a granddaughter with delays in her developmental milestones, Milly, age seven. Although Milly is a sweet child, she has an intellectual disability and requires assistance with her activities of daily living (such as dressing, bathing, feeding, and other hygiene tasks). Both Milly's mother and father are in prison on drug-related charges. In addition to Milly, Mrs. Thomas cares for her 72-year-old husband, who suffers from severe diabetes and cardiac conditions. Mrs. Thomas maintains the home and is the primary caregiver for both of her family members. Mr. Thomas's disability payment does not cover household expenses, so Mrs. Thomas also works part-time as a hairdresser, which requires her to be on her feet for several hours at a time. Because she has limited time to cook and grocery shop, she has resorted to bringing home fast food for their meals and has gained about 15 pounds over the past two years. Her face is flushed, and her ankles appear swollen. However, she refuses to see the doctor for herself, exclaiming, "I feel OK, just a little tired and run down! Besides, who would take care of everyone if I were sick?"

Protective Factors: Social Supports

Although the number of grandparents in caregiving roles has increased over the past decades, these grandparents often report feeling alone in their experience. These feelings of isolation stem from the perception that their peers cannot relate to their experiences as parents again and the fact that they are expending energy on the demands and responsibilities associated with caregiving (Giarrusso, Silverstein, & Feng, 2000; Kelley, Whitley, Sipe, & Yorker, 2000). Thus, grandparents may have less available support within their established informal support networks.

Friendship groups, leisure pursuits, or affiliations (for example, with churches or voluntary groups) may no longer provide the level of support they did before the grandparents assumed the role of care provider.

Social support can serve as both a buffer and a moderator of stress for custodial grandparents. In a study of grandmothers raising grandchildren, the more social support available to grandmothers the better the levels of physical and mental well-being (Emrick & Hayslip, 1999). Those who had support available seemed to absorb some of the associated demands of care in more functional ways than those who had no available or reliable sources of assistance. As Hayslip and Kaminski (2005a) stated, "Social support appears to be crucial to the physical and mental health of custodial grandparents, as well as to their ability to cope with the demands of parenting" (p. 265).

Social support is also important for children who are in the care of their grandparents. Project Healthy Grandparents is a multidisciplinary program that promotes health and social support interventions for grandparents raising their grandchildren (Kelley, Yorker, Whitley, & Sipe, 2001). This intervention model has been replicated in several rural areas around Georgia. In one rural area, children in grandparent-headed families participated in group activities that provided them with the opportunity to be around other children who lived in similar family configurations. During the first outing, the program van drove into the driveway of a house that was set back from the road, and a grandmother and two young girls bounded toward it. Two sisters and the driver were already in the van, and as they waited for the newcomers to approach, one of the girls said to the other, "Oh look, they live with their grandmother too!" This sentiment exemplifies the differences that some children feel when they are raised by grandparents, as their family looks different than those of their peers.

Applying FAM in Assessment

FAM can be used to assess the biopsychosocial and spiritual functioning of individual members in grandparent-headed families. In addition, it can be used to assess the functioning of the family system, including the family's ability to meet caregiving requirements. Community factors, such as the resources available or the locations in which families live, are also considered. The following case study shows how to apply FAM to the case of a grandparent raising grandchildren.

Ms. Evans is a 67-year-old grandmother who is raising two of her grandchildren: Joya, age eight, and Damon, age 11. She has been their primary care provider for the past six years, since her daughter, Angela, was killed by the children's father, Clayton, in a drug-induced rage. Clayton claimed that Angela had been sleeping with other men and stabbed her multiple times in the family home. Both children were in the house at the time. Clayton is serving a life sentence for murder.

After the loss of her daughter, Ms. Evans brought the children to live with her. As a 61-year-old woman at that time, she was counting on spending four more years working as a grade school teacher and then retiring to spend time with her second husband, Bennie, age 70, whom she married at age 58.

Although the household has stabilized since the tragedy, there continue to be issues. Both grandmother and grandchildren are getting older, and Joya's and Damon's preadolescent phases are taxing the family. Because Ms. Evans and her husband have never parented together, they are having to adapt to each other's child-rearing styles, which are not always compatible. Ms. Evans is determined to raise the children with discipline so that they "don't repeat the mistakes that got Angela into trouble." Bennie, having been a somewhat wild young adult himself, believes that "sowing your oats early" allows children to settle into more responsible roles later in life. His parenting style is much more relaxed and fluid than his wife's.

As the children age, they are starting to ask more questions about their parents. In prison, Clayton has "found religion," and he is interested in connecting with his children. This has created difficulty and a schism within the family. Damon in particular wants a relationship with his father and has requested that he be able to visit him in prison. Ms. Evans becomes enraged when he brings up this topic and begins to cry. At one point, she screamed at Damon, "He's a monster! He stabbed my baby!" During these episodes, Joya also starts to cry and clings to her grandmother. Damon, who looks like his father, has started to become an outsider in the family and is spending more and more time with friends away from the home.

Biopsychosocial and Spiritual Functioning

From a biological perspective, no health issues have emerged for any of the Evans family members. However, caregivers are less likely to engage in positive, health-promoting habits, such as eating balanced meals and getting enough sleep and exercise (Kropf & Yoon, 2006). An assessment of physical health functioning should focus on these positive health strategies as well as on any problems. In addition, the health of the grandparents should be monitored to ensure that they receive care for any undiagnosed or untreated conditions. Preventing a health crisis is critical to maintaining homeostasis within the family.

Psychological assessment includes understanding emotional and cognitive functioning. Although the family as a whole experienced a devastating tragedy, individuals in the family experienced Angela's death from different developmental and role perspectives. Joya in particular seems to be exhibiting fears of reabandonment, as she has separation anxiety and sometimes clings to her grandmother. Loss and abandonment are traumatic events; however, the murder of one parent by the other has numerous outcomes that can impair development and functioning. Moreover, having lost her daughter in an off-time and tragic event, Ms. Evans exhibits extended and complicated grief. Research on parents of murdered children indicates that posttraumatic stress reactions continue to manifest for years after the event itself (Murphy, Johnson, & Lohan, 2002).

In the area of social-cultural functioning, several issues are present in the family. As the children enter adolescence, the grandparents' ability to understand teen development in contemporary society needs to be gauged. What current trends, such as clothing styles, music, or social relationships, define individuation for the children? These trends will be different than they were when Ms. Evans was parenting Angela. In addition, social workers should assess whether the family members have relationships with others in grandparent-headed families. It is also important for the entire family to come together in recreation or leisure pursuits in order to normalize the experience of being in a grandparent-headed family. In research on service and program needs for custodial grandparents, one grandparent stated, "We need to get together and have hot dogs, and let the grandchildren come. You know, get everyone together. That's what I would like" (King et al., 2009, p. 235).

The Family as a Social System

Several issues affect the functioning of the Evans family as a social unit. Membership issues are coming to the forefront of family life and functioning. Damon's desire for a relationship with his father is competing with the relationship he has established with Ms. Evans, who continues to mourn the loss of her daughter. Should the family include Clayton in a meaningful way? How can he be included given the level of grief surrounding the tragic death of Angela? In addition, how is Angela included within the family, given that she is still present in the lives of her children and parent? As Falck (1988) stated, death does not attenuate membership in a family, as the individual continues to have meaning and legacy within the context of social relationships.

In addition, who are the missing members who might have a more active role within the family? That is, does the family function as a closed system or as an open system that invites the involvement of other sources of support? Although Ms. Evans assumed the role of primary care provider when Angela died, are there other family members or sources of support who could be more involved? This might include extended family members who could be available for care sharing with Damon and Joya. For example, are there male cousins or uncles who could be positive role models for Damon as he enters his teen years? Does the family have problems involving extended members in the care-sharing experience?

Roles and role relationships also need to be assessed within the family. For multiple reasons, Ms. Evans serves as the primary parent in the family. Angela was her biological daughter, not Bennie's blood relation. Plus, their divergent parenting styles have created different parenting role structures for Ms. Evans and her husband. These are all important issues to assess.

In addition, the two children seem to hold different role relationships with Ms. Evans. Ms. Evans and Damon demonstrate a conflicted relationship, as they experience Clayton's involvement in the family differently. Ms. Evans and Joya experience a close relationship. Is Ms. Evans transmitting feelings of grief and loss surrounding her daughter into the grandmother–granddaughter relationship in problematic ways (for example, in the form of favoritism, overindulgence, hyperprotection)?

Finally, the entrance of children into the family has created a different vision for later life for Ms. Evans and her husband. How have these caregiving responsibilities affected the marital relationship? This issue is especially significant because the couple partnered after the typical period for raising children and did not expect to be in parenting roles again. How has the caregiving situation altered their goals for retirement, leisure pursuits as a couple, and other quality-of-life issues?

Community-Level Factors

Community resources are available to assist grandparents, but they might not exist in every location. What resources are available to support the Evans family in the caregiving role? Kolomer (2009) identified various support resources that have been documented to assist grandparents in their caregiving role. These include support and psychoeducational groups, case management programs, and technologically based resources that connect grandparents with others in similar circumstances.

In addition, what resources are available for the Evans children? Research on the experiences of children with a murdered parent suggests that Damon and Joya will need ongoing support to deal with the trauma surrounding their mother's death. Sadly, few children in this situation actually receive the ongoing therapeutic support needed to cope with the trauma of a parent's murder. Without intervention, these children are at risk for turning to violence themselves (Lewandowski, McFarlane, Campbell, Gary, & Barenski, 2004).

Applying REM in Individual Intervention: Enhancing Resilience and Minimizing Risk

Using the information gathered in the assessment process, interventions can be initiated to help grandparent-headed families maintain functioning. Intervention approaches may be appropriate for both the care providers and the children being raised in this type of family system. In addition, family-level interventions can help the family system with internal and external relationships.

Empowerment-Based Interventions

Intervention approaches can help grandparents feel more empowered in their roles as care providers. Many of these grandparents have been away from child rearing for numerous years, and children's experiences are different now than they were in previous generations. Empowerment-based interventions provide opportunities for custodial grandparents to feel more confident in their role.

These interventions use group models to foster empowerment behaviors among grandparents. Cox (2008) described an empowerment-based intervention in which grandparents assist one another in gaining competence and confidence through activities that build self-esteem, develop communication skills, educate them about child and adolescent issues, and provide a foundation for the grandparents' relationship with their grandchildren. Collins (2011) reported on an empowerment group for African American grandmothers that uses a faith-based approach. This model uses congregations to provide support and outreach to these caregivers.

The Phelps case study provides a good example of the need for an empowerment intervention. Ms. Phelps could use additional support and skill development in her relationship with Tiffany. This might take the form of learning effective communication skills, strategies for adolescent behavior management, or strategies for boundary management.

Stress Reduction

Because of the complexity of family situations that precipitate this caregiving arrangement, custodial grandparents often face a great deal of stress in their role. Support groups provide grandparents with a way to be with others in similar roles, to share experiences, to solve problems, and to be a source of mutual aid (Hayslip & Kaminski, 2005b; Kolomer, McCallion, & Overendyer, 2003; Waldrop & Weber, 2001). These groups may include structured content to assist grandparents with caregiving (for example, content on child and adolescent development and ways to handle behavioral issues). Typically, grandparents are given ample time to share their situations, concerns, and successes as part of the group process.

Although support groups are helpful, some grandparents are unable or unwilling to participate in this type of intervention. Other types of interventions have been developed to provide stress relief to these caregivers. For example, Strozier, Elrod, Beiler, Smith, and Carter (2004) developed and implemented a computer-based intervention. Caregivers ($N = 46$) were drawn from area kinship support groups to participate in a computer-based intervention to promote technology-based skill attainment and support for care providers. The intervention consisted of an eight-week computer training course that promoted higher-level computer skills. In addition, an audio-based intervention containing eight modules that provided information specifically for custodial grandparents was developed (Kropf & Wilks, 2003). This intervention was designed to be flexible enough that grandparents could access it at their convenience.

Both the Evans and Bolton families are good candidates for participation in a grandparent support group. During support group sessions, they can discuss the challenges within the family and receive support from others in similar circumstances. Also, the children may have the opportunity to interact and socialize with other grandchildren in the group. This can normalize their family configuration and help the children feel that they are not different because they live with their grandparents.

Health-Based Interventions

The health of the grandparent caregiver is critical to maintaining family functioning. Grandparents' health concerns are a major source of stress, as grandparents worry about what will happen if they become ill or incapacitated (King et al., 2009). As a result, grandparents may use avoidance coping and resist seeing health care providers. In addition, they may prioritize family resources for the children and expend less on taking care of themselves. This situation can lead to undiagnosed conditions that can compromise the custodial grandparent's health and the caregiving arrangement.

Several health-based interventions for grandparents exist. One is Project Healthy Grandparents, mentioned previously (Kelley et al., 2001). In this program, student nurses under the supervision of a nursing faculty member are assigned to work with grandparents on a monthly basis. To reduce the stress on the grandparent, the student nurses travel to the family home and take vital signs, monitor medication adherence, and provide health-related information. This type of intervention increases the probability that health problems will be diagnosed and treated.

Other interventions stress good nutritional practices for families. Kicklighter, Whitley, Kelley, Lynch, and Melton (2009) tested an in-home nutrition and physical activity intervention to promote positive health practices among grandparents raising grandchildren. The participants reported that a major motivator for changing poor practices was to be healthier for their grandchildren. After the intervention, the participants reported engaging in higher levels of physical activity and making healthier food choices.

A primary intervention for Ms. Phelps is to help her regain and maintain better health. She has several health concerns, including diabetes and hypertension. Left untreated, these conditions can lead to serious and even life-threatening situations. In addition, the stress that she is experiencing as a result of Tiffany's behavior needs to be addressed, as this is only adding to her health problems. Mrs. Thomas also exhibits untreated symptoms. Because of her dual responsibility to provide care and augment the family income, she is under a great deal of stress. Her weight gain, poor nutrition, and lack of self-care are all cause for concern about her health.

Person-in-Environment Congruence

As part of the caregiving model of practice, the congruence between the family and the environment needs to be assessed. When grandparents are raising grandchildren, a host of different linkages straddle multiple service networks, including schools, physical and behavioral health care systems, and legal systems. This section highlights some of these goodness-of-fit issues.

Case Management

Case management practice is critical for grandparents because of the multiple systems many of these families are involved in. Kolomer (2009) described several evidence-based case management models that provide support to custodial grandparents. These programs lead to greater access to resources for the families, decreased isolation, higher levels of mastery in caregiving roles, and lower levels of caregiver depression.

Grandparents often are unaware of the caregiving resources that are available and may have limited experience interacting with child welfare or educational systems. Myers et al. (2002) described a case management system for rural grandparents. Many of these caregivers had low levels of education and were unprepared to deal with their grandchildren's school-related issues. Case managers assisted the care providers in working with teachers and accessing opportunities at school, such as extracurricular activities for the children. Case managers also helped these families interact with other service providers, such as health care personnel.

Physical Environment Factors

Many grandparents face issues related to housing and neighborhood safety. Grandparent caregiving disproportionately affects lower income households (Minkler, 1999). In fact, one study indicated that 14 percent of grandparent-headed households lived in public housing, and three out of 10 grandparent-headed households were living in overcrowded conditions (Fuller-Thomson & Minkler, 2003). For many grandparent-headed families, however, moving is not an option because of limited finances and poor health. Grandparents may also not want to move from their residence for other reasons, such as proximity to their support network, attachment to their home, or familiarity with the neighborhood.

A few areas have constructed housing specifically for grandfamilies. The first such structure was built outside of Boston in 1998 and is called the GrandFamilies House. It includes 26 apartment units specifically designed to meet the needs of both older adults and young children. Programs for the children are available on-site. The majority of the initial residents were African American families who had previously lived in Section 8 housing (Gottlieb, Silverstein, Bruner-Canhoto, & Montgomery, 2000). Without this option, many of the grandparents would have been stuck in neighborhoods that were unsafe and unsuitable for raising children. One grandmother said, "Where I was living before was a lot of drug activity around there and it was a bad neighborhood. . . . I was too glad to get a nice place for me and my grandkids" (p. 10). Other communities that have built similar housing structures include Hartford, Buffalo, Chicago, Phoenix, Detroit, and Baton Rouge.

Collective Efficacy and Human Capital

Use of REM also promotes and strengthens ties between individuals and families who experience similar conditions or life challenges as a community collective. Because custodial grandparents are dispersed across geographic and political lines, efforts are under way to use their shared experience to promote social policy. Efforts to bridge service networks for these families are also being made, as many families are involved with disparate service systems (for example, health, mental health, child welfare, and education systems). Beyond engaging in case management activities to help link families to services, it is important to use more macropractice approaches to highlight problems with service delivery.

Sponsored by a coalition of organizations that represent child welfare, aging, and intergenerational issues, the GrandRally is a collective efficacy intervention that harnesses family experiences to create positive social change for grandfamilies. During this annual event, grandparents march on the U.S. Capitol to raise awareness of grandfamily issues (Goyer, 2011). The event provides opportunities for grandparents to interact with elected officials using the experience of raising grandchildren. Through this effort, grandparents achieve a higher level of visibility in their communities as they make their experiences known to social policy makers.

Another example of collective efficacy is mobilization within local communities. J. Miller, Bruce, Bundy-Fazioli, and Fruhauf (2010) described a community strategy to develop goals and initiatives to help support local grandparents. Caregivers themselves contributed in this effort and helped develop ways to support others in their caregiving roles. Through this collective action, stronger bonds were created between custodial grandparents within the community.

Policy-Based Changes

Although programs for grandparents have begun to emerge across the United States, there continues to be a dearth of policies at the federal level. C. Smith and Beltran (2000) identified three priority areas for national policy regarding grandfamilies: subsidized guardianships, medical and educational consent laws, and housing policies. Most grandparents raise their grandchildren informally—that is, without going through child welfare placement requirements or adoption. As a result, decision making and consent can be difficult, as the grandparents are not recognized as the children's legal guardians. Policy changes would make this situation easier for grandparents to navigate.

Because grandparent-headed families represent diverse backgrounds, policies need to take into account cultural and kinship differences. Kropf and Kolomer (2004) provided several examples of policies that create hardships for some families. For example, some states require that kinship families adhere to the same rules and regulations as foster care families (Kolomer, 2000). These requirements are viewed as intrusive by some, especially African Americans, who perceive this as the government intervening in their family life. Given the long history of oppression in their culture, some African Americans choose to forego involvement with formal services, even though this means they will receive less assistance and support from formal structures.

In summary, grandparent-headed families are now part of social work programs in health, mental health, and educational settings. In fact, grandparents may have responsibility for multiple grandchildren, and many stay in this role for several years. Given age-related changes, these care providers benefit from participating in supportive programs that connect them to other custodial grandparents. The experiences of the grandparents in this chapter's case studies demonstrate that this role involves numerous challenges. Yet grandparents demonstrate resilience in caring for grandchildren and filling a parenting role when the biological parent is unavailable.

CHAPTER TEN

Caregiving with Lesbian, Gay, Bisexual, Transgender, and Questioning Clients

Lesbian, gay, bisexual, transgender, and questioning (LGBTQ) clients encounter a variety of caregiving issues across the life course. This chapter suggests ways for social workers to adapt and use caregiving models and practice skills differentially with this group, which includes diverse individuals, family forms, and communities. Like other chapters in this book, this one takes a life course perspective and addresses caregiving issues for both younger and older generations. Two case studies illustrate the complexity in caregiving for this population.

The first case, that of 15-year-old Michael, discusses the risks an LGBTQ youths may face, such as bullying and rejection by family or friends. It also outlines interventions and programs that can promote self-esteem and resilience. The emphasis in assessment and intervention in adolescence is on identity formation. Michael's case outlines the social care worker's roles in outreach, education, and treatment.

The chapter also explores LGBT older adults as a cohort or generation that has undergone its own sociocultural experiences. These individuals often had to overcome the effects of a lifetime of adverse societal messages about their sexual or gender identity (Cohen & Murray, 2006). In the second case study, Bert and Peter are older gay men, and their caregiving situation highlights an attempt to obtain equal access to the network of aging services and benefits. Their stories illustrate particular assessment, case management, and advocacy approaches in social work practice.

Using a Social Care Approach

Incidence

The Williams Institute at the University of California, Los Angeles, School of Law (G. Gates, 2011), a sexual orientation law and public policy think tank, estimates that 9 million Americans (about 3.8 percent) identify as gay, lesbian, bisexual, or transgender. It is estimated that bisexuals make up 1.8 percent of the population, gays and lesbians 1.7 percent, and transgender adults 0.3 percent. The Williams Institute believes that these estimates may be conservative because people are sometimes reluctant to identify as LGBT owing to the perceived stigma.

The teen years are a time of identity formation, when youths and young adults may question their sexual and gender identity. Thus, the term "questioning." Various studies have reported that 3 percent to 6 percent of adolescent and postadolescent youths report same-sex attraction or identify as lesbian, gay, or bisexual (Cianciotto & Cahill, 2003). Although individuals identify as LGBT at different times in their life courses, studies indicate this identification process is starting earlier in life. The increased visibility of LGBT people may be prompting earlier identification among teens (Floyd & Stein, 2002). Since the 1980s, the typical age at which LGBT identification takes place has decreased from the early 20s to about 16 (Cianciotto & Cahill, 2003).

An estimated 2 million Americans age 50 or older identify as LGBT, with that number expected to double by 2030 (Fredriksen-Goldsen et al., 2011). Many will need aging services. Like other populations, LGBT families provide the majority of care to their loved ones. This chapter discusses the concerns LGBT older adults may have about receiving care without discrimination from outside their family.

LGBTQ Youths: Risks and Parenting Issues

Many LGBTQ youths are at risk for emotional and health problems. For example, recent research has confirmed that although approximately 40 percent of homeless teens self-identify as gay or lesbian, relatively few resources are specifically designed to meet their needs (see "LGBTQ Youth Facts" on page 181). "These youths have either run away or been thrown out of their homes. Many may become involved in prostitution and other abusive behaviors in order to survive" (Lambda, n.d.). An unknown number may end up in the child welfare system:

> Although providers and agencies serving out-of-home youth have observed that lesbian, gay, bisexual, transgender (LGBT) adolescents are disproportionately over-represented among youth in out-of-home care, the actual proportion of the nearly 750,000 children served in foster care each year (U.S. Department of Health and Human Services [HHS], 2009) who identify as LGBT is not known. In fact, the LGBT population in foster care has been called an "invisible population." (Gallegos et al., 2011, p. 227)

According to a study sponsored by CSWE and Lambda Legal, the problem of invisibility can be compounded when social workers lack the knowledge and resources necessary to practice effectively with the LGBTQ population (J. I. Martin et al., 2009). Furthermore, foster parents may lack training and be "fearful" of caring for LGBTQ youths (Clements & Rosenwald, 2008). Private social care

LGBT Youth Facts

- It is estimated that in the U.S., a teen takes their own life every 5 hours because they are gay, bisexual, transgender, or lesbian, and cannot deal with the added stresses that society puts upon them.
- Several studies have found that approximately 40% of homeless "street" teens self-identify as gay/lesbian yet there are relatively few resources specifically aimed at meeting their needs.
- Homeless LGBT teens face increased risk for a variety of health and emotional problems.
- GLB youths are two to three times more likely to attempt suicide than non-gay teens, according to a 1989 U.S. Department of Health and Human Services study.
- The same study found that 30 percent of successful teen suicides are by gay or lesbian youths.
- LGBT youths are attacked at alarmingly high rates nationwide.
- Queer youths are more likely to be attacked physically.
- Queer youths are at increased risk for drug/alcohol problems and dropping out of school.
- An estimated 40% of street kids are lesbian or gay. These youths have either run away or been thrown out of their homes. Many get involved with prostitution and other abusive behaviors as a way of surviving.
- Many bisexual, gay and lesbian youths drop out of school due to harassment or low self-esteem, and fear of "being found out."
- Studies have found that more than 25% of gay and lesbian youths have severe drug and alcohol problems.
- Those who believe they don't know someone who is gay are more likely than those who do to reject equal rights for, and equal treatment of, LGBT people.
- Early exposure to diversity and sexuality issues helps to reduce prejudice and homophobia, including internalized homophobia which often leads to self-destructive behaviors.
- Teenagers and young adults are among the leading perpetrators of anti-gay violence.

Source: Reprinted from *Lesbigay Youth Facts,* by Lambda, n.d., retrieved from http://www.lambda.org/youth.htm#youth facts

organizations are teaming up with public services to help resolve this situation and other risks faced by these youths. Social work practitioners in the child welfare system, school systems, and other settings that serve children and youths must have knowledge and skills to work with LGBTQ children and adolescents.

Parents may need support and education when their son or daughter identifies as LGBTQ. Parents who are raising gay or lesbian children report that they perceive a stigma because of their child's identification, worry about losing close relationships with others, and fear for the physical well-being and safety of their child (Conley, 2011). In particular, mothers seem to harbor fears about their child's safety issues, but both parents report more fear about the safety of a gay son than a lesbian daughter. Family support is a protective factor for LGBTQ individuals, especially in the process of self-acceptance. In an Israeli study of gay men, family acceptance was positively related to self-esteem and adjustment (Elizur & Ziv, 2001). Research on parental reactions to a son's or daughter's sexual identity is mixed, and reactions may become more accepting over time as a result of support and additional knowledge about sexual identity development (Savin-Williams, 2001). Even highly religious parents may come to accept their child's identification as gay or lesbian while concurrently holding beliefs that homosexuality is a sin (Freedman, 2008). Parenting a child who is gay or lesbian is complex, and interventions can assist parents with understanding and supporting their son or daughter.

Older LGBT Population

In later life, older adults often require support, and most rely on informal sources such as family and friends (see chapter 4). When older adults are LGBT, however, the nature and experience of care may be unique. In a qualitative study of post-caregiving experiences in a same-sex relationship, unsupportive family, friends, and professionals added to the sense of stress and strain experienced by the care provider (Hash, 2002). Conversely, the encouragement and involvement of both informal and formal supports was helpful in reducing the stress of care.

In LGBT caregiving, a unique aspect of using formal services is dealing with the disclosure of sexual identity to providers:

> Both the anticipation of discrimination and actual experiences of discrimination in health care services contribute to great tension and represent a challenge to the possibility of coming out to health care providers in order to receive appropriate care. This represents a significant challenge to seniors and their spousal/partner caregivers. (Brotman et al., 2007, p. 490)

Sadly, one coping mechanism is for older LGBT individuals to "re-closet," that is, to conceal their sexual identity to formal service providers even after they have previously lived a life of relatively open identification. At a time in the life course that involves myriad other assaults on their identity (for example, loss of functioning and loss of social roles), this additional stress can have a detrimental effect on the mental and emotional health of LGBT adults.

Care Sharing: Programs for the LGBTQ Population

To serve LGBTQ individuals using a social care approach, social workers need to be aware of existing, but not highly visible, services and programs. Programs for LGBTQ youths are structured to reduce the negative experiences of violence and bullying and create safer physical and emotional environments. Programs for older adults support family relationships and promote access to health and social services.

LGBTQ Youths

The following federal programs, listed on the HHS (2012) Web site, illustrate some of the approaches directed at this population of adolescents.

Anti-bullying Efforts. In 2011, HHS collaborated with five other departments (Education, Agriculture, Defense, Interior, and Justice) to establish a federal task force on bullying. HHS also announced a cross-departmental National Action Alliance for Suicide Prevention, with a wide range of public and private partners, to coordinate suicide prevention efforts, particularly among at-risk groups, such as LGBTQ youths. HHS also launched a new Web site (http://www.StopBullying.gov), which contains a section specifically for LGBTQ youths.

Improvements in Foster and Adoptive Care. To help address barriers to permanency in foster care and well-being for LGBTQ foster youths, who are disproportionately represented in the foster care population, in 2012 HHS awarded a $3.3 million grant to the Los Angeles LGBT Center. This is one of the largest federal grants ever awarded to an organization serving primarily LGBTQ individuals. It will help reduce the barriers encountered by prospective and current foster and adoptive parents who are LGBTQ, allowing for more sexual minority youths to be adopted.

Services for Runaway and Homeless Youths. HHS requires that all organizations serving runaway and homeless youths be equipped to serve LGBTQ youths. HHS also allows service providers who serve homeless and runaway youths to apply for funds to serve primarily LGBTQ youths. Moreover, HHS has initiated a process of improving data collection among homeless and runaway LGBTQ youths through the Runaway and Homeless Youth Management Information System.

In addition to these federal programs, nonprofit and community organizations are involved in creating safe communities for LGBTQ children and youths. These efforts may take the form of professional and community partnerships. Although some of these organizations are targeted directly at LGBTQ youths, others target risk situations (such as bullying) and promote higher levels of acceptance for these children and youths within the community.

Lambda Legal. In 2008, NASW partnered with Lambda Legal, a nonprofit organization dedicated to reducing homophobia, inequality, and hate crimes against gay, lesbian, and transgender people. One of the ways the two organizations hoped to promote nonviolence was through training-the-trainer workshops for child welfare workers to improve the care and treatment of LGBTQ youths in the foster care system.

At a 2013 training workshop in Louisiana, Carmen Weisner, executive director of the NASW Louisiana Chapter, said, "We are undertaking this project because LGBT youth are particularly vulnerable to physical or emotional abuse, depression, rape, unethical 'conversion therapies,' prostitution, substance abuse and suicide"

(Malai, 2013). Using a social care approach, the chapter is working with several entities in the state—including the Louisiana Court Appointed Special Advocates, the Louisiana Department of Children and Family Services, and the Court Improvement Project within the state supreme court—to get the training initiative out to as many people as it can across various demographic categories, targeting social workers especially.

Family Acceptance Project. The Family Acceptance Project, a nonprofit agency that provides social support for LGBTQ youths, is housed at the César E. Chávez Institute at San Francisco State University. Founded in 2002, the project was created to research parents', families', and caregivers' reactions and adjustment to an adolescent's coming out and LGBTQ identity; develop training and assessment materials for health, mental health, and school-based providers as well as child welfare, juvenile justice, and family service workers and community service providers who work with LGBTQ youths and families; advance resources to strengthen families to support LGBTQ children and adolescents; and develop a new model of family-related care to improve health and mental health outcomes for LGBTQ adolescents.

PFLAG. In 1972, Jeanne Manford walked with her son, Morty, down Christopher Street in New York City in the precursor to the Gay Pride Parade. When she marched in that parade, she carried a hand-lettered sign that said "Parents of Gays Unite in Support for Our Children." Numerous parade participants begged her to talk with their parents about accepting their son or daughter as gay or lesbian. Manford's placard framed the mission of PFLAG (PFLAG, 2013b). The organization was formally founded in 1973 for parents, families, friends, and straight allies as an LGBT equality movement. Today, there are 350 chapters across the United States and 11 countries worldwide (PFLAG, 2013a). Such organizational efforts illustrate the power of advocating for client access to social work services.

Older LGBT Adults

Support for same-sex marriage varies across the United States. To date, 19 states and the District of Columbia issue marriage licenses to same-sex couples (Human Rights Campaign, n.d.). It is not known how federal policy will be implemented for same-sex families now that the U.S. Supreme Court has declared the Defense of Marriage Act unconstitutional. But, because of the uneven nature of same-sex marriage legality across the nation and gaps in the interpretation of legal marriage status, some federal government policies and programs are being written to ensure that same-sex married couples are able to enjoy the rights and privileges afforded to heterosexual married couples. Some examples of programs are described here.

Social Security. On September 20, 2013, the U.S. Social Security Administration posted a message urging same-sex couples to apply for spousal Social Security benefits. However, the administration has not officially done the same for potential spousal benefits. Same-sex couples are being urged by the Social Security Administration to apply for spousal Social Security benefits even if the state in which they live does not recognize same-sex marriage.

Hospital Visitation. In 2010, a Presidential Memorandum on Hospital Visitation directed HHS to initiate rule making to ensure that hospitals receiving Medicare or Medicaid payments respect the rights of patients to designate visitors, regardless of sexual orientation, gender identity, or any other nonclinical factor. On November 17, 2010, HHS issued the final rule affirming those rights.

Advance Directives. The 2010 Presidential Memorandum also called for new guidelines to facilitate hospitals' compliance with existing regulations allowing patients to designate who they want to make medical decisions on their behalf through advance directives. The Centers for Medicare and Medicaid Services are on track to issue these guidelines as decisions about legal rights remain in question.

Affordable Care Act. The Affordable Care Act is helping to improve access to health care for all Americans, including individuals in the LGBT community. Studies have shown that health disparities related to sexual orientation and gender identity are due in part to lower rates of health insurance coverage and a lack of cultural competency in the health care system. As HHS implements the Affordable Care Act, it will pay close attention to the unique health insurance needs of LGBT populations and continue to include LGBT health experts on Affordable Care Act and other advisory boards, as appropriate.

Aging Services. In 2010, HHS funded the nation's first national technical assistance resource center to support public and private organizations serving the unique needs of LGBT older adults. HHS also published a toolkit for providing respectful and inclusive services for diverse communities, including LGBT populations.

Stigmatized and Politicized Caregiving Context

Because of the stigmatized political environment surrounding LGBT issues, a social care approach for people who are LGBT must include the various social supports described previously. The stigma against members of the LGBT community developed through perceived negative interactions with the group historically. Even today, when some political and social gains have been made, there continues to be social oppression against those who are LGBTQ. Therefore, LGBT clients are likely to have experienced discrimination attributable to *homophobia*, or a range of negative attitudes toward them simply because they are LGBT. Unfortunately, people who are LGBTQ may experience homophobia in any social system across their life course, including schools, houses of worship, financial or health care institutions, and even social service venues. Therefore, as the NASW *Code of Ethics* suggests, social care workers may need to be on alert to and work to combat discriminatory practice (NASW, 2008).

Furthermore, violence against people who are LGBT has occurred in every state of the union. A 2010 intelligence report from the Southern Poverty Law Center examined Federal Bureau of Investigation data on national hate crimes from 1995 to 2008 (Potok, 2010). Findings showed that LGBT people were "far more likely than any other minority group in the United States to be victimized by violent hate crime" and to face stigma (Potok, 2010). At the same time, many people who are LGBT have long advocated against such stigma and discrimination. In 1969, when police raided the Stonewall Inn, a gay bar in New York City, LGBT customers decided to fight, sparking the Stonewall Riots, an event that is considered the beginning of the modern LGBT rights movement. LGBT protesters' slogan was "Gay Power." They felt that this was the start of a "revolution." Another important advocacy action occurred in 1973, when the American Psychiatric Association decided to declassify homosexuality as a psychiatric disorder.

A more recent decision to fight LGBT stigma and discrimination is the repeal of "Don't Ask, Don't Tell." "Don't Ask, Don't Tell" was a U.S. military policy that banned discrimination of gays who did not reveal their sexual orientation and barred openly gay people from entering the military. On July 6, 2011, a federal appeals court barred further enforcement of the U.S. military's ban on openly gay service. This ban was officially revoked on September 20, 2011.

Although progress has been made in achieving civil rights for gays, the achievement of equal status under the law lags. For example, current federal laws, including the Civil Rights Act of 1964 and the Age Discrimination Act of 1979, protect employees from discrimination in the workplace on the basis of race, national origin, sex, religion, disability, pregnancy, and age, but not sexual orientation. The Employment Non-Discrimination Act, which would prohibit discrimination in hiring and employment on the basis of sexual orientation or gender identity by civilian, nonreligious employers with at least 15 employees, has been introduced in every Congress since 1994 except the 109th but has not yet passed.

Social workers who work in many different life settings can prepare themselves to be part of the solution, helping clients to overcome the cumulative risks associated with increased environmental stress. Not only can social care workers intervene to prevent the magnification of environmental risks, they can attempt to foster client resiliency by building on natural healing processes that overcome stigma (Garmezy, 1974).

Applying FAM in Assessment

This case example involves an adolescent, Michael, who is questioning his sexual identity. He has experienced some bullying and threats from peers and is struggling with feeling alone and alienated from others. Mrs. Hobson, the school social worker, has worked to eradicate bullying and create a safe environment for LGBTQ youths.

Case Study: Gay Adolescence

Michael is a 15-year-old high school student. His family includes his mother, Joan (age 45); his father, Tom (age 47); his sister, Diane (age 13); and his brother, Jared (age 10). The family lives in the Midwest. Their rural community has witnessed a series of antigay acts of violence and the suicide of a young person. Several months ago, Michael himself received hate mail from a class member that said, "You better watch out." Michael has started to question his sexual orientation. He wonders about his family and their reaction if he were to say he is gay.

Dad is the disciplinarian of the family. Michael complained to his sister, Diane, that Dad makes all of the decisions. Mom "just goes along." Michael has recently begun his first semester at Abraham Lincoln High School. He is happy to have left his middle school, where his locker was often defaced and students jostled him in the hallways. But he is beginning to wonder if he is also not welcome at his high school because he seems unable to make new friends. For almost a year, he has felt like he just doesn't fit in anywhere and has been increasingly depressed. A few months ago, when Michael received the hate mail, he decided to trust his sister, Diane, with his fear of bullying. On Diane's urging, Michael decided to see the school social worker, Mrs. Hobson.

Following the violence in the community, the principal of the school and Mrs. Hobson researched support programs for LGBTQ youths. They found a study by Gallegos et al. (2011) that indicated that LGBTQ youths were reluctant to openly share their sexual orientation because they thought that people would neither understand nor accept them; they feared being judged or ridiculed and being the victims of violence.

The principal and Mrs. Hobson also visited the Family Acceptance Project Web site, which provides information about programs to decrease major health and related risks for LGBTQ youths, including suicide, substance abuse, HIV, and homelessness. Because Family Acceptance Project programs use "a culturally grounded approach to help ethnically, socially and religiously diverse families to decrease rejection and increase support for their LGBT children" (Family Acceptance Project, n.d.), the principal and Mrs. Hobson were able to get buy-in from the Abraham Lincoln Parents and Teachers Organization for after-school programs to support LGBTQ youths and their families.

Mrs. Hobson was chosen by the school principal to work with questioning youths who sought counseling. In addition to searching online for resources, she has attended Lambda Legal workshops, read American Psychological Association publications, and used an HHS Web site to find resources in her community (Find

Youth Info, n.d.). She has learned that questioning youths feel validated by gaining information on human behavior and sorting out their personal circumstance using a narrative approach. She hopes this approach will allow Michael to understand the challenges many LGBTQ teenagers face.

FAM Assessment

Biological Age. By all physical accounts, Michael is developing and functioning well as an adolescent male. He has had no major health problems to date and has had unremarkable physiological development. Although drugs and alcohol are risk factors for LGBTQ youths (Talley, Sher, & Littlefield, 2010), Michael has not started to use these substances.

However, Michael clearly struggles with his emerging sexual identity. He indicates that he feels conflicted about the negative views of gay youths. Mrs. Hobson shares with him that there is debate about what causes differences in sexual orientation. She shares the following statement from the American Psychological Association (2008):

There is no consensus among scientists about the exact reasons that an individual develops a heterosexual, bisexual, gay, or lesbian orientation. . . . Although much research has examined the possible genetic, hormonal, developmental, social, and cultural influences on sexual orientation, no findings have emerged that permit scientists to conclude that sexual orientation is determined by any particular factor or factors. (p. 2)

Psychological Age. Michael learns that during the teenage years youths make the transition from adolescence to adulthood, which culminates in the formulation of personal identity (Erikson, 1950). During adolescence, many feel confused about or start to question their sexual feelings and sexual orientation. Michael is relieved to learn that it is not unusual to struggle with his sexual orientation while at the same time seeking his adult identity (see "Identities" on page 189). He feels that his uncertainty has been normalized when he hears that this experience is shared by others around his age. Michael has also come to understand that adolescence is a time when youths in Western mainstream culture begin to seek autonomy from parents and family. He gleefully shares with Diane that many kids find that their dad is "a pain" sometimes.

Social Age. Goffman (1963), a renowned sociologist who studied stigmatized identity, would say that social age is defined by teenagers getting together to exchange opinions about other teenagers. Teens question their own identity and try and make sense of themselves and others by using categories and comparisons. For example, they try to acquire information about one another, sizing the players up. They ask whether others are "nerds" or "geeks." They may put other teens into categories on the basis of socioeconomic status or intelligence. In this manner, teenagers may eventually learn to deal with the demands of those with power and

Identities

- *Gender identity.* One's subjective sense of belonging to a particular sex—male or female.
- *Sexual orientation.* An enduring pattern of emotional, romantic, or sexual attraction to men, women, or both sexes.
- *Heterosexual identity.* Having emotional, romantic, or sexual attractions to members of the other sex.
- *Gay or lesbian identity.* Having emotional, romantic, or sexual attractions to members of one's own sex.
- *Bisexual identity.* Having emotional, romantic, or sexual attractions to both men and women.

Source: Adapted from *Answers to Your Questions: For a Better Understanding of Sexual Orientation and Homosexuality* (p. 1–6), by the American Psychological Association, 2008, Washington, DC: Author.

---

influence and with their own personal set of meanings. Unfortunately, Michael has come to understand that some teenagers will stigmatize others' personal identities, whether they appear to be "fat," "dumb," or "gay." Michael and Mrs. Hobson talk about protective factors that may buffer Michael from such abuse.

Michael's social age is also influenced by the extent of his social supports—family, friends, social groups, or school programs, such as the Family Acceptance Project. Michael's school now has a number of social support activities that he may choose to attend. However, Michael continues to be afraid of being ridiculed or rejected by his father if he should decide to come out. *Coming out* refers to several aspects of lesbian, gay, and bisexual people's experiences: self-awareness of same-sex attractions; the telling of one or a few people about these attractions; the widespread disclosure of same-sex attractions; and identification with the lesbian, gay, and bisexual community (American Psychological Association, 2008).

Mrs. Hobson reassures Michael that if he does come to realize that he is gay, he can choose the manner in which he shares this information with others. In the meantime, Michael says he will access more information about LGBTQ social groups and their missions online. The experience of being *mirrored*—that is, being exposed to others who are also gay or lesbian—is an important part of understanding and accepting sexual identity for adolescents (Swann & Anastas, 2003). Through online LGBTQ communities, Michael can access support and connection with others, even though he is not ready to come out within his school and rural community.

Spiritual Assessment. Michael tells Mrs. Hobson that he has recently been worried about being a "normal" kid, particularly because he has heard negative messages about "the wrong" kind of sexuality. Mrs. Hobson explains that opinions differ on what is considered normal. Michael now understands that several decades of research and clinical experience have led mainstream medical and mental health organizations to conclude that the differences in sexual orientation represent normal forms of human expression (American Psychological Association, 2009). These facts are reassuring to him, and he is now able to consider other messages. His depression begins to lift.

Michael worries about his sexual identity and his religious beliefs. His family is religious, and the church is an important institution within his community. Sadly, the teachings of his religion label homosexuality a sin, and Michael feels confused about how his faith and sexual identity fit together.

Assessment of Family Functioning

System. Social care workers help families of diverse forms, all of which may be considered "a social system consisting of individuals who are related to each other by reasons of strong reciprocal affection and loyalties, comprising a permanent household or cluster of households that persist over time" (Terkelsen, 1980, p. 2) (see "Families" on page 190). To understand a family, one should not view each member in isolation. Rather, a change in any one member of the family brings about a change in the whole. Therefore, one can anticipate that as Michael finds his adult identity, there will be changes in his total family configuration. Perhaps at some later time, they will join him in a Family Acceptance Project program.

Families

- *Extended family.* A family that extends beyond the nuclear family, consisting of grandparents, aunts, uncles, and cousins all living nearby or in the same neighborhood. People in the same kinship line.
- *Family of choice.* A family that may or may not have legal status but includes same-sex partners in life.
- *Family of origin.* The family in which a person is born and grows up.
- *Nuclear family.* A family consisting of married female and male parents and dependent children living away from the extended family.
- *Self-defined family unit.* A group composed of individuals bound together by emotional relationships.
- *Traditional family.* A nuclear unit composed of blood relatives.

Source: Adapted from *Human Behavior: A Diversity Framework,* 2nd ed. (pp. 1–30), by R. R. Greene and N. P. Kropf, 2009, New Brunswick, NJ: Aldine Transaction Press; *Social Services for Senior Gay Men and Lesbians* (pp. 35–47), edited by J. K. Quam, 1997, New York: Haworth Press; and *Social Science Dictionary,* n.d., retrieved from http://www.socialsciencedictionary.com

Roles. Changes in a family system bring about modifications in roles. For example, as Michael reaches his adult identity, his highly structured, traditional family may change. How will Michael's mother and father as well as siblings Jared and Diane support his search for adult identity? One also might anticipate that the sister and brother relationships will remain strong.

Michael reports confusion about gender roles as related to his sexual identity. For example, he states that he would like to be a father one day but wonders how this can be possible if he's gay. He also states that he likes cars and backpacking and wonders how he can be gay and like those things. As a young adult, he is attempting to sort out the fit between the gender roles that are traditionally identified with being male and the possibility that he is gay. Clearly, Michael has some confusion about gender roles and sexual identity.

Development. Because the structure of U.S. families continues to undergo rapid and far-reaching changes, the idea that family development is fixed and sequential is increasingly being questioned (Laird, 1996). Germain (1994) argued that normative models—those that assume that development is a linear movement through sequential stages—were best suited for the nuclear families of the 1950s rather than the family forms, such as same-sex families, found in contemporary life. She contended that the concept of the life course is better able to embrace diversity and economic, political, and social variables. As a questioning youth, Michael's individual growth and the intersection with the social era of his development will affect his family of origin's future development in ways yet unknown.

Applying REM in Intervention

In addition to understanding family dynamics, social workers can understand caregiving among LGBT people within the context of risk and resilience across the life course. Therefore, social care workers may want to explore how REM assessment lends itself to better understanding the risks and resiliency aspects of a client family's functioning.

Summary of REM Assessment

Risks. Michael's risks may include rejection by his family, school bullying, and hate crimes. Maladaptive coping strategies (such as alcohol or drug use and acting out sexually) are also risks. Michael's treatment with Mrs. Hobson has hopefully reduced his risks for depression and suicide. Yet he still has work to do, as he may later want to sort out his relationship with family members who may or may not be supportive of him. Mrs. Hobson knows that conflicts in belief systems must be resolved if family resilience is to be maintained. She has asked Michael to keep in touch about future needs in this regard.

Protective Factors. Michael has discovered that he has several protective factors that act as buffers against negative and homophobic reactions. He enjoys his schoolwork. He is glad to understand that he has an important, close bond with his sister and that peer support is available at his school if he wants it.

Resilience. Resilience can be fostered by helping a client get in touch with his or her own strengths and ability to face homophobia. To accomplish this task, the practitioner must be realistic about his or her own self-awareness, empathy, and readiness to accept LGBTQ clients. Because of her genuineness and continued "engagement in career-long learning" (CSWE, 2012, p. 3), Mrs. Hobson is better prepared to foster Michael's resiliency.

Mrs. Hobson has tapped into several elements of REM to assist Michael in his quest for identity. Michael is now able to acknowledge his vulnerability, collaborate in self-change, and plan for his future. He has accepted that his questioning of his sexual orientation was a source of stress. By recognizing that he does not have to come out at this or any other time, he has taken more control of his own situation. Mrs. Hobson has given Michael resources for change and has reassured him that the teenage years are a time of questioning. Hopefully, this has strengthened Michael's problem-solving abilities.

Aging in the LGBT Population

Over the next several decades, the U.S. population will grow increasingly older and more diverse. Although race and ethnicity have long been recognized as important sources of diversity in the older population, it was only in 2011 that the National Institutes of Health and the National Institute on Aging jointly funded an examination of LGBT aging and health issues (Fredriksen-Goldsen et al., 2011). The report from this project, *The Aging and Health Report: Disparities and Resilience among Lesbian, Gay, Bisexual, and Transgender Older Adults,* summarized the experiences of more than 2,500 LGBT adults across the nation ranging in age from 50 to 95. The report revealed that significant health disparities affect LGBT older adults as they age, including disability, physical and mental distress, victimization, discrimination, and lack of access to supportive aging and health services (see "LGBT Older Adults: Aging and Health Findings" on page 193 for other findings).

The challenges facing LGBT elders intensify as these individuals age into the long-term care system, which is often unwelcoming. Older LGBT adults fear that they will be separated from partners and other close relationships. They may also worry about the availability of both informal and formal supports as they age. Inadequate staff training at agencies that offer services for older adults is another concern. Older LGBT adults may fear having to go back into the closet to survive in long-term care settings.

LGBT Older Adults: Aging and Health Findings

- Nearly one-half of LGBT older adults have a disability, and nearly one-third report depression.
- Most LGBT older adults (91 percent) engage in wellness activities.
- Almost two-thirds have been victimized three or more times.
- Thirteen percent have been denied health care or received inferior care.
- More than 20 percent do not disclose their sexual or gender identity to their physician.
- About one-third do not have a will or durable power of attorney for health care.
- LGBT older adults need the following services: senior housing, transportation, legal services, and social events.

Source: Adapted from *The Aging and Health Report: Disparities and Resilience among Lesbian, Gay, Bisexual, and Transgender Older Adults* (pp. 22–27), by K. I. Fredriksen-Goldsen, H.-J. Kim, C. A. Emlet, A. Muraco, E. A. Erosheva, C. P. Hoy-Ellis, et al., 2011, Seattle: Institute for Multigenerational Health.

The following case exemplifies why practitioners need to be conversant in the knowledge, attitudes, and skills for effective and ethical means of working with LGBT elders. Skills include offering culturally and linguistically appropriate services and improving the collection of data on sexual orientation and gender identity to better identify and address health disparities (Auldridge & Espinoza, 2013).

Case Study: Gay Aging

This case study presents the situation of an aging couple as health-related changes create a need to receive formal services. From a care-sharing perspective, the case exemplifies how insensitive and culturally incongruent care can create a hostile environment and add to the stress of care. Fictitious names are used. However, the case is based on a true story reported in the mainstream media.

Bert is a 71-year-old African American research analyst, and Peter is a 68-year-old white book editor. They live in the San Francisco and have been partners for 35 years. Although they are community gay rights advocates, they are increasingly apprehensive about encountering discrimination as they grow older and more dependent on strangers for care.

Bert and Peter lived through an era when it was particularly dangerous to come out. They risked losing employment, family, and friends and even risked becoming victims of violence if others became aware of their sexual identity. Although they could have become habituated to living a closeted existence, Bert and Peter came out early in their adulthood as a political and social force. Both lived through the Stonewall era (mentioned earlier in the chapter) and decided to reside in one of the nation's most gay-friendly cities. These collective efforts have contributed to Bert and Peter's resiliency.

However, Bert had an unfortunate and painful experience after his back operation. One element of his physical therapist's home treatment harkened back to an era Bert and Peter thought they had left behind decades ago. "He [the physical therapist] took it upon himself to decide to pray for us," said Peter. "He wanted to clear the demons out of me and my partner." Bert and Peter ordered the therapist out of their home and complained to the agency that provided the service. The agency director told them that this breach of professional ethics would be reviewed and addressed. When they needed resources in the future, Peter and Bert decided to find services through their social work case manager, Ellen, who they knew "advocate[d] for human rights and social and economic justice" (CSWE, 2012, p. 5). In her role as case manager, Ellen had become aware that far too many LGBT older adults do not trust traditional health and social service agencies, preferring to seek out services specifically dedicated to gay and lesbian clients (Grossman, D'Augelli, & Dragowski, 2007). As a result, Ellen used only culturally sensitive, family-centered case management techniques, and she had become proficient in collecting data and conducting outreach to underserved populations.

Furthermore, Bert and Peter shared their experience with others in the LGBT community. Through their collective action, the local organization of LGBT seniors sent the care agency a letter that specified that other LGBT older adults would not use its services unless corrective action was taken. The letter indicated that sensitivity training for the agency staff seemed essential.

According to Woolf (1998), barriers to services are compounded when a generation of LGBT older adults like Bert and Peter has faced past discriminatory practices. In this case, Bert and Peter stood up for themselves and did not succumb to being pushed back into the closet. In addition, they took action to prevent others from undergoing these painful experiences.

Interventions to Enhance Collective Efficacy and Human Capital

Role of the Family-Centered Case Manager

As a case manager, Ellen aims to help Peter and Bert maintain their collective efficacy as a family, as outlined in chapter 1. Ellen is action oriented, is opposed to injustice, is not neutral (about discrimination), and links policy to her practice. She uses empowerment techniques with Peter and Bert to foster the problem-solving capacities that allow them to continue to advocate for themselves as much as possible.

Fostering Family Resilience

When social care workers address family and community resilience, their focus shifts to a systemic, relational perspective. In particular, their interest lies in the natural resources, patterns of functioning, and capabilities that enable families to manage crises (Greene, 2007). Studies have shown that the experience of combating discrimination and getting involved in advocacy can be transformative, as some people become increasingly resilient (Greene, Cohen, Gonzalez, & Lee, 2009). Therefore, Ellen has asked Peter and Bert to review their advocacy (civil rights) history to learn how they were able to positively face and overcome oppression and discrimination. She thus provides them with the message that they should stay hopeful, stay involved, and continue to contribute to the resiliency of their community.

Resilient LGBT Community

Despite the barriers to service provision faced by LGBT older adults, 90 percent of the participants in the study by Fredriksen-Goldsen et al. (2011) indicated that they felt good about belonging to their communities, with many having at least moderate levels of social support. Most engaged regularly in wellness activities (91 percent) and moderate physical activity (82 percent). Many attended spiritual or religious services or activities (38 percent), with bisexual men and transgender older adults most likely to participate. In addition to contributing to collective efficacy, these strengths likely act as protective factors in terms of physical and mental health, counteracting the unique challenges that LGBT older adults face (Fredriksen-Goldsen et al., 2011).

However, the aging LGBT community is resilient in other ways as well. For example, older LGBT adults have reported that if they needed to relocate from their own home, they would prefer to live in a gay and lesbian retirement facility (Neville & Henrickson, 2010). Joining these communities involves relocating, and social workers can help residents establish new relationships and ties. Social workers can also help potential residents make decisions about whether this type of community is a good fit for their later life plans and needs.

In summary, sexual identity, sexual orientation, and gender identity are all forms of diversity that affect the experience of care provision at points across the life course. As the age at which LGBT individuals come out decreases, a greater number of parents will be involved in raising LGBTQ sons or daughters. Sadly, these youths can face serious threats to their health and well-being, including emotional and physical attacks. Family support is crucial to assist these youths with their identity development.

At the other end of the life course, caregiving can also be challenging. The current cohort of older LGBT adults was raised in a time when their sexual identity was considered sinful, immoral, or a sign of mental illness. Many may carry these negative messages into their later lives and continue to feel secretive about their identity. In addition, aging and health care services may be hostile and unwelcoming to these older adults. As a result, some who would benefit from services may not access them for fear of rejection or attempted conversion.

From a social care perspective, social work practitioners need to be aware of this form of diversity. Interventions can help LGBTQ individuals and promote more supportive environments. The It Gets Better campaign for youths is one example of a program that promotes resilience among young LGBTQ individuals (see http://www.itgetsbetter.org). Social workers have critical roles in assisting the LGBTQ population, their families, and the larger society in supporting individuals and families at multiple points in the life course.

CHAPTER ELEVEN

Immigrant Families:
Caregiving Transitions

People migrate to the United States—leaving behind a country, language, and culture familiar to them—for many reasons. When they arrive in this country, families will find new policies and norms governing the ways in which members provide care for one another. These unfamiliar policies can cause varying levels of distress but also offer opportunity (Fong & Greene, 2009).

This chapter discusses refugees who seek asylum from persecution and presents the cases of Harry and Lena from Russia and Sarah and John from Cambodia. These stories illustrate the complex factors driving immigration and show how the United States is often seen as a place of safety in which to begin a new life. Although the status of undocumented immigrants is a topic of concern, it is beyond the scope of this chapter. However, we do discuss immigrants' contribution to the human capital of the communities in which they live.

The chapter also focuses on some of the difficulties and solutions that immigrants find as they go through resettlement transitions, including employment and mental health issues. It further addresses the resilience of these new Americans as they face caregiving challenges.

Models and theoretical approaches presented in previous chapters are once again combined in this chapter to address therapeutic goals. To better explain cultural transitions among immigrants, we supplement the models applied in early chapters with frameworks adopted from the cross-cultural literature: the dual perspective of Delores Norton (1978) and the culturagram of Elaine Congress (1994). These frameworks can provide additional culturally sensitive techniques for social care workers assisting immigrant families.

Using a Social Care Approach

Incidence

Because the United States is the largest resettlement country in the world, accepting more immigrants than all other nations combined, aiding immigrants who come

TABLE 11.1
Inflow of New Legal Permanent Residents: Top Five Sending Countries, 2012

Country	Immigrants Sent in 2012	Region	Immigrants Sent in 2012
Mexico	146,406	Americas	407,172
China	81,784	Asia	429,599
India	66,434	Africa	107,241
Philippines	57,327	Europe	81,671
Dominican Republic	41,566	All immigrants	1,031,631

Source: Monger, R. & Yankay, J. (2013, March). *U.S. Legal Permanent Residents: 2012.* Office of Immigration Statistics, Annual Flow Report.

to the United States is truly social care in action, involving many complex private–public partnerships and innovative caregiving alternatives (E. Patrick, 2004). According to the Office of Immigration Statistics in the U.S. Department of Homeland Security, there were 1,031,631 immigrants to the United States in 2012 (Monger & Yankay, 2013) (see Table 11.1). Latin Americans and Asians currently constitute the largest groups of immigrants.

The number of people around the world fleeing their country for a better or safer life elsewhere is increasing at an alarming rate. The United Nations High Commissioner for Refugees (UNHCR) (n.d.) estimated there were 28.8 million refugees around the world at the end of 2012. Moreover, according to the U.S. Census, six states received the majority of immigrants: California, New York, Texas, Florida, New Jersey, and Illinois. This represents a shift away from the East Coast metropolitan areas noted in previous census data (Chiswick & Miller, 2004).

In 2013, the largest percentages of immigrants were found in areas close to the Mexican border, in southern Florida, in the West, and in large cities, such as New York City, Chicago, Atlanta, and Washington, DC. Latin Americans were mainly located in the states that border Mexico and in Florida. Asians were the largest immigrant group in Hawaii. In Alaska, Russian immigrants were most numerous. As we will see, information about where immigrants settle in the United States is important to social care workers because these communities can be tapped for their social support networks (GeoCurrents, 2010).

Immigrants Seeking Economic Opportunity

Immigrants seeking economic opportunity in the United States must meet several conditions before they can immigrate. They must apply for an immigration visa and be sponsored by either a relative or an employer who requires their work skills.

They must also acquire a green card, which allows them to live legally in the United States as long as they retain their work status.

Shifting labor force areas are also part of the changing immigration picture. In the 1930s, for example, the first immigrants to the United States from Mexico came to work on farms and ranches. Today, according to the *Washington Post*, because the Mexican economy is on the rise, U.S. farmers and ranchers do not have sufficient immigrant workers (Plumer, 2013). High-tech companies are also seeking employees.

Refugees Seeking Asylum

Refugees are people who have been displaced and are given special permission to come to the United States. Their lives may be disrupted by famine, war, civil conflict, or persecution. They fear persecution based on race, religion, nationality, membership in a particular social group, or public opinion (D. C. Martin & Yankay, 2013).

Refugees who apply for asylum in the United States follow a distinct process. The asylum process is initiated by the president, who establishes the U.S. refugee admissions ceiling in consultation with Congress and the State Department. Individuals seeking asylum are usually referred to the U.S. Refugee Admissions Program by UNHCR, a nongovernmental organization, or a U.S. embassy. Qualifying family members of designated nationalities may refer their relatives so that they can be reunited.

Most applicants are first interviewed by the Commissioner for Refugees. If the UNHCR refers a case to the United States, the prospective immigrant will then interview with staff of a resettlement support center working on behalf of the State Department and then with staff of the Department of Homeland Security. Currently, only the Department of Homeland Security can make the final decision about whether a person will be accepted for resettlement in the United States.

Federal Agencies

In addition to the State Department, several federal agencies are involved in immigration concerns. Following a National Security Council–led interagency process started in 2010, for example, the Office of Refugee Resettlement in HHS and the Bureau of Population, Refugees, and Migration in the State Department instituted quarterly placement consultation meetings with a broad spectrum of resettlement stakeholders to share a variety of data, including state-by-state employment rates, health insurance access, average housing costs, and state minimum wages (HHS, 2014). The Office of Refugee Resettlement's goal for coordinated placement is to facilitate and ensure refugee self-sufficiency and integration into U.S. society.

Volunteer Nongovernmental Agencies

Volunteer agencies, mostly faith- or community-based organizations, are essential to the refugee resettlement process. The case studies in this chapter illustrate how refugees are assigned to volunteer nongovernmental organizations that assist them on their arrival in the United States. The major nongovernmental organizations involved consider caring for resettling refugees as part of their core mandate.

The most active agencies include the U.S. Conference of Catholic Bishops, Lutheran Immigrant Aid Society, International Rescue Committee, World Relief Corporation, Immigrant and Refugee Services of America, Hebrew Immigrant Aid Society, Church World Service, Domestic and Foreign Missionary Service of the Episcopal Church of the USA, Ethiopian Community Development Center, and International Catholic Migration Commission. As discussed later, the State Department gives reception and placement (R&P) grants to various agencies according to the number of refugees for whom they are responsible during a given period.

Stigmatized and Politicized Caregiving Context

The United States is often referred to as a nation of immigrants, yet immigrants to America often face prejudice and discrimination. Refugees may be seen as standing apart from or causing disruption to the social fabric of the host country. That is, refugees may be both welcomed and stigmatized and their caregiving context politicized (Duke Global Health Institute, 2012). Moreover, the convergence of the terrorist attacks of September 11, 2001, changing U.S. demographics, and recent election results has repoliticized U.S. immigration policy.

Immigration debate may increase as Congress goes through the process of deciding which refugee groups should have priority in migrating to the United States. Deciding refugee priority when there is strife in a particular region of the world can become contentious, with special interest groups arguing the extent of a particular refugee group's humanitarian concerns. Starting in the 1970s, for example, Haitian refugees arrived in Miami by makeshift boats to escape oppression in their home country. Their arrival was met with mixed reactions, and often they were arrested and returned to Haiti. On October 21, 1998, after much debate, the Haitian Refugee Immigration Fairness Act was belatedly enacted by Congress to protect certain nationals of Haiti who had long been residing in the United States, often undercover. This is just one example of the complexity of and politics behind U.S. immigration law and policy.

Hidden immigrants, especially those whose appearance or dress does not conform to that of the mainstream population, can live in fear. At the same time, immigrant groups like the Haitians have established social networks using businesses, such as groceries, bakeries, and restaurants. We will later see how immigrants contribute to individual, family, and community well-being.

Columbia University Policy Report

Despite many humanitarian efforts, immigration services have not been substantially revised since 1980. In 2010, the U.S. Office of Refugee Resettlement asked the

Columbia University School of International and Public Affairs to write a report on the challenges facing the immigration system (Brick et al., 2010). The report concluded that revised U.S. legislation is needed to

- address conflicting policy goals
- provide adequate funding to all aspects of the resettlement process
- remove obstacles to coordination and planning
- establish monitoring and evaluation processes

New immigration law must address these four inadequacies as well as many other vexing issues, including the problem of immigrants with undocumented status.

Refugee Resettlement: A Case Management Function

Case Management

According to NASW, case management is a component of many social work jobs, and a significant number of practitioners spend more than half of their time on case management tasks (Whitaker, Weismiller, & Clark, 2006). Case management may be defined differently according to one's job description but generally includes planning, coordinating, and using therapeutic skills. It includes many of the same elements of social work practice, such as engaging and assessing the client, setting mutual goals, implementing interventions in the care plan, obtaining resources, reassessing or evaluating the client situation, and achieving closure.

In the tradition of a care-sharing philosophy, agencies that receive an R&P grant from the State Department are expected to provide the following services to people like Harry, Lena, and their children (see the following case study):

- *Sponsorship:* prearrival resettlement planning (including placement)
- *Reception upon arrival:* support with basic needs for at least 30 days, including housing, furnishings, food, and clothing
- *Community orientation:* referral to social service providers (in the areas of health care, employment, and so forth)
- *Case management and tracking* for 90 to 180 days

Case Study

Harry, Lena, their children (Joseph, age 14; Irving, 12; and Anna, 10), and Grandpa Alex (age 75) immigrated in 1991 to Silver Spring, Maryland, from Minsk, then in USSR, where they were members of the marginalized Jewish minority. This marginalization had not always existed; they remembered that their great-grandparents had once been part of a flourishing ethnic community: At the time of the 1897 census under the Russian Empire, Jews such as Harry and Lena's great-grandparents made up the largest ethnic group in Minsk, constituting 52 percent of the population. But by the end of the Nazi occupation and Holocaust, ethnic Jews made up less than 10 percent of the population. After World War II, anti-Semitism continued under Soviet rule. By 1999, only 1 percent of the population was Jewish.

Harry and his family were allowed to immigrate thanks to the Lautenberg Amendment enacted by Congress in November 1989 as part of the Foreign Operations Appropriations Act for fiscal year 1990. The Lautenberg Amendment required the executive branch to establish refugee priority processing categories for Soviet Jews, evangelical Christians, and members of the Ukrainian Catholic Church or the Ukrainian Orthodox Church who were facing persecution in their home country (Gindin, 2013).

The process of case management began with the case manager engaging the family in relationship building. Harry and his family were resettled by Jewish Social Services of Greater Washington, DC, and Elsa was assigned as their social worker. In anticipation of their arrival, Elsa began prearrival planning, or constructing a service plan. She first became more familiar with the culture of the family, learning that people from the USSR generally mistrusted official agencies and officials. She realized that her transparency would be important to the family.

Elsa's first task was to deliver appropriate resources and services. Having a network of volunteers and community agencies was critical to her social care approach. She contacted a real estate company that collaborated with Jewish Social Services of Greater Washington, DC, to find an apartment for the family near public transportation and a cluster of other Russian émigrés.

Volunteers were called together and organized to furnish the family's apartment. The community donated items and shopped for new ones. After the family's time of arrival had been verified, a group of volunteers met them at Dulles Airport. The next day, a volunteer took the family to a grocery store, attending to the basics and each member's likes and dislikes. The following day, male and female volunteers went to department stores with the family looking for what Anna called "those modern U.S. fashions"—jeans.

Social workers in all roles are increasingly accountable for delivering cost-effective services. Because the State Department gives every family three months to become self-sufficient and be removed from their R&P grant, one of Elsa's most important case management tasks was to secure jobs for Harry and Lena. Elsa compiled a list of potential job openings and found Harry, an engineer, work at a biotech firm located on a bus line. Lena, a teacher, was secured a job as a teacher's aide at a local Hebrew school.

Joseph, Irving, and Anna were assigned volunteer tutors who took them to their respective schools and coordinated homework assignments. Once the children were proficient in English and knew their way around the neighborhood, they would attend school on their own. These are traditional case management and care-sharing activities.

Elsa's next task was to orient the family to their community. This process included an introduction to nearby parks, movies, and religious institutions, such as the synagogue and senior center. She then evaluated her progress in meeting the family's needs. As she assessed the progress of her service delivery, she became concerned with the effect of resettlement policy on the lives of her clients. She wanted to evaluate gaps in services and the changes necessary to make them more effective and accessible.

When Elsa met with the family for termination interviews, she learned that the younger family members were enjoying their lives in Silver Spring. However, Grandpa Alex was reclusive and seemed to be depressed. He told the family that he "wished he was still in Minsk, where he had friends." Here in the United States, he thought only about "joining his wife," who had died three years earlier.

Once Grandpa's depression was revealed, Elsa invited Grandpa to the agency to determine his need for mental health services. A volunteer translator was used to facilitate the interview, during which Elsa confirmed that Grandpa was indeed depressed. Yet she soon became aware of a potential barrier to Grandpa receiving mental health services. Because he mistrusted U.S. institutions and did not believe in mental health difficulties, Grandpa said that he had "no interest in mental health treatment." Elsa sought a bicultural solution.

Biculturalism assumes that every individual is part of two systems: the smaller system of his or her immediate environment and the larger societal system of the more distant or mainstream environment. This concept is known as the "dual perspective" (see Figure 11.1). Although various characteristics of the two systems exist side by side, the systems may or may not be congruent and may cause conflict for those on the edge of two cultures (Chestang, 1984; S. Miller, 1980). Therefore, an evaluation from the dual perspective involves an assessment "of these disparate systems and determining where [or if] the major source of stress [between the two systems may] lie" (Norton, 1978, p. 7). Elsa's assessment led her to understand that Grandpa was estranged from local support networks. She sought out a group of Russian older adults at the Jewish Community Center, where Grandpa could find social support. With the help of the bilingual translator, who transported him to the center, Grandpa gradually became integrated into the Jewish Community Center group, in which one of the main topics of conversation was the "bad" influence of American youths.

Applying FAM in Assessment

Because many immigrants have faced trauma and adversity, there is concern about the mental health services available to them and the cultural sensitivity of those services. According to the Duke Global Health Institute (2012), by 2030 mental health issues will be among the top difficulties refugees are trying to solve. The

FIGURE 11.1
Dual Perspective

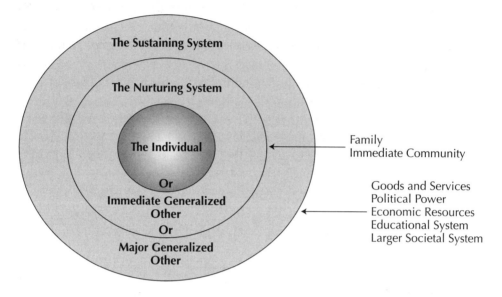

Source: Adapted from *The Dual Perspective: Inclusion of Ethnic Minority Content in Social Work Curriculum* (p. 5), by D. G. Norton, 1978, New York: Council on Social Work Education.

case of Sarah and her family illustrates this situation and provides assessment and intervention strategies.

Case Study

Sarah and her husband, John, met on a forced collective labor farm in Cambodia in 1974. They married and came to the United States in 1980, receiving case management services from Catholic Family Services in Long Beach, California. About that time, Congress initiated a special immigration status for those who lived in the geographical area affected by the Vietnam conflict. The married couple was among hundreds of thousands of refugees from the Khmer Rouge Cambodian Communist regime who fled to America. Many in this group resettled in California. (As of 2005, approximately 3 million Cambodians were living in the United States [Pfeifer, 2006].)

As in the case of Harry and his family, volunteers and community groups worked together with Sarah and John's case manager to deliver services. The couple had two children and successfully settled in to the Cambodian American community.

However, in 2003, the family returned to Catholic Family Services to obtain mental health services for Sarah from their former case manager, Rachel. Because

Cambodian refugees were frequently served by her agency, Rachel, a clinical social worker, had become familiar with the genocide in Cambodia, in which an estimated 1.7 to 2.5 million people had been killed or starved to death. She knew that the helping process in the United States was influenced by these terrifying historical events. She knew that the Khmer Rouge regime was known for its forceful separation of families, relocation of people to collective farms (labor camps), removal of privately owned property, and torture of suspected government agitators. In addition, Rachel learned that during the Khmer Rouge regime,

> everyone was deprived of their basic rights. People were not allowed to go outside their cooperative. The regime would not allow anyone to gather and hold discussions. If three people gathered and talked, they could be accused of being enemies and arrested or executed. . . . Family relationships were also heavily criticized. People were forbidden to show even the slightest affection, humor or pity. (Dy, 2007, p. 15)

Rachel also knew that refugees who have experienced trauma may have increased need for mental and physical health care.

Sarah told Rachel that she had been in a state of constant worry since she had read about the establishment of the Extraordinary Chambers in the Courts of Cambodia. The purpose of the chambers, established in 2006 by the United Nations and the Cambodian Documentation Center, was to adjudicate crimes against humanity, war crimes, and genocide and to provide justice to the Cambodian people who were victims of the Khmer Rouge regime. Sarah and many others like her were reexperiencing these past traumatic events. Sarah was concerned that her distress, which involved nightmares, was having negative effects on her children, Mark (age 27) and Kim (age 29). The family decided to seek counseling together.

FAM Assessment

Family-Centered Interviews. Sarah and her family came to the agency with Sarah as the self-designated client. Rachel interviewed the family together but focused on Sarah's complaints. The recognition of the family as a system and treatment unit of choice is central to FAM. The model emphasizes the interdependence among family members as well as the dynamics of the family and societal change. This means that Rachel evaluated and treated the family as an organizational whole in past and current societal contexts (Greene, 2008c). Rachel also kept in mind that behavior considered acceptable or functional in one culture may not be perceived that way in another.

Biological Age. Sarah, who had always been an energetic worker, told Rachel that she was feeling tired constantly. She had been to the doctor, who had found no physical basis for her fatigue. As a result, Sarah and her family had decided to seek out Rachel, the former resettlement worker, who took on a therapeutic role.

Psychological Age. Rachel asked Sarah what she thought was causing her present difficulties. This subjective approach to interviewing is important to refugees who struggle with whether their difficulties rest with them as a personal problem or are related to their past experience with political events (Gorman, 2001). Sarah said that she had recently been experiencing sleeplessness and anxiety and believed that her mental distress was a matter that needed to be resolved with the help of her family.

Sarah's response was in keeping with the fact that many ethnic groups frequently assume a relational perspective to development of the self. A *relational perspective* to human development sees an individual's psychological growth as "a process of differentiation and separation in relationships rather than disengagement and separation from relationships" as one matures (Genero, 1998, p. 33). Thus, Sarah was most comfortable receiving social care in a family format.

Social Age. To assess Sarah's social age, Rachel asked questions to explore her bicultural competence and relationship with social networks. From Sarah's description of her life in the United States, Rachel concluded that Sarah appeared at ease with her bicultural status as a Cambodian American.

Bicultural competence is the ability to alternate and integrate cultural forms that people need to validate the acceptability of living in two communities (Genero, 1998). Thus, Sarah, who was bicultural, felt effective and well grounded in both her ethnic and mainstream cultures (La Fromboise, Coleman, & Gerton, 1993).

Sarah's family had social networks among Cambodians and other social groups, particularly the young people with whom Mark and Kim went to school. The presence of social supports was an important part of the family's adjustment to the United States, and the family spoke warmly about their friends.

Spiritual Assessment. Sarah and her family were Buddhist. They found that this gave a spiritual dimension to their family that usually fostered peace and tranquility. However, Sarah's story revealed that the practice of *ancestor worship*, or the custom of venerating deceased ancestors who are considered still a part of the family (Ancestor worship, n.d.), had occasioned Sarah's anxiety about the death of her parents during the Khmer Rouge regime. This was important information for the intervention process.

Assessment of Family Functioning

System. Ethnic minority families put *familism,* or "the perceived strength of family bonds and the sense of loyalty to the family," as a top priority (Luna et al., 1996, p. 267). Cambodians follow in this tradition, often living in three-generation households, and tend to emphasize the extended family as a unit or collective rather than each individual (Chan & Kim, 2003). The family's shifting membership, including births, marriages, or deaths; the changing status of the members in relationship to one another; and the challenges to a family's adaptational capacity at each stage are at the heart of family functioning (Carter & McGoldrick, 2005).

In addition, the cultural tradition of *filial piety*, or the belief that children should respect and take care of their parents, is often followed (Lee & Sung, 1998). Rachel observed that Mark and Kim were solicitous of Sarah's needs and wanted to understand her anxieties. This attention was a major aspect of Sarah's healing process.

Roles. Cambodian families generally have a more hierarchical family structure than mainstream U.S. families. This may be typified by men appearing to have more power and privilege. However, research studies have revealed that women often make decisions about how to spend money and discipline children (Gorman, 2001). When exploring role differentiation in the family, Rachel learned that this was the case in Sarah's family.

Development. From taking a family life course history, Rachel understood that the nature of Sarah and John's family in the United States had evolved over time. When they first arrived, Sarah and John received training for employment, job and housing locations, and an orientation to the Long Beach community. Later, their children attended school, bringing home many of the behaviors of U.S. teenagers. Thus, the process of socialization to the United States was a major aspect of the whole family's development.

Socialization. Socialization involves preparing children through the teaching and learning of traditional beliefs, values, and standards of behavior necessary to assume adult roles and obligations of society (Boykin & Toms, 1985). Socialization usually begins in a person's family and continues as youngsters interact with major societal socialization agents, such as schools, the mass media, and the world of work. However, adults are also socialized into new roles as they enter novel and unfamiliar situations. In the case of immigrant families, all members undergo the process of socialization at various rates, accounting for variations in assimilation.

Sarah and her family members exhibited differences in *assimilation*, or the degree to which people take on the mainstream culture. Because Sarah and John came from rural areas of Cambodia, when they arrived in the United States they needed information about customs necessary for living in Long Beach. In contrast, their children were more *acculturated*, or immersed in the mainstream culture, listening to American music and going to community college to prepare for employment. However, they retained the cultural values associated with familism.

Cultural Sensitivity: The Culturagram and Healing Strategies

As described previously, case managers begin their assessment of refugee clients by being aware of the challenges and solutions they may have faced in the resettlement transition. A social worker's information about the immigration process can also be supplemented by clients' stories using Elaine Congress's (1994) culturagram, which depicts the factors that influence adaptation to life among new Americans, including holidays celebrated, languages spoken, and health beliefs held (see Figure

11.2). Together, the immigrant family answers the questions on the culturagram as a method of telling their stories and of sorting out chosen family issues.

For example, Sarah's family stories demonstrated that events before migration can still influence family functioning. Rachel learned that Sarah's family was high school educated and as a consequence was a target of the Khmer Rouge regime. Individuals who wore eyeglasses were rounded up for relocation, and Sarah (who wore glasses) was sent to a reeducation camp. She was separated from the other members of her family of origin, who died of starvation in another labor camp. This explained why Sarah felt that she had not had the opportunity to give her parents proper respect. Mark and Kim suggested that they light a candle at the Dalai Lama's Temple at the Dharma Center located in Long Beach. This suggestion had a therapeutic effect.

Rachel also learned that having been in a labor camp did not have the same effect on Sarah as it did on John. As Sarah revisited her story, Mark and Kim, who were

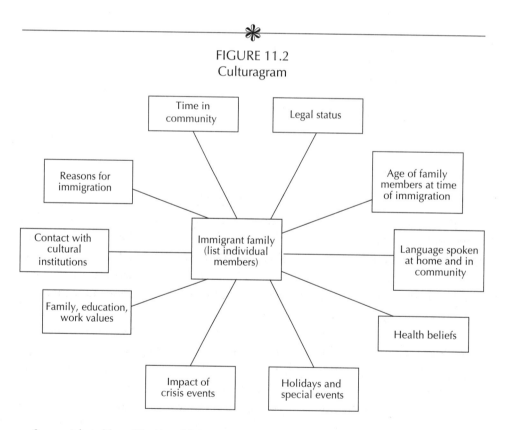

FIGURE 11.2
Culturagram

Source: Adapted from "The Use of Culturagrams to Assess and Empower Culturally Diverse Families," by E. P. Congress, 1994, *Families in Society, 75,* p. 533.

now old enough to understand what had happened before they were born in the United States, came to understand their mother's travails. This contributed to reaffirming Sarah's brave escape from the labor camp in Cambodia.

Applying REM in Intervention

The family-centered narrative approach to FAM assessment contributed to Sarah's family cohesion and resilience. This section presents the major tenets of the narrative approach used to gather the family story. It then summarizes Sarah's and her family's risks, protective factors, and resilience factors.

Narrative Resilience-Enhancing Treatment

Narrative approaches to treatment are part of the social construction school of thought and were used to reconstruct Sarah's family story. *Restorying*, or reframing a family story, allows for new, more positive meanings of past negative events. Because Sarah and her family had traumatic events in their background, the practice principles incorporated into this school of thought are appropriate.

Rachel, their clinical social worker, attempted to foster the family's resilience by

- focusing on both individual and societal or political events
- emphasizing the family's subjective account of difficult life events
- listening to the family members' difficulties as they perceived them and encouraging them to describe, explain, or account for their circumstances in their own terms
- exploring and seeking new meanings of traumatic life events (Gergen, 1985a, 1985b).

Summary of REM Assessment

Risk. Risks are those factors that might put a family in jeopardy. Sarah, John, Mark, and Kim had faced various risks across the life course. These included Sarah and John separating from their families of origin, working in a labor camp, resettling in America, and establishing new roots. Mark and Kim had experienced living in a bicultural environment. When the family members assessed how they had overcome these past events, they realized that they had much strength.

Protective Factors. One of the ways in which Sarah's family had overcome past difficult events and maintained resilience was by preserving cultural values from their country of origin. This served as a protective factor and promoted ethnic pride. Another protective factor was their strong support system.

Resilience. Among the resilience factors displayed by Sarah and her family were communicating well with family members, maintaining a stable organization, and retaining a positive belief system (Walsh, 1998). By retaining cultural beliefs, Rachel and her family contributed to their own natural healing processes.

REM Outcomes

Sarah and her family showed that they could meet two important therapeutic outcomes expected in the REM approach: (1) adapting to extraordinary circumstances (Fraser, 1997) and (2) maintaining "continuity of one's personal narrative and a coherent sense of self following traumatic events" (Borden, 1992, p. 135).

Not all families are willing to discuss traumatic life events, and practitioners should respect this. Because of Sarah's and her family's willingness to disclose these events, there were several positive outcomes related to the family belief system. The value of familism and ancestor worship was affirmed; the family life cycle and belief in familial piety were upheld; past adversity was better understood, giving the Cambodian crisis more meaning and making it comprehensible and manageable; and a sense of family coherence and stability was restored (Block & Gebeloff, 2009).

Collective Efficacy and Human Capital in Immigrant Populations

Assessing resilience requires that practitioners understand the mutual influences of the various systems in which clients participate: family, school, peers, work, neighborhood, community, and the larger society. At the same time, practitioners must evaluate whether families and communities can be considered resilient in their own right. This type of adaptation is sometimes known as *collective efficacy*, defined as social cohesion among neighbors combined with their willingness to intervene on behalf of the common good (Sampson, Raudenbush, & Earls, 1997). As seen in the following example of economic development, collective efficacy is actualized in immigrant communities as they engage in activism and belongingness (Carroll & Rosson, 1996).

Communities that have large immigrant populations may have fewer resources because of poverty and lack of available services. However, research on collective efficacy and immigrant communities indicates that stronger social ties and networks have an advantageous effect on health and social functioning (Browning & Cagney, 2003). Residents of neighborhoods with more social connections had better health outcomes and better educational attainment. An important reason for families to leave their homelands is to find better opportunities. In social work practice, interventions that strengthen the human capital within these communities will have a potentially better outcome for raising children and caring for older adults and those with disabilities.

Human capital grows when communities foster the interconnectedness of people, reinforce their assets, and augment community institutions. The Councils of Economic Advisers (2007, 2013) under both George W. Bush and Barack Obama have reported that the work of immigrants contributes greatly to the growth of human capital and the expansion of the economy (see "Highlights from the Council of Economic Advisers of George W. Bush, 2007" on page 211):

Highlights from the Council of Economic Advisers of George W. Bush, 2007

1. On average, U.S. natives benefit from immigration. Immigrants tend to complement (not substitute for) natives, raising natives' productivity and income.
2. Careful studies of the long-term fiscal effects of immigration conclude that it is likely to have a modest, positive influence.
3. Skilled immigrants are likely to be especially beneficial to natives. In addition to contributions to innovation, they have a significant positive fiscal impact.

General Points

- *Immigrants are a critical part of the U.S. workforce and contribute to growth in productivity and technological advancement.* They make up 15% of all workers and even larger shares of certain occupations, such as construction, food services, and health care. Approximately 40% of PhD scientists working in the United States were born abroad.[1]
- Many immigrants are entrepreneurs. The Kauffman Foundation's index of entrepreneurial activity is nearly 40% higher for immigrants than for natives.[2]
- Immigrants and their children assimilate into the U.S. culture. For example, although 72% of first-generation Latino immigrants use Spanish as their predominant language, only 7% of the second generation are Spanish dominant.[3]
- Immigrants have lower crime rates than natives. Among men ages 18 to 40, immigrants are much less likely than natives to be incarcerated.[4]
- Immigrants slightly improve the solvency of pay-as-you-go entitlement programs such as Social Security and Medicare. The 2007 OASDI (Old Age, Survivors & Disability Insurance) Trustees Report indicated that an additional 100,000 net immigrants per year would increase the long-range actuarial balance by about 0.07% of taxable payroll.[5]
- The long-term impact of immigration on public budgets is likely to be positive. Projections of future taxes and government spending are subject to uncertainty, but a careful study published by the National Research Council estimated that immigrants and their descendants would contribute about $80,000 more in taxes (in 1996 dollars) than they would receive in public services.[6]

Source: Excerpted from *Immigration's Economic Impact,* by Council of Economic Advisers, 2007, retrieved from georgewbush-whitehouse.archives.gov/cea/cea_immigration_062007.html

[1]Pfeifer, M. E. (2006, October 28). U.S. Census releases 2005 American Community Survey data for Southeast Asian Americans. *Asian American Press.* Retrieved from http://www.hmongstudies.org/2005ACSArticle.html

[2]Fairlie, R. W. (2006). *Kauffman index of entrepreneurial activity: National report, 1996–2005.* Retrieved from http://www.kauffman.org/what-we-do/research/kauffman-index-of-entrepreneurial-activity

[3]Pew Hispanic Center/Kaiser Family Foundation. (2002, December). *2002 National Survey of Latinos.* Retrieved from http://www.pewhispanic.org/2002/12/17/2002-national-survey-of-latinos/

[4]Butcher, K. F., & Piehl, A. M. (2005) *Why are immigrants' incarceration rates so low? Evidence on selective immigration, deterrence, and deportation.* Cambridge, MA: National Bureau of Economic Research. Retrieved from http:www.nber.org/papers/w13229

[5]Social Security Administration. (n.d.). *A summary of the 2013 annual reports.* Retrieved from http://www.socialsecurity.gov/OACT/TRSUM/index.html

[6]Smith, J., & Edmonston, B. (Eds.). (1997). *The new Americans: Economic, demographic, and fiscal effects of immigration.* Washington, DC: National Research Council, National Academies Press.

Immigrants increase the size of the population and thus of the labor force and customer base, making an important contribution to economic growth. . . . Immigrants work in diverse industries and occupations. While they represent 16 percent of the workforce, they account for more than 20 percent of workers in agriculture, construction, food services, and information technology. They are agricultural laborers, domestic workers, and cabdrivers as well as health care workers, computer software engineers, and medical scientists. (Council of Economic Advisers, 2013, p. 1)

Immigrants also contribute to the development of community infrastructure, which in turn expands human capital. For example, Houston, Texas, was home to an estimated 2,160,821 Korean Americans in 2012. Their collective action has created, among other things, a chamber of commerce, a Korean community center, restaurants, hair salons, a Web site, a community learning center that provides general equivalency diplomas, and churches, illustrating the power of the social care approach to community building.

Finally, in the words of President Obama during his 2013 State of the Union speech,

We define ourselves as a nation of immigrants. That's who we are—in our bones. The promise we see in those who come here from every corner of the globe, that's always been one of our greatest strengths. It keeps our workforce young. It keeps our country on the cutting edge. And it's helped build the greatest economic engine the world has ever known. (Obama, 2013)

CHAPTER TWELVE

Caregiving and Care Sharing:
The Social Environment of Family Life

This book has explored various caregiving situations and contexts. Looking at the contents, it is clear that caregiving takes place across the life course. Depending on the situation and reasons for care, families experience different sources of stress and challenges with their roles. Within the various chapters, family case studies were provided to illustrate both the uniqueness and similarities of different caregiving contexts. Although the families in the case studies faced struggles, resilience, love, and joy were part of all their stories. As a social work practitioner, it is important to remember that all these experiences are part of caregiving.

The purpose of this book is to highlight aspects of caregiving and provide practice models and frameworks to use in assessing and intervening with families. Practice models based on an integration of the ecological perspective (Bronfenbrenner, 1979), family system dynamics (Carter & McGoldrick, 2005), and the stress process model (Lazarus & Folkman, 1984) were presented. FAM (Greene, 2008a) is a practice model for determining individuals' capacities to perform effectively in social roles and function within the environment. In using this model, the practitioner can assess the caregiver's capacity to provide care, the requirements of the care recipient, and the resources available within the family. REM (Greene, 2007), a model that identifies sources of risk and resilience and those aspects of caregiving that may make care provision difficult, was also presented. In practice, social workers can intervene to enhance the family's resilience or ability. Protective factors are those conditions that help with coping or adaptation, such as social support. The chapters also included attention to the goodness of fit of families within their environment. Case management interventions identify caregiving need and link families to resources or work to address gaps in service provision. Additionally, collective responses that can work to change the social environment for caregiving families were featured, and human capital issues were presented as an aspect of community functioning. These macropractice issues focus on ways that the social environment can be modified to support families more effectively in their roles.

However, families do not perform caregiving tasks in isolation. Caregiving involves relationships between both the informal caregivers (for example, family and close friends) and formal care systems. This is the foundation of the care-sharing aspect of the book—that informal and formal support systems must be able to work together and complement each other. Unfortunately, that does not always happen, and gaps may exist or tension may develop between the family and service providers. In an ideal situation, roles for all members of a care team—what the family and friends can do and how practitioners and service providers can provide support— would be articulated.

In this final chapter, the social environment of caregiving is explored more fully. Various questions will be addressed including, What are the sources of tension between the informal and formal support systems? What occurs over time in caregiving families, and how does this influence the type of services needed? What social policies affect family care? Finally, the chapter will conclude by looking into the future and outlining some directions in caregiving and care sharing.

What Are Problems in Care Sharing?

As the chapters indicate, providing someone with care involves time, energy, and resources. Intuitively, one would imagine that families would enthusiastically embrace help and assistance. However, this does not always happen, and families struggle with situations without adequate support.

As the chapters discussed, families may not be using the services and resources that can provide them assistance with caregiving responsibilities. Why don't families use the available services, professionals, or other forms of support that can be helpful in this area? Can these resources be offered and arranged in ways that would be more acceptable and helpful to families? What are some of the ways to promote a care-sharing approach?

Culturally Sensitive Practice Approaches

Cultural issues and experiences of care may promote or inhibit care sharing. The chapters provide examples of situations in which assistance from formal service providers was provided in ways that were incongruent with families' values and experiences. Applying social work competencies to family care (see chapter 2), practitioners need to do the following:

- *Engage diversity and difference in practice.* Families have particular cultural patterns and values, and these affect the experience of care. Practitioners who work with families need to assess and intervene in culturally competent ways.
- *Respond to contexts that shape practice.* Changing demography and social experiences affect families and their caregiving needs. Emerging family forms

(for example, grandparents raising grandchildren and military veterans returning home) create new contexts for caregiving supports.

- *Advance human rights and social and economic justice.* Caregiving is a shared experience, as health and social programs, policies, and resource allocation affect the ability of families to provide care. Oppressive structures and regulations that do not take into account the cultural contexts of families hinder this ability and create stress.

The various chapters also include examples of the ways that practitioners and service providers are helpful to families and the presence of insensitivities that create distance. Chapter 10, on LGBTQ care provision, for example, presents the case of Bert and Peter, two older gay men who lived in San Francisco. After Bert had had a back operation, the first physical therapist who came to their home prayed for the couple—to "clear the demons" from them. As a consequence, the couple discontinued service with the therapy agency. But they were able to secure another physical therapist who provided assistance to the couple in a culturally sensitive way. With this new therapist, Bert and Peter were treated with dignity and as a family coping with a health transition.

A second example of culturally insensitive services was provided in chapter 8, on caregiving for people with HIV/AIDs. In the case study of Anita, the grandmother who was raising her grandson, the case manager assessed her caregiving competence on the basis of her age and not her abilities. This example showed how a particular bias about who is able (and who is not able) to provide care influences evaluations and assessment.

Life Course Perspective

Caregiving happens across the life course, and families will require different services and supports at different points. Resources may exist for families at one point that may not exist at another point. Chapters 5 and 6, on caregiving for people with IDD and mental health issues, demonstrate this situation well. Families are often the primary sources of support for people who have either a psychiatric or intellectual disability. However, the experiences of care are different for a child than they are for an adult. Additionally, the experience of caring for an older adult may include new challenges and experiences. A major transition in care occurs when a parent is no longer able to provide primary care provision for a son or daughter with a psychiatric or intellectual disability. Supports for transitions in the family life course are critical. Practitioner competencies that relate to a life course perspective include the following:

- *Apply knowledge of human behavior and the social environment.* The person-in-environment framework provides the lens for understanding family caregiving. Practitioners need to understand life course issues, family subsystems, the effect of care on internal family relationships, and the relationship of the family to other systems in the environment.

- *Apply critical thinking to inform and communicate professional judgments.* Social workers must be able to understand how caregiving situations change across the life course. In particular, how do these changes affect all aspects of family life? Practitioners need to be able to help families identify particular risk situations and solve the problems faced.

The life course perspective considers an individual's biopsychosocial and spiritual development and family transitions over time, but it also intersects with the geographic, social, economic, and historical contexts of the day (Elder 1978; Haraven, 1978). This is why each chapter pays considerable attention to how care varies with the societal factors of time and place. For example, chapter 8, on caregiving for people with HIV/AIDs, illustrates how caregiving can be different in San Francisco, Washington, DC, and Africa.

Care-sharing approaches must also include the experience of the individual receiving care. What are the transitions that the individual experiences? From a life course perspective, individual changes can precipitate experiences that affect caregiving. The Grogan family case study in chapter 5, on caregiving for people with IDD, provides an example. The parents' employment comes into question as their son with an intellectual disability (Kevin) matures. Like other adolescents, including his siblings, Kevin may desire additional contact with friends who are his age. What opportunities does Kevin have to be with others and have a social life outside his family? Are there ways to assist him with friendship opportunities?

Unresponsive Service Systems

Care sharing is also difficult because of the way that social service systems are created. As discussed, service systems are often fragmented, and this creates additional difficulties for families that require services from multiple sectors. Social work competencies that address service system issues are as follows:

- *Engage in policy practice to advance social and economic well-being and to deliver effective social work services.* Policies can either provide support to families in their caregiving roles or create challenges that lead to stress. Part of social work with caregivers is to advocate for just and equitable services.
- *Engage, assess, intervene, and evaluate with individuals, families, groups, organizations, and communities.* To be an effective practitioner, social workers must be able to work with multiple systems. In addition, practitioners need to work between systems by, for example, making appropriate referrals and serving as an advocate for a family. Social workers may also work at the community level to mobilize caregivers to collective action or mutual aid.

Challenges that individuals and families face cannot always be addressed by the service provided by one service delivery system. Uncoordinated and disconnected services can lead to frustration, isolation, and increased caregiver stress (Sadavoy, Meier, & Ong, 2004). Instead of decreasing caregiver stress, ineffective services create additional barriers and challenges that add to the difficulties experienced by caregiving families.

The amount of funding provided to health and social services in our country illustrates the lack of coordination and inequality of resources among service systems. Figure 12.1 provides a comparison of health care and social service expenditures by various countries. As the graph, indicates, the United States trails several other countries in combined expenditures on health and social welfare. In other countries, a greater amount is spent on social welfare programs, with fewer dollars targeted to health services. In the United States, however, about twice as much is spent on health as on social programs. This imbalance presents challenges to

✳

FIGURE 12.1
Health Care Investment Comparison by Country

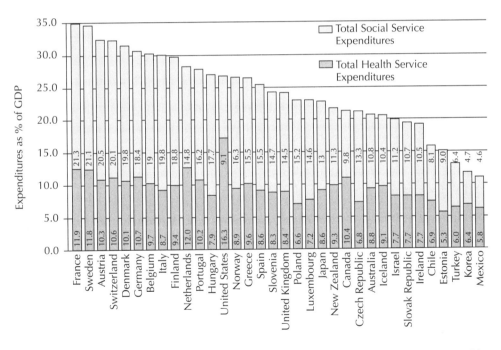

Source: Reprinted from "US Health Care Paradox: How Spending More Is Getting Us Less," by E. Bradley and L. A. Taylor, 2013, seminar presented at the 141st American Public Health Association Annual Meeting, Boston.

families, and as discussed in the chapters, poor health outcomes are one consequence of care provision.

Sadly, service professionals often do not include caregivers as members of treatment teams. Although caregivers may have invaluable information and experience to share with formal care providers, their knowledge and information may be overlooked or viewed as unimportant. Care providers who perceive that they are a part of a collaborative process report higher levels of satisfaction with services (Perreault et al., 2012).

Affordable Care Act: Hope for Caregivers?

Social policy shapes the environment of family care and the incentives for care-sharing approaches. Throughout this book, various health care issues have been addressed because a primary reason for care is the poor health and functioning of the care recipient. However, health care is also crucial for the care provider, as the physical and emotional demands of care may compromise their health and well-being as well.

In 2013–2014, the United States experienced a seismic shift in the way that health care is delivered. The Affordable Care Act was implemented with the goals of providing greater access, more coordinated care, and expanded health care coverage. This new health care orientation diverges from the United States' previous fragmented and disparate health services. The Affordable Care Act moves from an acute care and disease-focused model to a person-centered and coordinated care model (Golden, 2011). Although outcome research on the new law is in the nascent stages, the expectation is that additional coverage will benefit both individuals and their care providers. In this way, implementation of the Affordable Care Act can be a method for promoting care sharing to family caregivers.

The Affordable Care Act has exciting new opportunities for social workers. It not only increases access to affordable health care services, but also places additional emphasis on the social environment. Whereas social workers have always stressed the connection between physical and social functioning, the medical community has now also begun to pay attention to the social environment of those receiving health care services. For example, a national study of primary care physicians and pediatricians reported that 85 percent believe that unmet social needs (for example, adequate housing, transportation, and access to nutritious food) contribute to poor health statuses for Americans (Robert Wood Johnson Foundation, 2011). Furthermore, 80 percent of these physicians do not believe that they have the capacity to address these needs, and this gap impedes their ability to deliver quality health care. Clearly, this area is one in which social workers have necessary knowledge and skills to help improve health care outcomes.

With changes in financing, structure, and organization of health care, social workers will have increased opportunities to play pivotal roles in service delivery. Andrews, Darnell, McBride, and Gehlert (2013) identified four major areas in which social workers are well suited to advance the goals established by the Affordable Care Act.

1. Social workers understand individuals within the contexts of their physical and social environments. These influences have an effect on health, psychosocial well-being, and functioning. As a result, social workers play important roles in understanding transitions in care, capability of care providers, and adequacy of the environment to support care provision.

2. Social workers' orientation to a systems approach provides a lens for seeing how various resources and needs intersect and affect health. As analyzed within the various chapters of this book, services and programs used by individuals and families often span multiple networks. In addition, caregivers have their own involvements, which are affected by their care provision role (for example, employment and civic ties). Social workers understand how coordination between these various networks is needed to provide an effective care-sharing experience.

3. Social workers have an evidence-based approach to practice and select interventions that have the highest level of demonstrated efficacy. In addition, practice includes evaluating the outcome of interventions, treatments, and programs. In this way, social workers can advance knowledge and practice about those approaches that provide support and assistance to individuals and their care providers.

4. Although the Affordable Care Act aims to expand health care coverage, attention to the uninsured is still necessary. Approximately 29 million Americans will continue to lack health insurance after the Affordable Care Act is implemented (Congressional Budget Office, 2012). With a historic and fundamental value of social and economic justice, social workers will be able to identify those individuals who continue to be uninsured and document the disadvantaged conditions of these individuals.

Social work skills and roles are particularly relevant for this new health care environment. With social work's legacy in case management, practitioners' abilities to bridge and link individuals, families, and services are essential. In particular, navigator and assister roles are opportunities to help individuals decide on the best form of coverage, make the best use of their coverage, and "bend the cost curve" to bring down overall costs (Darnell, 2013). With the implementation of the Affordable Care Act, social workers have vital roles in the new orientation to health care that are consistent with our professional mission and mandate to provide effective services to promote well-being (Golden, 2011).

One part of the Affordable Care Act that was not implemented was the Community Living Assistance Services and Supports (CLASS) Act. Championed by the late Ted Kennedy, these provisions would have provided voluntary long-term care insurance (Wiener, 2012). Although the program had the potential to provide families with another option for care, the high cost of the premiums (about $300 per month) would have contributed to low enrollment and a lack of fiscal stability over time (Greenlee, 2011). In late 2011, HHS Secretary Kathleen Sebelius (2011) announced that the program would be discontinued. Advocates for older adults and those with disabilities were particularly disappointed with this outcome, as the option could have provided additional support to those who required care within their homes and communities.

Moving Forward: Next Steps in Supporting Family Care

Numerous social and political changes are currently shaping the delivery of social work services. Greene (2005a) identifies several, such as changing demographics; changes in service delivery systems, including privatization and use of technology; and the stress of empirically based services. These changes affect how social work practice is configured (see "Changing Social Work Practice" on page 220). In regard to work with caregivers, social workers will be part of more interdisciplinary teams, involved with family-centered care models, and responsible for developing new

---

Changing Social Work Practice

Changing social, economic, and political realities affect the nature of social work. The reconfiguration of social work involves the following:

- Blurring of professional boundaries and training across disciplines
- Participating in community-based and family-centered care
- Differentiating practice to work with diverse groups
- Acting as interchangeable members of health and mental health teams
- Enacting performance-based outcome measures and evaluating effectiveness of practice
- Seeking new revenue streams
- Aiming for cost-effectiveness and cost containment
- Increasing use of technology
- Forging new community partnerships
- Collapsing the boundaries between education and practice

Source: Adapted from "Redefining Social Work for the New Millennium: Setting a Context," by R. R. Greene, 2005, *Journal of Human Behavior in the Social Environment, 11,* pp. 37–54.

---

sources of revenue and cost-effective program models for caregiving families. With these new realities, additional challenges will be part of the future agenda for supporting families in their caregiving roles.

Family-Centered Care

A family-centered care (FCC) model is most identified with health and medical practice. *FCC* is "an approach to health-care based on mutually beneficial partnerships among patients, families, and healthcare professionals" (B. Johnson, 2000, p. 138). FCC has the dual focus of attending to the patient's physical and psychosocial health and the family's needs and concerns (Kovacs, Bellin, & Fauri, 2006). The FCC model was based on the following set of assumptions (Weissbourd, 1994):

- The most effective approach to families emanates from a perspective of health and well-being.
- The capacity of parents to raise their children effectively is influenced by the parents' own development.
- Child-rearing techniques and values are influenced by cultural and community values and mores.
- Social support networks are essential to family well-being.
- Information about child development enhances parents' capacity to respond appropriately to their children.
- Families that receive support become empowered to advocate on their own behalf.

Although this set of assumptions specifically addresses the care that parents provide children, it could easily be broadened to address care provision at different points in the life course as well.

In addition to acute health concerns, FCC can assist with transitions that occur across the life course. End-of-life decisions and transitions can be particularly difficult for caregivers and may involve new services and service providers, such as hospice or palliative care. FCC practice provides relief to caregivers and assists with an understanding of the end-of-life trajectory (Kovacs et al., 2006). Securing needed resources, such as respite care or transportation, is one way to support care providers. Caregivers may also benefit from information that can help with their role in, for example, pain management and the dying process itself. For caregivers who have been in their role for a long time, assistance can also come after the death itself, when they work to create a new chapter in their life.

Labor Force and Employment Issues

In addition to their caregiving responsibilities, care providers assume other significant roles. In the case studies, employment issues surfaced as a source of both stress and resources for caregivers and families (see, for example, the Grogan family case study in chapter 5). The nature of care may create difficulties in the labor force, there may be inflexibility in the workplace, or no alternative for care may be available during the caregiver's work time.

This issue seems particularly salient for female caregivers, who often have to make adjustments in this area. In a national study, caregiving was related to decreased labor force participation for women, but not for men (Lee & Tang, 2013). The decision to leave the workplace comes with costs for the family and caregiver, including decreased financial resources, fewer benefits (including pension and Social Security credits) for their own later years, and none of the intrinsic rewards of having a job. Although some caregivers leave the labor force voluntarily, with positive outcomes in their individual and family functioning, others experience less favorable outcomes.

Public policies about employment and caregiving need to change in the United States to support female workers who have responsibility for the well-being of family members. One possibility is increasing incentives for employers to offer more flexible employment options that would allow individuals to hold part-time or flexible-time employment (Scharlach, 1994). Additionally, more liberal family or unpaid leave policies could provide caregivers with greater options to stay in the labor force (Pavalko & Henderson, 2006). A study examining cross-national comparisons reported large variance across countries as related to caregiving policy. Not surprising, Scandinavian countries had the most integrated systems of care and provided women with the greatest options and choices. The study concluded with the statement:

> Relieving women of their informal caregiving roles and enabling them to *share these roles* [italics added] with formal care providers and other resources might increase the participation of women in the labor force and thereby enhance the economic development of societies. (Jang, Avendano, & Kawachi, 2012, p. 25)

Families and Transitions

Caregiving involves numerous transitions that involve individual and family adjustments. At these junctures, families often require some assistance in recalibrating and establishing a new level of homeostasis. Social workers may need to be involved in helping the families with new tasks and roles, as well as linking them to new resources that can provide care-sharing assistance.

Several of the case situations involved transition issues. One example is the Grogan family (chapter 5), whose son Kevin had an intellectual disability, was non-ambulatory, and was reaching adolescence. The Grogan's care plan for Kevin was no longer sufficient. Transitions also affected Philip and his parents (chapter 6) as Philip's lifelong psychiatric disability became more challenging for his older parents to care for. Grandparents who are raising their grandchildren (chapter 9) face numerous transitions as well, for example, when they begin their role as caregiver or when parents reenter the situation either temporarily or permanently. At these junctures, families need help to establish a new family structure, realign roles and dynamics, and acknowledge the emotions that accompany these situations.

Social work practitioners need to be aware of how transitions affect family caregiving arrangements. Some care provision takes place over extended periods, and reassessment of functioning needs to occur regularly to determine changing needs. Research to identify the junctures and present particular risks for families should be undertaken. In addition, programs must consider these transition issues in service delivery. Several questions need to be included in an assessment:

1. What are the needs of caregivers as changes occur in the family?
2. How do these changes affect the family relationships? Are there sources of stress and strain? Are new resources that can be used to meet family needs available?
3. How do these transitions affect the care recipient? What physical, emotional, and spiritual changes occur?
4. How do these changes affect family resources? Are there existing resources that no longer address family needs? What resources are needed now?
5. What systems can help with care sharing with the family? Can formal or informal resources be tapped as partners in the caregiving task?

These questions will help practitioners consider how transitions in the family affect multiple levels of functioning.

Conclusions

This book has covered several important topics related to family caregiving. Although caregiving situations vary in many ways, some consistent messages and themes have emerged across the chapters. As a social work practitioner, you will need to individualize each caregiver and family situation. At the same time, some essential overarching principles can help you understand the experience of care with your clients.

Principle 1:
Care Provision Is a Normative Part of Family Life
and Takes Place across the Life Course

Parenting is often considered the primary type of caregiving, and all mothers and fathers know that having baby is a joyful but demanding task. As the examples in this book indicate, some families, such as those that include a son or daughter with a disability, have responsibility for care well beyond the usual time of parenting.

For some parents, their caregiving role is unending and extended into adulthood. Caregiving is also part of family life when an injury, illness, or disability occurs later in the life course. Parents who care for wounded military veterans or sons or daughters with chronic illnesses (such as diabetes or HIV) and grandparents who step in when parents cannot care for their children are examples of people moving into a caregiving role later in life. Although caregiving may take different forms, the family is the most basic unit in our society to assume care when it is needed.

Principle 2:
Caregiving Involves Both Stresses and Rewards

The chapters provided numerous examples of the stresses that caregivers experience. Caregiving tasks can take a toll on care providers' physical, emotional, and social functioning. Too often, caregivers prioritize their caregiving tasks to the detriment of their own health and well-being. An important area for social work intervention is to help caregivers manage self-care even as they provide for the well-being of the care recipient.

Although stresses exist, caregivers experience joys and rewards in their role. Unfortunately, these experiences are often not part of an assessment and therefore are not considered in social work interventions. For example, an older parent of an adult child with a disability may be challenged by the physical tasks associated with care. Yet this relationship may also be a source of companionship and support. The positive aspects of care need to be recognized in understanding the caregiving dynamic.

Principle 3:
In Addition to Care Provision, Caregivers Assume Other
Roles That Require Their Time, Attention, and Resources

Often, the stress of caregiving results from competing demands on caregivers' time. Few caregivers assume only this role; most have other family relationships that require time and attention, are employed and have job demands, and have other commitments, such as involvement in voluntary or civic organizations. Caregivers may feel overwhelmed when trying to keep all these "balls in the air" and become stressed or depressed. At this point, the caregiver might seek social work services to try and manage all these roles.

Principle 4:
Families Benefit from Care Sharing with Formal and Informal Supports

This book has used the term "care sharing" to describe a collective approach to care provision (see chapter 1). While this sounds intuitive, in reality care sharing does not occur for numerous reasons. Care sharing should be a source of support and relief for families. However, relationships with services can be a source of stress and challenge if families do not receive the type of support needed for their circumstances.

Social workers can promote care sharing in several ways. First, case management skills can link families with available resources. Second, practitioners can identify informal sources that can help the family, such as faith communities that provide outreach to those in their congregations who are in caregiving roles. Third, social workers can be involved in community organizing that brings together caregivers from several families, who can share resources and provide mutual aid to each other. Finally, practitioners can advocate to expend public support for care and increase options for families.

This book aimed to provide you with a practice framework for understanding caregiving that can improve your effectiveness as a practitioner. The initial chapters provided a context for care and an integrated model for viewing individual, family, and community contexts of care provision. The remaining chapters provided information about different caregiving configurations and case studies that illustrated the experiences of some families.

Given the number of changes in family life over the last few decades, today's social work practitioners in all types of roles will work with caregiving families. Regardless of your career path, you will most likely have some involvement with families that face challenges in caring for someone who has limitations in functioning. We hope the contents of and the experiences of the families in the book will help you understand caregiving families in your practice area.

References

AARP. (2007). *Home safety: How well does your home fit your needs?* Retrieved from http://www.aarp .org/livable-communities/info-2014/make-your-home-a-safe-home.html

AARP. (n.d.). *GrandFacts*. Retrieved from http://www.aarp.org/relationships/friends-family/grand facts-sheets/

Ackerman, N. W. (1958). *The psychodynamics of family life.* New York: Basic Books.

Ackerman, N. W. (1970). *Family process.* New York: Basic Books.

Administration for Community Living. (2013). *Administration on Intellectual and Developmental Disabilities (AIDD): The Developmental Disabilities Assistance and Bill of Rights Act of 2000.* Retrieved from http://www.acl.gov/Programs/AIDD/DDA_BOR_ACT_2000/p2_tI_subtitleA.aspx

Administration on Aging. (2011). *A profile of older Americans: 2011.* Retrieved from http://www.aoa .gov/aoaroot/aging_statistics/Profile/2011/4.aspx

Administration on Aging. (2012). *A profile of older Americans: 2012.* Retrieved from http://www.aoa .gov/Aging_Statistics/Profile/2012/3.aspx

Administration on Aging. (2013). *Aging statistics.* Retrieved from http://www.aoa.gov/aoaroot/aging_ statistics/index.aspx

Aged & Community Services Australia. (n.d.). *Beacon Hill Village, Boston.* Retrieved from http:// www.agedcare.org.au/what-we-do/housing-retirement-living/innovative-housing-solutions/ beacon-hill-village

Agosta, J., & Melda, K. (1995). Supporting families who provide care at home for children with disabilities. *Exceptional Children, 62,* 271–282.

Aguirre, J. C. (2012, July 27). Cost of treatment still a challenge for HIV patients in U.S. [Web log post]. *Shots: Health News from NPR.* Retrieved from http://www.npr.org/blogs/health/2012/07/ 27/157499134/cost-of-treatment-still-a-challenge-for-hiv-patients-in-u-s

Almasy, S. (2012, October 29). *The toll of war now includes more amputees.* Retrieved from http:// www.cnn.com/2012/05/27/us/amputee-veterans-come-home

American Association on Intellectual and Developmental Disabilities. (2013). *Frequently asked questions on intellectual disabilities.* Retrieved from http://aaidd.org/intellectual-disability/definition/ faqs-on-intellectual-disability#.Ui479z_ehsk

American Diabetes Association. (2014, June 20). *Symptoms.* Alexandria, VA: Author. Retrieved from http://www.diabetes.org/diabetes-basics/symptoms/

American Psychological Association. (2008). *Answers to your questions: For a better understanding of sexual orientation and homosexuality.* Washington, DC: Author.

American Psychological Association. (2009). *Report of the APA Task Force on Appropriate Therapeutic Responses to Sexual Orientation.* Washington, DC: Author.

American Psychological Association. (2010, November 9). *APA survey raises concern about health impact of stress on children and families.* Retrieved from http://www.apa.org/news/press/releases/2010/11/stress-in-america.aspx

American Psychological Association. (2012, January 11). *Stress in America: Our health at risk.* Retrieved from http://www.apa.org/news/press/releases/stress/2011/final-2011.pdf

American Psychological Association, Presidential Task Force on Military Deployment Services for Youth, Families, and Service Members. (2007, February). *Psychological needs of U.S. military services members & their families: A preliminary report.* Retrieved from http://www.ptsd.ne.gov/publications/military-deployment-task-force-report.pdf

Ancestor worship. (n.d.) In *Merriam-Webster's online dictionary* (11th ed.). Retrieved from http://unabridged.merriam-webster.com/unabridged/ancestor%20worship

Andersson, C., & Mattsson, E. (2001). Adults with cerebral palsy: A survey describing problems, needs, and resources, with special emphasis on locomotion. *Developmental Medicine & Child Neurology, 43*(2), 76–82.

Andrews, C. M., Darnell, J. S., McBride, T. D., & Gehlert, S. (2013). Social work and implementation of the Affordable Care Act. *Health & Social Work, 38*, 67–71.

Angel, J. L., Jiménez, M. A., & Angel, R. J. (2007). The economic consequences of widowhood for older minority women. *Gerontologist, 47*, 224–234.

Antonovsky, A. (1979). *Health, stress and coping.* San Francisco: Jossey-Bass.

Antonovsky, A. (1987). *Unraveling the mystery of health: How people manage stress and stay well.* San Francisco: Jossey-Bass.

Arieti, S. (1955). *Interpretation of schizophrenia.* New York: Brunner.

Ashish, K., Perlin, J., Kizer, K. W., & Dudley, R. A. (2003). Effect of the transformation of the Veterans Affairs health care system on the quality of care. *New England Journal of Medicine, 348*, 2218–2227.

Auldridge, A., & Espinoza, R. (2013). *Health equity and LGBT elders of color: Recommendations for policy and practice.* Thousand Oaks, CA: Sage Publications.

Austin, C. D., DesCamp, E., Flux, D., McClelland, R. W., & Sippert, J. (2005). Community development with older adults in their neighborhoods: The Elder Friendly Communities Program. *Families in Society, 86*, 401–409.

AVERT. (2013). *Worldwide HIV and AIDS statistics.* Retrieved from http://www.avert.org/worldstats.htm

Bailey, D., & Koney, K. M. (2000). *Strategic alliances among health and human service organizations: From affiliations to consolidations.* Thousand Oaks, CA: Sage Publications.

Baird, A., John, R., & Hayslip, B., Jr. (2000). Custodial grandparenting among African Americans: A focus group perspective. In B. Hayslip, Jr., & R. Goldberg-Glen (Eds.), *Grandparents raising grandchildren: Theoretical, empirical, and clinical perspectives* (pp. 125–144). New York: Springer.

Banach, M. M., Iudice, J. J., Conway, L. L., & Couse, L. J. (2010). Family support and empowerment: Post autism diagnosis support group for parents. *Social Work with Groups, 33*(1), 69–83.

Bandura, A. (1982). Self-efficacy mechanism in human agency. *American Psychologist, 37*, 122–147.

Bandura, A. (1995). Exercise of personal and collective efficacy in changing societies. In A. Bandura (Ed.), *Self-efficacy in changing societies* (pp. 1–45). New York: Cambridge University Press.

Bandura, A. (1997). *Self-efficacy: The exercise of control.* New York: Worth Publishers.

Barrett, D. L., Secic, M., & Borowske, D. (2010). The Gatekeeper Program: Proactive identification and case management of at-risk older adults prevents nursing home placement, saving healthcare dollars program evaluation. *Home Healthcare Nurse, 28*(3), 191–197.

Barrett, P., Hale, B., & Butler, M. (2014). Caring for a family member with a lifelong disability. In *Family care and social capital: Transitions in informal care* (pp. 75–90). Amsterdam: Springer.

References

Bartels, S. (2003). Improving the system of care for older adults with mental illness in the United States. *American Journal of Geriatric Psychiatry, 11,* 486–497.

Barusch, A. S. (2013). Age-friendly cities: A social work perspective. *Journal of Gerontological Social Work, 56*(6), 465–472.

Basham, K. (2008). Homecoming as safe haven or the new front: Attachment and detachment in military couples. *Clinical Social Work Journal, 36,* 83–96.

Beck, E., Britto, S., & Andrews, A. (2007). *In the shadow of death: Restorative justice and death row families.* New York: Oxford University Press.

Bengtson, V. L., Giarrusso, R., Silverstein, M., & Wang, H. (2000). Families and intergenerational relationships in aging societies. *Hallym International Journal of Aging, 2*(1), 3–10.

Bengtson, V. L., Rosenthal, C., & Burton, L. (1990). Families and ageing: Diversity and heterogeneity. In R. H. Binstock & L. George (Eds.), *Handbook of ageing and social sciences* (3rd ed., pp. 263–287). San Diego: Academic Press.

Bertalanfy, L. (1968). *General systems theory: Human relations.* New York: Braziller.

Bielefeld, W., Scotch, R. K., & Thielmann, G. S. (2000). National mandates and local nonprofits: Shaping a local delivery system of HIV/AIDS services. In F. M. Cox, J. L. Erlich, J. Rothman, & J. E. Tropman (Eds.), *Strategies in community organization* (pp. 329–336). Itasca, IL: Peacock.

Bigby, C. C., Ozanne, E. E., & Gordon, M. M. (2002). Facilitating transition: Elements of successful case management practice for older parents of adults with intellectual disability. *Journal of Gerontological Social Work, 37*(3–4), 25–43.

Birren, J. E. (1969). The concept of functional age, theoretical background. *Human Development, 12,* 214–215.

Blatt, B., & Kaplan, F. (1966). *Christmas in purgatory: A photographic essay on mental retardation.* Retrieved from http://pds15.egloos.com/pds/200907/07/96/Xmas-Purgatory.pdf

Block, M., & Gebeloff, R. (2009, March 10). Remade in America: Immigration explorer. *New York Times.* Retrieved from http://www.nytimes.com/interactive/2009/03/10/us/20090310-immigration-explorer.html

Blow, A., MacInnes, M. D., Hamel, J., Ames, B., Onaga, E., Holtrop, K., et al. (2012). National Guard service members returning home after deployment: The case for increased community support. *Administration and Policy in Mental Health, 39,* 383–393.

Blumer, H. (1969). *Symbolic interactionism: Perspective and method.* Englewood Cliffs, NJ: Prentice Hall.

Blundo, R., Greene, R. R., & Riley, J. (2012). Promoting resilience among returning veterans. In R. R. Greene (Ed.), *Resiliency: An integrated approach to practice, policy, and research* (2nd ed., pp. 307–334). Washington, DC: NASW Press.

Bobrow, J., Cook, E., Knowles, C., & Vieten, C. (2013). Coming all the way home: Integrative community care for those who serve. *Psychological Services, 10*(2), 137.

Boehm, W. W. (1958). The nature of social work. *Social Work, 3,* 10–18.

Boehm, W. W. (1959). *Objectives for the social work curriculum of the future: Social work curriculum study.* New York: Council on Social Work Education.

Bonanno, G. A. (2004). Loss, trauma, and human resilience: Have we underestimated the human capacity to thrive after extremely adverse events? *American Psychologist, 59,* 20–28.

Bond, G. R., Drake, R. E., Mueser, K. T., & Latimer, E. (2001). Assertive community treatment for people with severe mental illness: Critical ingredients and impact on patients. *Disease Management & Health Outcomes, 9,* 141–159.

Borden, W. (1992). Narrative perspectives in psychosocial intervention following adverse life events. *Social Work, 37,* 125–141.

Boszormenyi-Nagy, I., & Spark, G. (1973). *Invisible loyalties*. New York: Harper & Row.

Botsford, A. L. (2000). Integrating end of life care into services for people with an intellectual disability. *Social Work in Health Care, 31*(1), 35–48.

Bowen, E. A. (2013). AIDS at 30: Implications for social work education. *Journal of Social Work Education, 49*(2), 265–276.

Bowen, G. L., & Martin, J. A. (2011). The resiliency model of role performance for service members, veterans, and their families: A focus on social connections and individual assets. *Journal of Human Behavior in the Social Environment, 21*(2), 162–178.

Bowen, G. L., Martin, J. A., & Mancini, J. A. (2013). The resilience of military families: Theoretical perspectives. In M. A. Fine & L. D. Finchan (Eds.), *Handbook of family theories: A content-based approach* (pp. 417–436). New York: Routledge.

Bowen, G. L., Martin, J. A., Mancini, J. A., & Nelson, J. P. (2001). Civic engagement and sense of community in the military. *Journal of Community Practice, 9*(2), 71–93.

Boykin, A. W., & Toms, F. D. (1985). Black child socialization: A conceptual framework. In H. P. McAdoo & J. L. McAdoo (Eds.), *Black children* (pp. 33–52). Beverly Hills, CA: Sage Publications.

Boyle, C. A., Boulet, S., Schieve, L. A., Cohen, R. A., Blumberg, S. J., Yeargin-Allsopp, M., et al. (2011). Trends in the prevalence of developmental disabilities in US children, 1997–2008. *Pediatrics, 127*, 1034–1042.

Braddock, D., Hemp, R., Rizzolo, M. C., Haffer, L., Tanis, E. S., & Wu, J. (2011). *The state of the states in developmental disabilities, 2011.* Washington, DC: American Association on Intellectual and Developmental Disabilities.

Bradley, E., & Taylor, L. A. (2013, November). US health care paradox: How spending more is getting us less. Seminar presented at the 141st American Public Health Association Annual Meeting, Boston.

Brick, R., Cushing-Savvi, A., Elshafie, S., Krill, A., Scanion, M., & Stone, M. (2010). *Refugee resettlement in the U.S.: An examination of the challenges and proposed solutions.* New York: Columbia University Press.

Bride, E. B., & Figley, C. R. (2009). Secondary trauma and military veteran caregivers. *Smith College Studies for Social Work, 79*, 314–329.

Brody, E. (1985). Parent care as normative family stress. *Gerontologist, 25*, 19–29.

Bronfenbrenner, U. (1979). *The ecology of human development.* Cambridge, MA: Harvard University Press.

Bronfenbrenner, U. (1990). Discovering what families do. In D. Blankenhorn, S. Bayme, & J. B. Elshtain (Eds.), *Rebuilding the nest: A new commitment to the American family* (pp. 27–38). New York: Family Service America.

Bronski, M. (2003, November 14). *Rewriting the script on Reagan: Why the president ignored AIDS.* Retrieved from http://forward.com/articles/7046/rewriting-the-script-on-reagan-why-the-president/

Brotman, S., Ryan, B., Collins, S., Chamberland, L., Cormier, R., Julien, D., et al. (2007). Coming out to care: Caregivers of gay and lesbian seniors in Canada. *Gerontologist, 47*, 490–503.

Browning, C. R., & Cagney, K. A. (2003). Moving beyond poverty: Neighborhood structure, social processes, and health. *Journal of Health and Social Behavior, 44*, 552–571.

Buckley, W. (1968). Society as a complex adaptive system. In W. Buckley (Ed.), *Modern systems research for the behavioral scientist* (pp. 490–511). Chicago: Aldine.

Bumiller, E. (2012, September 19). One year later, military says gay policy is working. *New York Times*, p. A17.

Bureau of Labor Statistics. (2013, June 13). Persons with a disability: Labor force characteristics summary [Press release]. Retrieved from http://www.bls.gov/news.release/disabl.nr0.htm

References

Burnette, D. (1997). Grandparents raising grandchildren in the inner city. *Families in Society, 78*, 489–501.

Burns, T., Catty, J., Dash, M., Roberts, C., Lockwood, A., & Marshall, M. (2007). Use of intensive case management to reduce time in hospital in people with severe mental illness: Systematic review and meta-regression. *British Medical Journal, 335*(7615), 336.

Burton, L. M. (1992). Black grandparents rearing children of drug-addicted parents: Stressors, outcomes, and social service needs. *Gerontologist, 32*, 744–751.

Burton, L. M., & Dilworth-Anderson, P. (1991). The intergenerational family roles of aged Black Americans. *Marriage & Family Review, 16*(3/4), 311–330.

Bush, N., Bosmajian, C. P., Fairall, J. M., McCann, R. A., & Ciulla, R. P. (2011). Afterdeployment.org: A Web-based multimedia wellness resource for the postdeployment military community. *Professional Psychology: Research and Practice, 42*, 455–462.

Butler, R. N. (1963). The life review: An interpretation of reminiscence in the aged. *Psychiatry, 26*, 65–76.

Butler, R. N. (1975). *Why survive? Being old in America.* New York: Harper & Row.

Cagney, K. A., Browning, C. R., & Wen, M. (2005). Racial disparities in self-rated health at older ages: What difference does the neighborhood make? *Journal of Gerontology: Social Sciences, 60B*, S181–S190.

Calhoun, L. G., & Tedeschi, R. G. (2006). *Handbook of posttraumatic growth: Research and practice.* Mahwah, NJ: Erlbaum.

Cappadocia, M. C., Weiss, J. A., & Pepler, D. (2012). Bullying experiences among children and youth with autism spectrum disorders. *Journal of Autism and Developmental Disorders, 42*(2), 266–277.

Cardoso, J. B., & Thompson, S. J. (2010). Common themes of resilience among Latino immigrant families: A systematic review of the literature. *Families in Society, 91*, 257–265.

Carroll, J. M., & Rosson, M. B. (1996, December). Developing the Blacksburg Electronic Village. *Communications of the ACM, 39*(12), 69–74.

Carter, A., Briggs-Gowan, M., & Davis, N. (2004). Assessment of young children's social-emotional development and psychopathology: Recent advances and recommendations for practice. *Journal of Child Psychology and Psychiatry, and Allied Disciplines, 45*(1), 109–134.

Carter, B., & McGoldrick, M. (Eds.). (1999). *The expanded family life cycle: Individual, family, and social perspectives* (3rd ed.). Boston: Allyn & Bacon.

Carter, B., & McGoldrick, M. (Eds.). (2005). *The expanded family life cycle: Individual, family, and social perspectives* (3rd ed.). Boston: Allyn & Bacon.

Centers for Disease Control and Prevention. (2007, June 21). *Living with HIV: Treatment.* Retrieved from http://www.cdc.gov/hiv/living/

Centers for Disease Control and Prevention. (2010, March 10). *CDC analysis provides new look at disproportionate impact of HIV and syphilis among U.S. gay and bisexual men.* Retrieved from http://www.cdc.gov/nchhstp/newsroom/2010/msmpressrelease.html

Centers for Disease Control and Prevention. (2011a). *HIV surveillance report, 2009* (Vol. 21). Retrieved from http://www.cdc.gov/hiv/topics/surveillance/resources/reports

Centers for Disease Control and Prevention. (2011b). HIV surveillance—United States, 1981–2008. *Morbidity and Mortality Weekly Report, 60*, 689–693.

Centers for Disease Control and Prevention. (2011c, January 26). Number of Americans with diabetes rises to nearly 26 million [Press release]. Retrieved from http://www.cdc.gov/media/releases/2011/p0126_diabetes.html

Centers for Disease Control and Prevention. (2011d). Vital signs: HIV prevention through care and treatment—United States. *Morbidity and Mortality Weekly Report, 60*, 1618–1623.

Centers for Disease Control and Prevention. (2012a, November 27). *HIV among youth: Protecting a generation.* Retrieved from http://www.cdc.gov/Features/vitalsigns/hivAmongYouth/

Centers for Disease Control and Prevention. (2012b). *Key findings: Trends in the prevalence of developmental disabilities in U.S. children, 1997–2008.* Retrieved from http://www.cdc.gov/ncbddd/features/birthdefects-dd-keyfindings.html

Centers for Disease Control and Prevention. (2012c). *Specific conditions.* Retrieved from http://www.cdc.gov/ncbddd/developmentaldisabilities/specificconditions.html

Chan, J. (2008). A profile of respite providers in New South Wales. *Journal of Disability, Development & Education, 589,* 289–302.

Chan, J., Merriman, B., Parmenter, T., & Stancliffe, R. (2012). Rethinking respite policy for people with intellectual and developmental disabilities. *Journal of Practice and Policy in Intellectual Disabilities, 9,* 120–126.

Chan, J., & Sigafoos, J. (2000). A review of family and child characteristics related to the use of respite care in developmental disability services. *Child and Youth Forum, 29,* 27–39.

Chan, S., & Kim, A. U. (2003). *Not just victims: Conversations with Cambodian community leaders in the United States.* Chicago: University of Illinois Press.

Chandra, A., Acosta, J., Meredith, L. S., Sanches, K., Stern, S., Uscher-Pines, L., et al. (2010, February). *Understanding community resilience in the context of national health security.* Santa Monica, CA: Rand Health.

Chang, B. H., Stein, N. R., Trevino, K., Stewart, M., Hendricks, A., & Skarf, L. M. (2012). Spiritual needs and spiritual care for veterans at end of life and their families. *American Journal of Hospice and Palliative Medicine, 29,* 610–671.

Chapin, R., & Cox, E. O. (2001). Changing the paradigm: Strengths-based and empowerment or oriented social work with frail elders. *Gerontological Social Work Practice: Issues, Challenges, and Potential, 36,* 165–179.

Chappell, N., & Funk, L. M. (2011). Social support, caregiving, and aging. *Canadian Journal on Aging, 30,* 355–370.

Chaskin, R. J. (2001). Building community capacity: A definitional framework and case studies from a comprehensive community initiative. *Urban Affairs Review, 36,* 291–323.

Chen, W. Y., & Lukens, E. (2011). Well being, depressive symptoms, and burden among parent and sibling caregivers of persons with severe and persistent mental illness. *Social Work in Mental Health, 9,* 397–416.

Chestang, L. W. (1984). Racial and personal identity in the Black experience. In B. W. White (Ed.), *Color in a White society* (pp. 83–94). Silver Spring, MD: NASW Press.

Child Welfare League of America. (n.d.). *Kinship care: About the program.* Retrieved from http://www.cwla.org/programs/kinship/kinshipaboutpage.htm

Chiswick, B. R., & Miller, P. W. (2004). *Where immigrants settle in the United States* [Discussion Paper No. 1231]. Bonn, Germany: Institute for the Study of Labor.

Choi, N. G., & Mayer, J. (2000). Elder abuse, neglect, and exploitation. *Journal of Gerontological Social Work, 33*(2), 5–25.

Christopoulos, K. A., Kaplan, B., Dowdy, D., Haller, B., Nassos, P., Roemer, M., et al. (2011). Testing and linkage to care outcomes for a clinician-initiated rapid HIV testing program in an urban emergency department. *AIDS Patient Care & STDs, 25,* 439–444.

Cianciotto, J., & Cahill, S. R. (2003). *Education policy: Issues affecting lesbian, gay, bisexual and transgender youth.* New York: National Gay and Lesbian Task Force Policy Institute.

Clayton, L. (2012). Jill Biden announces NASW's commitment to Joining Forces initiative. *NASW News, 57*(8), 1.

References

Clements, J. A., & Rosenwald, M. (2008). Foster parents' perspectives on LGB youth in the child welfare system. *Journal of Gay & Lesbian Social Services, 19*(1), 57–69.

Cohen, C. I. (2003). Introduction. In C. I. Cohen (Ed.), *Schizophrenia into later life* (pp. xiii–xx). Washington, DC: American Psychiatric Publishing.

Cohen, C. I., & Ibrahim, F. (2012). Serving elders in the public sector. In H. L. McQuistion, W. E. Sowers, J. M. Ranz, & J. M. Feldman (Eds.), *Handbook of Community Psychiatry* (pp. 485–502). New York: Springer.

Cohen, H., & Murray, Y. (2006). Older lesbian and gay caregivers: Caring for families of choice and caring for families of origin. In R. R. Greene (Ed.), *Contemporary issues in life care* (pp. 275–298). New York: Haworth Press.

Coie, J. D., Watt, N. F., West, S. G., Hawkins, J. D., Asarnow, J. R., Markman, H. J., et al. (1993). The science of prevention: A conceptual framework and some directions for a national research program. *American Psychologist, 48*, 1013–1022.

Collins, J. (1998). The complex context of American military culture: A practitioner's view. *Washington Quarterly, 21*(4), 213–228.

Collins, W. L. (2011). A strengths-based support group to empower African American grandmothers raising grandchildren. *Social Work & Christianity, 38*, 453–466.

Congress, E. P. (1994). The use of culturagrams to assess and empower culturally diverse families. *Families in Society, 75*, 531–540.

Congressional Budget Office. (2012). *Estimates for the insurance coverage provisions of the Affordable Care Act updated for the recent Supreme Court decision.* Washington, DC: Author.

Conley, C. L. (2011). Learning about a child's gay or lesbian sexual orientation: Parental concerns about societal rejection, loss of loved ones, and child well being. *Journal of Homosexuality, 58*, 1022–1040.

Coontz, S. (2006). *Marriage, a history: How love conquered marriage.* New York: Penguin.

Corman, J. M. & Kingson, E. R. (1996). Trends, issues, perspectives, and values for the aging of the baby boom cohort. *Gerontologist, 36*, 15–26.

Council of Economic Advisers. (2007, June 20). *Immigration's economic impact.* Retrieved from georgewbush-whitehouse.archives.gov/cea/cea_immigration_062007.html

Council of Economic Advisers. (2013). *The economics of commonsense immigration reform from the economic report of the president.* Washington, DC: Author.

Council on Social Work Education. (2008). *Educational policy and accreditation standards.* Alexandria, VA: Author.

Council on Social Work Education. (2010). *Advanced military social work practice guidelines.* Alexandria, VA: Author.

Council on Social Work Education. (2012, August). *Educational policy and accreditation standards* [Updated online version]. Retrieved from http://www.cswe.org/File.aspx?id=41861

Country Doctor. (2010, October 22). Continuity of care starts with caring [Web log post]. *KevinMD .com.* Retrieved from http://www.kevinmd.com/blog/2010/10/continuity-care-starts-caring.html

Covan, E. K. (1998). Caresharing: Hiding frailty in a Florida retirement community. *Health Care for Women International, 19*(5), 423–439.

Cox, C. (2008). Empowerment as an intervention with grandparent caregivers. *Journal of Intergenerational Relationships, 6*(4), 465–477.

Cox, C., Brooks, L. R., & Valcarcel, C. (2000). Culture and caregiving: A study of Latino grandparents. In C. Cox (Ed.), *To grandmother's house we go and stay: Perspectives on custodial grandparents* (pp. 215–233). New York: Springer.

Cranford, P. G. (2008). *But for the grace of God: The inside story of the world's largest insane asylum* [ePub version]. Retrieved from http://www.lulu.com/shop/dr-peter-g-cranford/but-for-the-grace-of-god-the-inside-story-of-the-worlds-largest-insane-asylum/ebook/product-20706162.html

Crowther, M. R., Parker, M. W., Achenbaum, W. A., Larimore, W. L., & Koenig, H. G. (2002). Rowe and Kahn's model of successful aging revisited: Positive spirituality—The forgotten factor. *Gerontologist, 42,* 613–620.

Cummings, S. M., & Kropf, N. P. (2009a). Formal and informal support for older adults with severe mental illness. *Aging and Mental Health, 13,* 619–627.

Cummings, S. M., & Kropf, N. P. (Eds.). (2009b). *Handbook of psychosocial interventions with older adults: Evidence-based treatment.* London, England: Routledge.

Cummings, S. M., & Kropf, N. P. (2011). Aging with a severe mental illness: Challenges and treatments. *Journal of Gerontological Social Work, 54*(2), 175–188.

Cummings, S. M., Kropf, N. P., Cassie, K. M., & Bride, B. (2004). Evidence-based treatment for older adults. *Journal of Evidence-Based Social Work, 1*(4), 53–81.

Cummings, S. M., & MacNeil, G. (2008). Caregivers of older clients with severe mental illness: Perceptions of burdens and rewards. *Families in Society, 89,* 51–59.

Daatland, S. O. (1983). Care systems. *Aging and Society, 3*(Pt. 1), 21–33.

Darnell, J. S. (2013). Navigators and assisters: Two case management roles for social workers in the Affordable Care Act. *Health & Social Work, 38,* 123–126.

Dawson, G., Ashman, S. B., & Carver, L. J. (2000). The role of early experience in shaping behavioral and brain development and its implications for social policy. *Development and Psychopathology, 12,* 695–712.

DC Appleseed. (2006, September 24). *HIV in the nation's capital: Improving the District of Columbia's response to a public health crisis.* Retrieved from http://www.dcappleseed.com/wp-content/uploads/2013/08/ReportCard2.0.pdf

Demers, A. (2011). When veterans return: The role of community in reintegration. *Journal of Loss and Trauma, 16*(2), 160–179.

Department of Health. (n.d.). *Adult Social Care Outcomes Framework 2014 to 2015.* Retrieved from https://www.gov.uk/government/topics/social-care

Derose, K. P., Dominguez, B., Plimpton, J. H., & Kanouse, D. E. (2010). Project New Hope: A faith-based effort to provide housing for persons with HIV/AIDs. *Journal of HIV/AIDS & Social Services, 9*(1), 90–105.

de Winter, C. F., Bastiaanse, L. P., Hilgenkamp, T.I.M., Evenhuis, H. M., & Echteld, M. A. (2012). Overweight and obesity in older people with intellectual disability. *Research in Developmental Disabilities, 33,* 398–405.

Diacosvvas, A. P., & Specjal, A. (2012, January). *The meaning of personal sacrifice and its impact on combat trauma recovery of Iraq/Afghanistan veterans: Individual, community, and national resilience and the relations among them.* Paper presented at Trauma through the Life Cycle from a Strengths Perspective, Hebrew University, Jerusalem. Retrieved from http://traumaconference.huji.ac.il/presentations/Psirakis_Diacosvvas.pdf

Diamond, P. M., Wang, E. W., Holzer, C. E., Thomas, C., & Cruser, D. A. (2001). The prevalence of mental illness in prison. *Administration and Policy in Mental Health, 29,* 21–40.

Dilworth-Anderson, P., Williams, I. C., & Gibson, B. E. (2002). Issues of race, ethnicity, and culture in caregiving research: A 20-year review (1980–2000). *Gerontologist, 42,* 237–272.

Dolgoff, R., & Feldstein, D. (2008). *Understanding social welfare: A search for justice* (8th ed.). Boston: Pearson.

References

Drake, R. E., Green, A. I., Mueser, K. T., & Goldman, H. H. (2003). The history of community mental health treatment and rehabilitation for persons with severe mental illness. *Community Mental Health Journal, 39*(5), 427–440.

Drukker, M., Kaplan, C., Feron, F., & van Os, J. (2003). Children's health-related quality of life, neighbourhood socio-economic deprivation and social capital: A contextual analysis. *Social Science & Medicine, 57*, 825–841.

Duke Global Health Institute. (2012, May 2). *Addressing a stigmatized health issue among Bhutanese refugees*. Retrieved from https://globalhealth.duke.edu/media/news/addressing-stigmatized-health-issue-among-bhutanese-refugees

Duncan, B. L., Solovey, A. D., & Rusk, G. S. (1992). *Changing the rules: A client directed approach to therapy*. New York: Guilford Press.

Dunkin, J. J., & Anderson-Hanley, C. (1998). Dementia caregiver burden. *Neurology, 51*, 553–560.

Duran, B., Harrison, M., Shurley, M., Foley, K., Morris, P., Davidson-Stroh, L., et al. (2010). Tribally-driven HIV/AIDS health services partnerships: Evidence-based meets culture-centered interventions. *Journal of HIV/AIDS & Social Services, 9*(2), 110–129.

Dy, K. (2007). *A history of democratic Kampuchea (1975–1979)*. Phnom Penh, Cambodia: Documentation Center of Cambodia.

Dyck, D. G., Short, R., & Vitaliano, P. P. (1999). Predictors of burden and infectious illness in schizophrenia caregivers. *Psychosomatic Medicine, 61*, 411–419.

Dykens, E. M. (2005). Happiness, well-being, and character strengths: Outcomes for families and siblings of persons with mental retardation. *Mental Retardation, 43*(5), 360–364.

Elder, G. H. (1978). History, family, and the life cycle. In T. K. Haraven (Ed.), *Transitions and the family life course in historical perspective* (pp. 17–64). New York: Academic Press.

Elder, G. H., Gimbel, C., & Ivie, R. (1991). Turning points in life: The case of military service and war. *Military Psychology, 3*(4), 215–231.

Elizur, Y., & Ziv, M. A. (2001). Family support and acceptance, gay male identity formation, and psychological adjustment: A path model. *Family Process, 40*, 125–144.

Emrick, M., & Hayslip, B., Jr. (1999). Custodial grandparenting: Stresses, coping skills, and relationships with grandchildren. *International Journal of Aging and Human Development, 48*(1), 35–62.

Erikson, E. H. (1950). *Childhood and society*. New York: W. W. Norton.

Fair, E., Williams, K., & Janis, T. (2013, March 16). A war, before and after, part 1 [Web log post]. *Opinionator*. Retrieved from http://opinionator.blogs.nytimes.com/2013/03/16/a-war-before-and-after/

Falck, H. (1988). *Social work: The membership perspective*. New York: Springer.

Family Acceptance Project. (n.d.). Retrieved from http://familyproject.sfsu.edu/

Family Caregiver Alliance. (2004). *Caregiving in the U.S.—National Alliance for Caregiving*. Retrieved from http://www.caregiving.org/data/04finalreport.pdf

Family Caregiver Alliance. (2012, December 31). *Selected caregiver statistics*. Retrieved from http://www.caregiver.org/caregiver/jsp/content_node.jsp?nodeid=439

Farran, C., Miller, B., Kaufman, J., Donner, D., & Fogg, L. (1999). Finding meaning through caregiving: Development of an instrument for family caregivers of persons with Alzheimer's disease. *Journal of Clinical Psychology, 55*, 1107–1125.

Farris, K. D. (2007). The role of African-American pastors in mental health care. *Journal of Human Behavior in the Social Environment, 14*(1–2), 159–182.

Federal Interagency Forum on Aging Related Statistics. (2012). *Older Americans 2012: Key indicators of well-being*. Retrieved from http://www.agingstats.gov/agingstatsdotnet/Main_Site/Data/2012_Documents/Docs/EntireChartbook.pdf

Federal Reserve Bank of Dallas. (2008). Banks building markets by building communities. *Banking and Community Perspectives, Issue 1.* Retrieved from http://www.dallasfed.org/assets/documents/cd/bcp/2008/bcp0801.pdf

Feinberg, L. F., Reinhard, S. C., Houser, A., & Choula, R. (2011). *Valuing the invaluable: 2011 update—The growing contributions and costs of family caregiving.* Washington, DC: AARP Policy Institute.

Fenning, R. M., & Baker, J. K. (2012). Mother–child interaction and resilience in children with early developmental risk. *Journal of Family Psychology, 26,* 411.

Fields, J., O'Connell, M., & Downs, B. (2001). *Grandparents in the United States, 2001.* Washington, DC: U.S. Census Bureau, Housing and Household Economic Statistics Division. Retrieved from http://www.census.gov/population/www/socdemo/grandparents2001SIPP.pdf

Figley, C. F. (Ed.). (1995). *Compassion fatigue: Coping with secondary traumatic stress disorder in those who treat the traumatized.* New York: Brunner/Mazel.

Find Youth Info. (n.d.) *Map my community.* Retrieved from http://www.findyouthinfo.gov/maps/map-my-community

Floyd, F. J., & Stein, T. S. (2002). Sexual orientation identity formation among gay, lesbian, and bisexual youths: Multiple patterns of milestone experiences. *Journal of Research on Adolescence, 12*(2), 167–191.

Fong, R., & Greene, R. R. (2009). Resettlement. In R. R. Greene (Ed.), *Resiliency theory: An integrated framework for practice, research, and policy* (2nd ed., pp. 147–165). Washington, DC: NASW Press.

Fowler, M. G., Gable, A. R., Lampe, M. A., Etima, M., & Owor, M. (2010). Perinatal HIV and its prevention: Progress toward an HIV-free generation. *Clinics in Perinatology, 37,* 699–719.

Frank, C., Kurland, J., & Goldman, B. (1978). *Tips for getting the best from the rest.* Baltimore: Jewish Family & Children's Service.

Frankl, A., & Gelman, S. (1998). *Case management: An introduction to concepts and skills.* Chicago: Lyceum.

Fraser, M. (1997). *Risk and resilience in childhood.* Washington, DC: NASW Press.

Fredriksen-Goldsen, K. I., Kim, H.-J., Emlet, C. A., Muraco, A., Erosheva, E. A., Hoy-Ellis, C. P., et al. (2011). *The aging and health report: Disparities and resilience among lesbian, gay, bisexual, and transgender older adults.* Seattle: Institute for Multigenerational Health.

Freedman, L. L. (2008). Accepting the unacceptable: Religious parents and adult gay and lesbian children. *Families in Society, 89,* 237–244.

Freire, P. (1990). *Pedagogy of the oppressed.* New York: Continuum.

Fuller-Thomson, E., & Minkler, M. (2003). Housing issues and realities facing grandparent caregivers who are renters. *Gerontologist, 37,* 406–411.

Fuller-Thomson, E., & Minkler, M. (2005). American Indian/Alaskan Native grandparents raising grandchildren: Findings from the Census 2000 Supplementary Survey. *Social Work, 50,* 131–139.

Fuller-Thomson, E., Minkler, M., & Driver, D. (1997). A profile of grandparents raising grandchildren in the United States. *Gerontologist, 37,* 406–411.

Furniss, T., Müller, J. M., Achtergarde, S., Wessing, I., Averbeck-Holocher, M., & Postert, C. (2013). Implementing psychiatric day treatment for infants, toddlers, preschoolers and their families: A study from a clinical and organizational perspective. *International Journal of Mental Health Systems, 7*(1), 12. Retrieved from http://www.ijmhs.com/content/7/1/12

Gallegos, A., White, C. R., Ryan, C., O'Brien, K., Pecora, P., & Preneka, T. (2011). Exploring the experiences of lesbian, gay, bisexual, and questioning adolescents in foster care. *Journal of Family Social Work, 14*(3), 226–236.

Garbarino, J. (1982). *Children and families in the environment.* New York: Aldine de Gruyter.

Gardner, E. M., McLees, M. P., Steiner, J. F., del Rio, C., & Burman, W. J. (2011). The spectrum of engagement in HIV care and its relevance to test-and-treat strategies for prevention of HIV infection. *Clinical Infectious Diseases, 52,* 793–800.

References

Gardner, L. I., Metsch, L. R., Anderson-Mahoney, P., Loughlin, A. M., del Rio, C., Strathdee, S., et al. (2005). Efficacy of a brief case management intervention to link recently diagnosed HIV-infected persons to care. *AIDS, 19,* 423–431.

Garity, J. (1997). Stress, learning style, resilience factors, and ways of coping in Alzheimer family caregivers. *American Journal of Alzheimer's Disease, 12*(4), 171–178.

Garmezy, N. (1974). The study of children at risk: New perspectives for developmental psychopathology. In E. J. Anthony & C. Koupernik (Eds.), *The child in his family: Children at psychiatric risk* (Vol. 3, pp. 77–97). New York: John Wiley & Sons.

Gates, G. J. (2011, April). *How many people are lesbian, gay, bisexual, and transgender?* Retrieved from the Williams Institute Web site, http://williamsinstitute.law.ucla.edu/wp-content/uploads/Gates-How-Many-People-LGBT-Apr-2011.pdf

Gates, R. M. (2009, October 26). *Mental health summit* [Speech]. Retrieved from Department of Defense Web site, http://www.defense.gov/speeches/speech.aspx?speechid=1391

Genero, N. P. (1998). Culture, resiliency, and mutual psychological development. In H. I. McCubbin, E. A. Thompson, A. I. Thompson, & J. A. Futrell (Eds.), *Resiliency in African-American families* (pp. 31–48). Thousand Oaks, CA: Sage Publications.

GeoCurrents. (2010, March). New York Times *"immigration explorer" interactive map.* Retrieved from http://www.nytimes.com/interactive/2009/03/10/us/20090310-immigration-explorer.html?module=Search&mabReward=relbias%3Ar

Gergen, K. J. (1985a). *Social constructionist inquiry: Context and implications.* New York: Springer.

Gergen, K. J. (1985b). The social constructionist movement in modern psychology. *American Psychologist, 40*(3), 266.

Germain, C. B. (1994). Emerging conceptions of family development over the life course. *Families in Society, 75,* 259–268.

Getachew, I. (2012, August 6). *Ethiopia, 6 August, 2012: More HIV-positive mothers deliver babies free of the virus.* Nairobi, Kenya: Eastern and South Africa Regional Office, UNICEF. Retrieved from http://www.unicef.org/esaro/5440_Ethiopia_more_babies_born_HIV_free.html

Gettings, R. M. (2012). *Forging a federal–state partnership.* Washington, DC: American Association on Intellectual and Developmental Disabilities.

Giarrusso, R., Silverstein, M., & Feng, D. (2000). Psychological costs and benefits of raising grandchildren: Evidence from a national survey of grandparents. In C. B. Cox (Ed.), *To grandmother's house we go and stay: Perspectives on custodial grandparents* (71–90). New York: Springer.

Gilligan, S. G., & Price, R. (1993) *Therapeutic conversations.* New York: Brunner/Mazel.

Gindin, W. S. (2013, June 19). Legacy and continued viability of Lautenberg Amendment. *Legal Intelligencer.* Retrieved from http://www.law.com/jsp/pa/PubArticlePA.jsp?id=1202607086104&slreturn=20131004161235#ixzz2jiJpVDK2

Giordano, T. P., Gifford, A. L., White, A. C., Suarez-Almazor, M. E., Rabeneck, L., Hartman, C., & Morgan, R. O. (2007). Retention in care: A challenge to survival with HIV infection. *Clinical Infectious Diseases, 44,* 1493–1499.

Goffman, E. (1961). *Asylums: Essays on the social situation of mental patients and other inmates.* New York: Doubleday.

Goffman, E. (1963). *Stigma: Notes on the management of spoiled identity.* New York: Prentice Hall.

Goffman, E., & Helmreich, W. B. (1961). *Asylums: Essays on the social situation of mental patients and other inmates* (Vol. 277). New York: Anchor Books.

Goldberg-Glen, R., Sands, R. G., Cole, R., & Cristofalo, C. (1998). Multigenerational patterns and internal structures in families in which grandparents raise grandchildren. *Families in Society, 79,* 477–489.

Golden, R. L. (2011). Coordination, integration, and collaboration: A clear path for social work in health care reform. *Health & Social Work, 36,* 227–228.

Goodman, C., & Silverstein, M. (2002). Grandparents raising grandchildren: Family structure and well-being in culturally diverse families. *Gerontologist, 42,* 676–689.

Gordon, E. W., & Song, L. D. (1994). Variations in the experience of resilience. In M. C. Wang & E. W. Gordon (Eds.), *Educational resilience in inner-city America: Challenges and prospects* (pp. 27–44). Hillsdale, NJ: Erlbaum.

Goreczny, A. J., Bender, E. E., Caruso, G., & Feinstein, C. S. (2011). Attitudes toward individuals with disabilities: Results of a recent survey and implications of those results. *Research in Developmental Disabilities, 32*(5), 1596–1609.

Gorman, W. (2001). Refugee survivors of torture: Trauma and treatment. *Professional Psychology, Research, and Practice, 32,* 443–451.

Gottlieb, A. G., Silverstein, N. M., Bruner-Canhoto, L., & Montgomery, S. (2000). *Life at GrandFamilies House: The first six months.* Retrieved from University of Massachusetts–Boston ScholarWorks Web site, scholarworks.umb.edu/cgi/viewcontent.cgi?article=1022&context=gerontologyinstitute_pubs

Goyer, A. (2010, December 20). *More grandparents raising grandkids.* Retrieved from AARP Web site, http://www.aarp.org/relationships/grandparenting/info-12-2010/more_grandparents_raising_grandchildren.html

Goyer, A. (2011, September 19). Grand day for a GrandRally [Web log post]. *AARP Blog.* Retrieved from http://blog.aarp.org/2011/09/19/grand-day-for-a-grandrally-2/

Green, J. W. (1999). *Cultural awareness in the human services: A multi-ethnic approach* (3rd ed.). Boston: Allyn & Bacon.

Greenberg, A. E., Hader, S. L., Masur, H., Young, A. T., Skillicorn, J., & Dieffenbach, C. W. (2009). Fighting HIV/AIDS in Washington, D.C. *Health Affairs, 28,* 1677–1687.

Greenberg, J. S., Greenley, J. R., & Brown, R. (1997). Do mental health services reduce distress in families of people with serious mental illness? *Psychiatric Rehabilitation Journal, 21*(1), 40–50.

Greene, R. R. (1986). *Social work with the aged and their families.* Hawthorne, NY: Aldine de Gruyter.

Greene, R. R. (2002). Holocaust survivors: A study in resilience. *Journal of Gerontological Social Work, 37*(1), 3–18.

Greene, R. R. (2005a). The changing family of later years and social work practice. In L. Kaye (Ed.), *Productive aging* (pp. 107–122). Washington, DC: NASW Press.

Greene, R. R. (2005b). Family life. In L. W. Kaye (Ed.), *Perspectives on productive aging: Social work with the new aged* (pp. 107–122). Washington, DC: NASW Press.

Greene, R. R. (2005c). Redefining social work for the new millennium: Setting a context. *Journal of Human Behavior in the Social Environment, 10*(4), 37–54.

Greene, R. R. (2007). *Social work practice: A risk and resilience perspective.* Monterey, CA: Brooks/Cole.

Greene, R. R. (2008a). *Human behavior theory and social work practice* (3rd ed.). New Brunswick, NJ: Aldine Transaction Press.

Greene, R. R. (2008b). Resilience. In T. Mizrahi & L. E. Davis (Eds.), *Encyclopedia of social work* (Vol. 3, 20th ed., pp. 526–531). Washington, DC: NASW Press.

Greene, R. R. (2008c). *Social work with the aged and their families.* New Brunswick, NJ: Aldine Transaction Press.

Greene, R. R. (2010). Family dynamics, the Nazi Holocaust, and mental health treatment. *Journal of Human Behavior in the Social Environment, 20*(4), 469–488.

Greene, R. R. (2012). *Resiliency theory: An integrated framework for practice, research, and policy* (2nd ed.). Washington, DC: NASW Press.

Greene, R. R., & Cohen, H. L. (2005). Social work with older adults and their families: Changing practice paradigms. *Families in Society, 86,* 367–373.

References

Greene, R. R., Cohen, H. L., Galambos, C. M., & Kropf, N. P. (2007). *Foundations of social work practice in the field of aging: A competency-based approach*. Washington, DC: NASW Press.

Greene, R. R., Cohen, H. L., Gonzalez, J., & Lee, Y. (2009). *Narratives of social and economic justice*. Washington, DC: NASW Press.

Greene, R. R., & Graham, S. (2009). Role of resilience among Nazi Holocaust survivors: A strength-based paradigm for understanding survivorship. *Family & Community Health, 32*(1), S75–S82.

Greene, R. R., & Jones, S. (2006). Introduction: The functional-age model of intergenerational treatment. In R. R. Greene (Ed.), *Contemporary issues in life care* (pp. 1–30). New York: Haworth Press.

Greene, R. R., & Kropf, N. P. (2009). *Human behavior: A diversity framework* (2nd ed.). New Brunswick, NJ: AldineTransaction Press.

Greene, R. R., & Kropf, N. P. (2011). *Competence: Select theoretical frameworks*. New Brunswick, NJ: Aldine Transaction Press.

Greene, R. R., & Livingston, N. (2012). Resilience: A social construct. In R. R. Greene (Ed.), *Resiliency: An integrated approach to practice, policy, and research* (2nd ed., pp. 63–94). Washington, DC: NASW Press.

Greene, R. R., & Ubel, M. (2007). Intervention continued: Providing care through case management. In R. R. Greene (Ed.), *Contemporary issues of care* (pp. 31–50). New York: Haworth Press.

Greenlee, K. (2011, October 14). Memorandum on the CLASS program to Secretary Sebelius. Retrieved from U.S. Department of Health and Human Services Web site, http://aspe.hhs.gov/daltcp/reports/2011/class/CLASSmemo.pdf

Greeno, C. G. (2013). Mental health: Overview. *Encyclopedia of Social Work*. Retrieved from http://socialwork.oxfordre.com/view/10.1093/acrefore/9780199975839.001.0001/acrefore-9780199975839-e-598?rskey=jm6aI4&result=1

Grossman, A., D'Augelli, A. R., & Dragowski, E. A. (2007). Caregiving and care receiving among older lesbian, gay, and bisexual adults. *Journal of Gay & Lesbian Social Services, 18*(3–4), 15–38.

Guilford, M., Naithani, S., & Morgan, M. (2006). What is "continuity of care"? *Journal of Health Services Research & Policy, 11*(4), 248–250.

Haraven, T. K. (1978). *Transitions and the family life course in historical perspective*. New York: Academic Press.

Harper, W. J., Hardesty, P. H., & Woody, D. J. (2001). Differentiating characteristics and needs of minority grandparent caregivers. *Journal of Ethnic and Cultural Diversity in Social Work, 9*, 133–150.

Hart, M. (1999). *Guide to sustainable community indicators* (2nd ed.). North Andover, MA: Hart Environmental Data.

Hash, K. (2002). Preliminary study of caregiving and post-caregiving experiences of older gay men and lesbians. *Journal of Gay & Lesbian Social Services, 13*(4), 87–94.

Hash, K., & Netting, F. E. (2009). It takes a community: Older lesbians meeting social and care needs. *Journal of Gay & Lesbian Social Services, 21*(4), 326–342.

Hatfield, A. B., & Lefley, H. P. (2000). Helping elderly caregivers plan for the future care of a relative with mental illness. *Psychiatric Rehabilitation Journal, 24*(2), 103–107.

Hawley, D. R., & DeHaan, L. (1996). Toward a definition of family resilience: Integrating life-span and family perspectives. *Family Process, 35*, 283–298.

Hayslip, B., Jr., & Kaminski, P. L. (2005a). Grandparents raising their grandchildren: A review of the literature and suggestions for practice. *Gerontologist, 45*, 262–269.

Hayslip, B., Jr., & Kaminski, P. L. (2005b). *Parenting the custodial grandchild: Implications for practice*. New York: Springer.

Hayslip, B., Jr., Shore, J., Henderson, C. E., & Lambert, P. R. (1998). Custodial grandparenting and the impact of grandchildren with problems on role satisfaction and role meaning. *Journal of Gerontology: Social Sciences, 53B*, S164–S173.

Health Resources and Services Administration. (n.d.). *About the Ryan White HIV/AIDS Program.* Retrieved from http://hab.hrsa.gov/abouthab/aboutprogram.html

Heller, T., & Caldwell, J. (2006). Supporting aging caregivers and adults with developmental disabilities in future planning. *Mental Retardation, 44*(3), 189–202.

Henry J. Kaiser Family Foundation. (2012a). *HIV/AIDS fact sheet.* Washington, DC: Author.

Henry J. Kaiser Family Foundation. (2012b). *Medicare spending and financing fact sheet.* Retrieved from http://kff.org/medicare/fact-sheet/medicare-spending-and-financing-fact-sheet/

Henry J. Kaiser Family Foundation. (n.d.). *Total Medicaid spending, FY 2012.* Retrieved from http://kff.org/medicaid/state-indicator/total-medicaid-spending/

Hill, K. (2012). Permanency and placement planning for older youth with disabilities in out-of-home placement. *Children and Youth Services Review, 34*, 1418–1424.

Hill-Weld, J. (2011). Psychotherapy with families impacted by intellectual disability, throughout the lifespan. *Advances in Mental Health and Intellectual Disabilities, 5*(5), 26–33.

Hinckson, E. A., Dickinson, A., Water, T., Sands, M., & Penman, L. (2013). Physical activity, dietary habits and overall health in overweight and obese children and youth with intellectual disability or autism. *Research in Developmental Disabilities, 34*, 1170–1178.

Hobson, L. (2007). Families caring for persons with HIV/AIDS. *Journal of Human Behavior in the Social Environment, 14*(1–2), 24–28.

Hollingsworth, W. G. (2011). Community family therapy with military families experiencing deployment. *Contemporary Family Therapy, 33*, 215–228.

Hooyman, N., Browne, C. V., Ray, R., & Richardson, V. (2002). Feminist gerontology and the life course: Policy, research and teaching issues. *Gerontology and Geriatrics Education, 22*(4), 3–26.

Hooyman, N., & Kayak, H. (2005). *Social gerontology* (4th ed.). Boston: Allyn & Bacon.

Huang, W. W., DeLambo, D. A., Kot, R. R., Ito, I. I., Long, H. H., & Dunn, K. K. (2004). Self-advocacy skills in Asian American parents of children with developmental disabilities: A pilot study. *Journal of Ethnic and Cultural Diversity in Social Work, 13*, 1–18.

Hudson, R. B. (1996). The changing face of aging politics. *Gerontologist, 36*, 33–35.

Huebner, A. J., Mancini, J. A., Bowen, G. L., & Orthner, D. K. (2009). Shadowed by war: Building community capacity to support military families. *Family Relations, 58*, 216–228.

Human Rights Campaign. (n.d.). *Maps of state laws and policies.* Retrieved from http://www.hrc.org/resources/entry/maps-of-state-laws-policies

Hutton, J. L., & Pharoah, P.O.D. (2002). Effects of cognitive, motor, and sensory disabilities on survival in cerebral palsy. *Archives of Disease in Childhood, 86*(2), 84–89.

Institute of Medicine. (1986). *Confronting AIDS: Directions for public health, health care, and research.* Washington, DC: National Academies Press.

Institute of Medicine. (2011). *HIV screening and access to care: Health care system capacity for increased HIV testing and provision of care.* Retrieved from http://www.iom.edu/Reports/2011/HIV-Screening-and-Access-to-Care-Health-Care-System-Capacity-for-Increased-HIV-Testing-and-Provision-of-Care.aspx

Institute of Medicine. (2013). *Returning home from Iraq and Afghanistan: Readjustment needs of veterans, service members, and their families.* Retrieved from http://www.iom.edu/Reports/2013/Returning-Home-from-Iraq-and-Afghanistan.aspx

Iraq Coalition Casualty Count. (n.d.). Retrieved from www.icasualties.org

Irish Social Care Gateway. (2005, July 22). *What is social care?* Retrieved from http://staffweb.itsligo.ie/gateway/asp/whatis.asp

References

Isserman, N., Greene, R. R., Bowen, S. P., Hollander-Goldfein, B., & Cohen, H. (2014). Intergenerational families of Holocaust survivors: Designing and piloting a family resilience template. *Journal of Evidence-Based Social Work, 11*(3), 256–268.

Janevic, M. R., & Connell, C. (2001). Racial, ethnic, and cultural differences in the dementia caregiving experience: Recent findings. *Gerontologist, 40*, 334–347.

Jang, S. N., Avendano, M., & Kawachi, I. (2012). Informal caregiving patterns in Korea and European countries: A cross-national comparison. *Asian Nursing Research, 6*(1), 19–26.

Janicki, M. P., Dalton, A. J., Henderson, C., & Davidson, P. W. (1999). Mortality and morbidity among older adults with intellectual disability: Health services considerations. *Disability & Rehabilitation, 21*(5-6), 284–294.

Jennings, J. (1993). Elderly parents as caregivers for their adult dependent children. *Social Work, 87*(5), 430–433.

Johnson, B. (2000). Family-centered care: Four decades of progress. *Families, Systems & Health: The Journal of Collaborative Family Healthcare, 18*(2), 137–156.

Johnson, E. I., & Waldfogel, J. J. (2002). Parental incarceration: Recent trends and implications for child welfare. *Social Service Review, 76*, 460–479.

Johnson, R. W., & Schaner, S. G. (2005a, July). Many older Americans engage in caregiving activities. *Perspectives on Productive Aging, 3*. Retrieved from the Urban Institute Web site, http://www.urban.org/UploadedPDF/311203_Perspectives3.pdf

Johnson, R. W., & Schaner, S. (2005b, September). *Value of unpaid activities by older Americans tops $160 billion per year.* Washington, DC: Urban Institute.

Joslin, D. (Ed.). (2002). *Invisible caregivers: Older adults raising children in the wake of HIV/AIDS.* New York: Columbia University Press.

Karimli, L., Ssewamala, F. M., & Ismayilova, L. (2012). Extended families and perceived caregiver support to AIDS orphans in Rakai district of Uganda. *Children and Youth Services Review, 34*, 1351–1358.

Kelley, S. J., Whitley, D. M., Sipe, T. A., & Yorker, B. C. (2000). Psychological distress in grandmother kinship care providers: The role of resources, social support and physical health. *Child Abuse & Neglect, 24*, 311–321.

Kelley, S. J., Yorker, B., Whitley, D. M., & Sipe, T. A. (2001). Multimodal intervention for grandparents raising grandchildren: Results of an exploratory study. *Child Welfare Journal, 80*(1), 27–50.

Kelly, T. B., & Kropf, N. P. (1995). Stigmatized and perpetual parents: Older parents caring for adult children with life-long disabilities. *Journal of Gerontological Social Work, 24*(1–2), 3–16.

Kessler, R. C., Chiu, W. T., Demler, O., & Walters, E. E. (2005). Prevalence, severity, and comorbidity of twelve-month DSM-IV disorders in the National Comorbidity Survey Replication (NCS-R). *Archives of General Psychiatry, 62*, 617–627.

Kicklighter, J. R., Whitley, D. M., Kelley, S. J., Lynch, J. E., & Melton, T. S. (2009). A home-based nutrition and physical activity intervention for grandparents raising grandchildren: A pilot study. *Journal of Nutrition for the Elderly, 28*(2), 188–199.

King, S., Kropf, N. P., Perkins, M., Sessley, L., Burt, C., & Lepore, M. (2009). Kinship care in rural Georgia communities: Responding to needs and challenges of grandparent caregivers. *Journal of Intergenerational Relationships, 7*(2–3), 225–242.

Kirchner, J. E., Farmer, M. S., Shue, V. M., Blevins, D., & Sullivan, G. (2011). Partnering with communities to address the mental health needs of rural veterans. *Journal of Rural Health, 27*, 416–424.

Kisor, A. J., & Kendal-Wilson, L. (2002). Older homeless women: Reframing the stereotype of the bag lady. *Affilia, 17*, 354–370.

Kizer, K. W., & Dudley, R. A. (2009). Extreme makeover: Transformation of the veterans health care system. *Annual Review of Public Health, 30*, 313–339.

Klein, D., & Jurich, J. (1993). Metatheory and family studies. In P. Boss, W. J. Doherty, W. R. LaRossa, W. R. Schimm, & S. K. Steinmetz (Eds.), *Sourcebook of family theories and methods: A contextual approach* (pp. 31–70). New York: Springer.

Knight, B. (1999). The scientific basis for psychotherapeutic interventions with older adults: An overview. *JCLP/In Session, 55*, 927–934.

Kolomer, S. R. (2000). Kinship foster care and its impact on grandmother caregivers. *Journal of Gerontological Social Work, 33*(3), 85–102.

Kolomer, S. R. (2009). Grandparent caregivers. In S. M. Cummings & N. P. Kropf (Eds.), *Handbook of psychosocial interventions with older adults: Evidence-based treatment* (pp. 308–331). London: Routledge.

Kolomer, S. R., & McCallion, P. (2005). Depression and caregiver mastery in grandfathers caring for their grandchildren. *International Journal of Aging and Human Development, 60*(4), 283–294.

Kolomer, S. R., McCallion, P., & Overendyer, J. (2003). Why support groups help: Successful interventions for grandparent caregivers of children with developmental disabilities. In B. Hayslip, Jr., & J. H. Patrick (Eds.), *Working with custodial grandparents* (pp. 111–126). New York: Springer.

Koop, C. E. (1986). *Surgeon general's report on acquired immune deficiency syndrome.* Washington, DC: U.S. Public Health Service.

Korthuis, P. T., Berkenblit, G. V., Sullivan, L. E., Cofrancesco, J., Cook, R. L., Bass, M., et al. (2011). General internists' beliefs, behaviors, and perceived barriers to routine HIV screening in primary care. *AIDS Education and Prevention, 23*(3), 70–83.

Kovacs, P. J., Bellin, M. H., & Fauri, D. P. (2006). Family-centered care: A resource for social work in end-of-life and palliative care. *Journal of Social Work in End-of-Life & Palliative Care, 2*(1), 13–27.

Kristof, N., & WuDunn, S. (2010). *Half the sky: Turning oppression into opportunity for women worldwide.* New York: Random House.

Kropf, N. P. (2006). Community caregiving partnerships promoting alliances to support care providers. *Journal of Human Behavior in the Social Environment, 14*(1–2), 327–340.

Kropf, N. P. (2013). Intergenerational relations. *Encyclopedia of Social Work.* Retrieved from http://socialwork.oxfordre.com/view/10.1093/acrefore/9780199975839.001.0001/acrefore-9780199975839-e-956?rskey=0DJi7g&result=1

Kropf, N. P., & Kolomer, S. S. (2004). Grandparents raising grandchildren: A diverse population. *Journal of Human Behavior in the Social Environment, 9*(4), 65–83.

Kropf, N. P., & Robinson, M. M. (2004). Pathways into caregiving for rural custodial grandparents. *Journal of Intergenerational Relationships, 2*(1), 63–77.

Kropf, N. P., & Wilks, S. (2003). Grandparents raising grandchildren. In B. Berkman & L. Harootyan (Eds.), *Social work and health care in an aging society* (pp. 177–200). New York: Springer.

Kropf, N. P., & Yoon, E. (2006). Social work practice with older adults as caregivers. In B. Berkman (Ed.), *Handbook of social work in aging* (pp. 355–362). New York: Oxford University Press.

Kurth, A. E., Celum, C., Baeten, J. M., Vermund, S. H., & Wasserheit, J. N. (2011). Combination HIV prevention: Significance, challenges and opportunities. *Current HIV/AIDS Reports, 8*(1), 62–72.

La Fromboise, T. D., Coleman, H.L.K., & Gerton, J. (1993). Psychological impact of biculturalism: Evidence and theory. *Psychological Bulletin, 114*, 395–412.

Laird, J. (1993). *Revisioning social work education: A social construction approach.* New York: Haworth Press.

Laird, J. (1996). Family-centered practice with lesbian and gay families. *Families in Society: The Journal of Contemporary Social Services, 77*(9), 559–572.

Lalor, K., & Share, P. (2013). Understanding social care. In K. Lalor and P. Share (Eds.), *Applied social care: An introduction for students in Ireland* (3rd ed., pp. 3–18). Dublin: Gill and Macmillan.

References

Lambda. (n.d.). *Lesbigay youth facts*. Retrieved from http://www.lambda.org/youth.htm#youth facts

Lawton, M. P. (1982). Competence, environmental press, and the adaptation of older people. In M. P. Lawton, P. G. Windley, & T. O. Byerts (Eds.), *Aging and the environment: Theoretical approaches* (pp. 33–59). New York: Springer.

Lawton, M. P., & Nahemow, L. (1973). Ecology and the aging process. In C. Eisdorf & M. P. Lawton (Eds.), *The psychology of adult development and aging* (pp. 619–674). Washington, DC: American Psychological Association.

Lazarus, R. S., & Folkman, S. (1984). *Stress, appraisal, and coping*. New York: Springer.

Lee, Y., & Sung, K. (1998). Cultural influences on caregiving burden: Cases of Koreans and Americans. *International Journal of Aging and Human Development, 46*(2), 125–141.

Lee, Y., & Tang, F. (2013). More caregiving, less working: Caregiving roles and gender difference. *Journal of Applied Gerontology* (in press). Doi:10.1177/0733464813508649

Lefley, H. P. (2003). Changing caregiving needs as persons with schizophrenia grow older. In C. Cohen (Ed.), *Schizophrenia into later life: Treatment, research, and policy* (pp. 251–268). Washington, DC: American Psychiatric Publishing.

Lentz, C. (2010). A Fulbright experience: Building relationships with Christians and Muslims with HIV/AIDS in Zambia. *Journal of Public Affairs Education, 17*(3), 407–416.

Letiecq, B. L., Bailey, S. J., & Kurtz, M. A. (2008). Depression among rural Native American and European American grandparents rearing their grandchildren. *Journal of Family Issues, 29*, 334–356.

Levine-Perkell, J., & Hayslip, B., Jr. (2002). Death and bereavement issues. In D. Joslin (Ed.), *Invisible caregivers: Older adults raising children in the wake of HIV/AIDS* (pp. 64–89). New York: Columbia Press.

Lewandowski, L. A., McFarlane, J., Campbell, J. C., Gary, F., & Barenski, C. (2004). "He killed my mommy!" Murder or attempted murder of a child's mother. *Journal of Family Violence, 19*(4), 211–220.

Lightfoot, E., Hill, K., & LaLiberte, T. (2011). Prevalence of children with disabilities in the child welfare system and out of home placement: An examination of administrative records. *Children and Youth Services Review, 33*, 2069–2075.

Longres, J. F. (1990). *Human behavior in the social environment*. Itasca, IL: Peacock.

Lowe, K. N., Adams, K. S., Browne, B., & Hinkle, K. (2012). Impact of military deployment on family relationships. *Journal of Family Studies, 18*(1), 17–27.

Lumby, J. (2010). Grandparents and grandchildren: A grand connection. *International Journal of Evidence-Based Healthcare, 8*(1), 28–31.

Luna, I., Ardon, E., Lim, Y., Cromwell, S., Phillips, L., & Russell, C. (1996). The relevance of familism in cross-cultural studies of family caregiving. *Western Journal of Nursing Research, 18*(3), 267–274.

Lutz, A. (2008). Who joins the military? A look at race, class, and immigration status. *Journal of Political and Military Sociology, 36*(2), 167–188.

MacLean, A., & Elder, G. H. (2007). Military service in the life course. *Annual Review of Sociology, 33*, 175–196.

Maimon, B., Browning, C. R., & Brooks-Gunn, J. (2010). Collective efficacy, family attachment, and urban adolescent suicide attempts. *Journal of Health and Social Behavior, 51*, 307–324.

Malai, R. (2013). Chapter helps spread NASWF-Lambda training statewide. *NASW News, 58*. Retrieved from http://www.socialworkers.org/pubs/news/2013/09/lgbtq-youth-in-foster-care.asp?back=yes

Marks, G., Gardner, L. I., Craw, J., & Crepaz, N. (2010). Entry and retention in medical care among HIV-diagnosed persons: A meta-analysis. *AIDS, 24*, 2665–2678.

Martin, D. C., & Yankay, J. E. (2013, April). *Refugees and asylees: 2012*. Washington, DC: U.S. Department of Homeland Security, Office of Immigration Statistics.

Martin, J. I., Messinger, L., Kull, R., Holmes, J., Bermudez, F., & Sommer, S. (2009). *Council on Social Work Education–Lambda Legal study of LGBT issues in social work.* Alexandria, VA: Council on Social Work Education.

Marx, P. (2012, October 8). Golden years. How will boomers handle retirement? Hire an expert. *New Yorker,* pp. 72–75.

Maslach, C., Jackson, S. E., & Leiter, M. P. (1996). *MBI: The Maslach Burnout Inventory: Manual.* Palo Alto, CA: Consulting Psychologists Press.

Maslow, A. H. (1968). *Toward a psychology of being.* New York: Van Nostrand.

Masten, A. (1994). Resilience in individual development: Successful adaptation despite risk and adversity. In M. C. Wang & E. W. Gordon (Eds.), *Educational resilience in inner-city America: Challenges and prospects* (pp. 3–25). Hillsdale, NJ: Erlbaum.

Matheson, L. (1996). The politics of the Indian Child Welfare Act. *Social Work, 41,* 232–235.

Maugans, J. E. (1994). *Aging parents, ambivalent baby boomers: A critical approach to gerontology.* Dix Hills, NY: General Hall.

Mayo Clinic. (2013, July 23). *Stress management: Know your triggers.* Retrieved from http://www.mayoclinic.com/health/stress-management/SR00031

Mayo Clinic. (2014, August 11). *HIV/AIDS.* Retrieved from http://www.mayoclinic.com/health/hiv-aids/DS00005

McCorkle, B. H., Rogers, E., Dunn, E. C., Lyass, A., & Wan, Y. (2008). Increasing social support for individuals with serious mental illness: Evaluating the Compeer model of intentional friendship. *Community Mental Health Journal, 44*(5), 359–366.

McCoy, V. A., & DeCecco, P. G. (2011). *Person-first language training needed in higher education.* Retrieved from http://counselingoutfitters.com/vistas/vistas11/Article_05.pdf

McFaul, M. (nd). *Returning veterans and their families in rural America: A brief lay of the land.* Boulder, CO: Western Interstate Commission on Higher Education. Retrieved from http://www.wiche.edu/info/grand_rounds/McFaulLayoftheLand.pdf

McNamee, S., & Gergen, K. J. (Eds.). (1992). *Therapy as social construction.* Newbury Park, CA: Sage Publications.

McNeal, C., & Perkins, T. (2007). Potential roles of Black churches in HIV/AIDS prevention. *Journal of Human Behavior in the Social Environment, 15*(2–3), 219–232.

McNutt, J. (2011). Is social work advocacy worth the cost? Issues and barriers to an economic analysis of social work political practice. *Research on Social Work Practice, 21,* 397–403.

Mellman, T. A., Miller, A. L., Weissman, E. M., Crismon, M. L., Essock, S. M., & Marder, S. R. (2001). Evidence-based pharmacologic treatment for people with severe mental illness: A focus on guidelines and algorithms. *Psychiatric Services, 52,* 619–625.

Memoli, M. A. (2011, September 20). Obama marks end of "Don't Ask, Don't Tell" policy. *Los Angeles Times.* Retrieved from http://articles.latimes.com/2011/sep/20/news/la-pn-obama-dont-ask-20110920

Mental health treatment for families: Supporting those who support our veterans: Hearing before the Subcommittee on Health of the Community on Veterans' Affairs, U.S. House of Representatives, 110 Cong. 1 (2008). Retrieved from http://www.gpo.gov/fdsys/pkg/CHRG-110hhrg41373/html/CHRG-110hhrg41373.htm

Meridith, L., Sherbourne, C. D., Gaillot, S., Hansell, L., Ritschard, H. V., Parker, A. M., & Wrenn, G. (2011). *Promoting psychological resilience in the U.S. military.* Santa Monica, CA: Rand Center for Military Health Policy Research.

MetLife Mature Market Institute. (2011). *The MetLife study of caregiving costs to working caregivers: Double jeopardy for baby boomers caring for their parents.* Westport, CT: Author.

References

Miles, D. (2008, May 1). *Gates works to reduce mental health stigma.* Washington, DC: U.S. Department of Defense, American Forces Press Service.

Miller, J., Bruce, A., Bundy-Fazioli, K., & Fruhauf, C. A. (2010). Community mobilization model applied to support grandparents raising grandchildren. *Journal of Extension, 48*(2). Retrieved from http://www.joe.org/joe/2010april/pdf/JOE_v48_2iw7.pdf

Miller, S. (1980). Reflections on the dual perspective. In E. Mizo & J. Delaney (Eds.), *Training for service delivery for minority clients* (pp. 53–61). New York: Family Service Association.

Minkler, M. (1999). Intergenerational households headed by grandparents: Contexts, realities, and implications for policy. *Journal of Aging Studies, 13*(2), 199–221.

Minkler, M., & Fuller-Thomson, E. (2005). African American grandparents raising grandchildren: A national study using the Census 2000 American Community Survey. *Journal of Gerontology: Social Sciences, 60B,* S82–S92.

Minkler, M., & Roe, K. M. (1993). *Grandmothers as caregivers: Raising children of the crack cocaine epidemic.* Newbury Park, CA: Sage Publications.

Minkler, M., Roe, K. M., & Price, M. (1992). The physical and emotional health of grandmothers raising grandchildren in the crack cocaine epidemic. *Gerontologist, 32,* 752–761.

Minuchin, S. (1974). *Families and family therapy.* Cambridge, MA: Harvard University Press.

Mizrahi, T., & Rosenthal, B. B. (2001). Complexities of coalition building: Leaders' successes, strategies, struggles, and solutions. *Social Work, 46,* 63–78.

Mohamed, S., Neale, M., & Rosenheck, R. A. (2009). VA intensive mental health case management in urban and rural areas: Veteran characteristics and service delivery. *Psychiatric Services, 60,* 914–921.

Monger, R., & Yankay, J. (2013, March). *U.S. legal permanent residents: 2012.* Washington, DC: U.S. Department of Homeland Security, Office of Immigration Statistics.

Mumola, C. J. (2000). *Incarcerated parents and their children* (Report No. NCJ 182335). Washington, DC: U.S. Department of Justice, Office of Justice Programs, Bureau of Justice Statistics.

Murphy, S. A., Johnson, L. C., & Lohan, J. (2002). The aftermath of the violent death of a child: An integration of the assessments of parents' mental distress and PTSD during the first 5 years of bereavement. *Journal of Loss and Trauma, 7*(3), 203–222.

Musil, C. M., Gordon, N. L., Warner, C. B., Zauszniewski, J. A., Standing, T., & Wykle, M. (2011). Grandmothers and caregiving to grandchildren: Continuity, change, and outcomes over 24 months. *Gerontologist, 51,* 86–100.

Myers, L. L., Kropf, N. P., & Robinson, M. M. (2002). Grandparents raising grandchildren: Case management in a rural setting. *Journal of Human Behavior in the Social Environment, 5*(1), 53–71.

National Alliance for Caregiving & AARP. (2009). *Caregiving in the U.S.* Retrieved from http://www.caregiving.org/data/Caregiving_in_the_US_2009_full_report.pdf

National Alliance for Caregiving & EmblemHealth. (2010, March). *Care for the family caregiver: A place to start.* Retrieved from http://www.caregiving.org/data/Emblem_CfC10_Final2.pdf

National Alliance for the Mentally Ill. (2001). *Mental health, mental illness, healthy aging: A NH guide for older adults and caregivers.* Concord, NH: Author.

National Alliance on Mental Illness. (2010). *Facts on children's mental health in America.* Retrieved from http://www.nami.org/Template.cfm?Section=federal_and_state_policy_legislation&template=/ContentManagement/ContentDisplay.cfm&ContentID=43804

National Alliance on Mental Illness. (n.d.). *Spending money in all the wrong places: Jails and prisons.* Retrieved from http://www.nami.org/Template.cfm?Section=Fact_Sheets&Template=/ContentManagement/ContentDisplay.cfm&ContentID=14593

National Association of Area Agencies on Aging. (2011, June). *The maturing of America—Getting communities on track for an aging population.* Retrieved from http://www.n4a.org/files/MOA_FINAL_Rpt.pdf

National Association of Social Workers. (2002). HIV/AIDS stigma: Making the connection to discrimination and prejudice. *World AIDS Day 2009.* Retrieved from http://www.socialworkers.org/practice/hiv_aids/AIDS_Day2002.pdf

National Association of Social Workers. (2008). *Code of ethics of the National Association of Social Workers.* Retrieved from http://www.naswdc.org/pubs/code/code.asp

National Association of Social Workers. (2012). *NASW HIV/AIDS Spectrum: Mental health training and education of social workers project.* Retrieved from http://www.naswdc.org/practice/hiv_aids/default.asp

National Association of Social Workers. (2013). *The certified hospice and palliative social worker (CHP-SW).* Retrieved from http://www.socialworkers.org/credentials/credentials/chpsw.asp

National Association of Social Workers. (n.d.). *Social workers in elected office.* Retrieved from http://www.naswdc.org/pace/state.asp

National Center for Biotechnology Information. (2013, March 8). Post-traumatic stress disorder. Retrieved from http://www.ncbi.nlm.nih.gov/pubmedhealth/PMH0001923/

National Center for PTSD. (2006). *A guide for families of military members.* Retrieved from http://www.ptsd.va.gov/public/ptsd-overview/reintegration

National Center for Veterans Analysis and Statistics. (2011). *America's women veterans: Military service history and VA benefit utilization statistics.* Washington, DC: Author. Retrieved from U.S. Department of Veterans Affairs Web site, http://www.va.gov/vetdata/docs/specialreports/final_womens_report_3_2_12_v_7.pdf

National Diabetes Education Program. (n.d.). *I have diabetes.* Retrieved from http://ndep.nih.gov/i-have-diabetes/index.aspx

National Institute of Diabetes and Digestive and Kidney Diseases. (2013, December 11). *Publications in Spanish.* Retrieved from National Diabetes Information Clearinghouse Web site, http://www.diabetes.niddk.nih.gov/spanish/

National Institute of Mental Health. (2012). *The numbers count: Mental disorders in America.* Retrieved from http://www.namigc.org/documents/numberscount.pdf

National Institute of Neurological Disorders and Stroke. (2014, June 3). *NINDS traumatic brain injury information page.* Retrieved from http://www.ninds.nih.gov/disorders/tbi/tbi.htm

National Institutes of Health. (2010). *Methods for prevention packages program (MP3 II).* Retrieved from http://grants.nih.gov/grants/guide/rfa-files/RFA-AI-10-005.html

National Institutes of Health. (2013, August). *The NIH almanac.* Retrieved from http://www.nih.gov/about/almanac/organization/NIMH.htm

National Public Radio. (2012, May 10). Faris family fights for their military marriage. *Talk of the Nation.* Retrieved from http:/www.npr.org/2012/05/10/152426651/faris-family-fights-for-their-military-marriage

National Survey on Drug Use and Health. (2012, April 15). *Physical health conditions among adults with mental illness.* Washington, DC: U.S. Department of Health and Human Services, Substance Abuse and Mental Health Services Administration.

Nduwimana, F. (2004). *The right to survive sexual violence: Women and HIV/AIDS.* Montreal: International Centre for Human Rights and Democratic Development.

Neville, S., & Henrickson, M. (2010). "Lavender retirement": A questionnaire survey of lesbian, gay and bisexual people's accommodation plans for old age. *International Journal of Nursing Practice, 16,* 586–594.

References

Newman, B., & Newman, P. R. (2005). *Development through life: A psychosocial approach.* Monterey, CA: Thomson Brooks/Cole.

Newman, S., & Goldman, H. (2008). Putting housing first, making housing last: Housing policy for persons with severe mental illness. *American Journal of Psychiatry, 165,* 1242–1248.

New York Times. (n.d.). Health guide: Stress and anxiety. Retrieved from http://health.nytimes.com/health/guides/symptoms/stress-and-anxiety/overview.html

Norris, F. H., Stevens, S. P., Pfefferbaum, B., Wyche, K. F., & Pfefferbaum, R. (2008). Community resilience as a metaphor, theory, and set of capacities and strategy for disaster readiness. *American Journal of Community Psychology, 41,* 122–150.

Norton, D. G. (1978). *The dual perspective: Inclusion of ethnic minority content in social work curriculum.* New York: Council on Social Work Education.

Obama, B. (2012, August 31). *Executive order: Improving access to mental health services for veterans, service members, and military families.* Retrieved from White House Web site, http://www.whitehouse.gov/the-press-office/2012/08/31/executive-order-improving-access-mental-health-services-veterans-service

Obama, B. (2013, January 29). State of the Union, 2013. Retrieved from White House Web site, http://www.whitehouse.gov/state-of-the-union-2013

Ochs, E., & Izquierdo, C. (2009). Responsibility in childhood: Three developmental trajectories. *Ethos, 37,* 391–413.

Ohmer, M. L., & Korr, W. S. (2006). The effectiveness of community practice intervention: A review of the literature. *Research on Social Work Practice, 16,* 132–145.

Orthner, D. K., & Rose, R. (2007). *Family readiness group involvement and adjustment among army civilian spouses.* Washington, DC: Army Research Institute for the Behavioral and Social Sciences.

Östman, M. (2004). Family burden and participation in care: Differences between relatives of patients admitted to psychiatric care for the first time and relatives of re-admitted patients. *Journal of Psychiatric and Mental Health Nursing, 11,* 608–613.

Ozarin, L. (1978). The pros and cons of case management. In J. Talbott (Ed.), *The chronic mental patient* (pp. 165–170). Washington, DC: American Psychiatric Association.

Ozawa, M. N., & Hong, B. E. (2006). Postretirement earnings relative to preretirement earnings: Gender and racial differences. *Journal of Gerontological Social Work, 47*(3–4), 63–82.

Pace, P. (2012). Coaching can be logical career move. *NASW News, 57,* 7.

Palmer, C. (2008). A theory of risk and resilience factors in military families. *Military Psychology, 20,* 205–217.

Parish, S. L., & Lutwick, Z. E. (2005). A critical analysis of the emerging crisis in long-term care for people with developmental disabilities. *Social Work, 50,* 345–354.

Parish, S. L., Pomeranz-Essley, A., & Braddock, D. (2003). Family support in the United States: Financing trends and emerging initiatives. *Mental Retardation, 41*(3), 174–187.

Parsons, T. (1951). *The social system.* New York: Free Press.

Patrick, E. (2004, June 1). *The U.S. Refugee Resettlement Program.* Retrieved from Migration Policy Institute Web site, http://www.migrationpolicy.org/article/us-refugee-resettlement-program

Patrick, J. H., & Tomczewsk, D. K. (2008). Grandparents raising grandchildren: Benefits and drawbacks? Custodial grandfathers. *Journal of Intergenerational Relationships, 5*(4), 113–116.

Patterson, J., & Garwick, A. W. (1998). Theoretical linkages: Family meanings and sense of coherence. In H. I. McCubbin, E. A. Thompson, A. I. Thompson, & J. E. Fromer (Eds.), *Stress, coping and health in families: Sense of coherence and resiliency* (pp. 71–90). Thousand Oaks, CA: Sage Publications.

Pavalko, E. K., & Henderson, K. A. (2006). Combining care work and paid work: Do workplace policies make a difference? *Research on Aging, 28,* 359–374.

Payne, B., Monk-Turner, E., Kropf, N. P., & Turner, C. (2010). The influence of aging, health, and community characteristics on happiness. *International Public Health Journal, 2*(2), 1–11.

Perreault, M., Rousseau, M., Provencher, H., Roberts, S., & Milton, D. (2012). Predictors of caregiver satisfaction with mental health services. *Community Mental Health Journal, 48*(2), 232–237.

Perron, B. (2002). Online support for caregivers of people with a mental illness. *Psychiatric Rehabilitation Journal, 26*(1), 70–77.

Pescosolido, B., Perry, B., Martin, J., McLeod, J., & Jensen, P. (2007). Stigmatizing attitudes and beliefs about treatment and psychiatric medications for children with mental illness. *Psychiatric Services, 58*, 613–618.

Pfeifer, M. E. (2006, October 28). U.S. Census releases 2005 American Community Survey data for Southeast Asian Americans. *Asian American Press.* Retrieved from http://www.hmongstudies.org/2005ACSArticle.html

PFLAG. (2013a). *About PFLAG.* Retrieved from http://community.pflag.org/page.aspx?pid=191

PFLAG. (2013b). *PFLAG's history.* Retrieved from http://community.pflag.org/page.aspx?pid=267

Phillips, S. D., Burns, B. J., Wagner, H. R., Kramer, T. L., & Robbins, J. M. (2002). Parental incarceration among adolescents receiving mental health services. *Journal of Child and Family Studies, 11*, 385–399.

Pinquart, M., & Sörensen, S. (2005). Ethnic differences in stressors, resources, and psychological outcomes of family caregiving: A meta-analysis. *Gerontologist, 45*, 90–106.

Plumer, B. (2013, January 29). We're running out of farm workers. Immigration reform won't help [Web log post]. *Wonkblog.* http://www.washingtonpost.com/blogs/wonkblog/wp/2013/01/29/the-u-s-is-running-out-of-farm-workers-immigration-reform-may-not-help

Poindexter, C. P. (1999). Promises in the plague: Passage of the Ryan White Comprehensive AIDS Resources Emergency Act as a case study for legislative action. *Health & Social Work, 24*, 35–41.

Poindexter, C. P. (2002). "Be generous of spirit": Organizational development of an AIDS service organization. *Journal of Community Practice, 10*(2), 53–70.

Poindexter, C. P. (2007). Management success and struggles for AIDS service organizations. *Administration in Social Work, 31*(3), 5–28.

Poindexter, C. P. (2008). Older persons parenting children who have lost a parent due to HIV. *Journal of Intergenerational Relationships, 5*(4), 77–95.

Poindexter, C. P. (2009). United States HIV policy from the human rights perspective. *Journal of HIV/AIDS Social Services, 8*, 127–143.

Poindexter, C. P., & Linsk, N. L. (1999). HIV-related stigma in a sample of HIV-affected older female African American caregivers. *Social Work, 44*, 46–61.

Popenoe, D. (1993). American family decline, 1960–1990: A review and appraisal. *Journal of Marriage and Family, 55*, 527–555.

Potok, M. (2010). *Anti-gay hate crimes: Doing the math.* Retrieved from the Southern Poverty Law Center Web site, http://www.splcenter.org/get-informed/intelligence-report/browse-all-issues/2010/winter/anti-gay-hate-crimes-doing-the-math

Pruchno, R. (1999). Raising grandchildren: The experiences of Black and White grandmothers. *Gerontologist, 39*, 209–221.

Putnam, R. D. (2000). *Bowling alone: The collapse and revival of American community.* New York: Simon & Schuster.

Quam, J. K. (Ed.). (1997). *Social services for senior gay men and lesbians.* New York: Haworth Press.

Rao, S. (2004). Faculty attitudes and students with disabilities in higher education: A literature review. *College Student Journal, 38*(2), 191–198.

Rawls, J. (1971). *A theory of justice.* Cambridge, MA: Harvard University Press.

Real Warriors. (n.d.). Tweets. Retrieved from http://www.twitter.com/realwarriors

References

Reamer, F. (2001). *Ethics education in social work*. Alexandria, VA: Council on Social Work Education.

Redfoot, D., Feinberg, L., & Houser, A. (2013, August). *The aging of the baby boom and the growing care gap: A look at future declines in the availability of family caregivers* [Insight on the Issues 85]. Washington, DC: AARP Public Policy Institute. Retrieved from http://www.aarp.org/content/dam/aarp/research/public_policy_institute/ltc/2013/baby-boom-and-the-growing-care-gap-insight-AARP-ppi-ltc.pdf

Reynolds, B. (1935). Rethinking social casework. *Family, 16*, 230–237.

Rhodes, S. L. (1980). A developmental approach to the life cycle of the family. In M. Bloom (Ed.), *Life span development* (pp. 30–40). New York: Macmillan.

Richardson, M., Cobham, V., McDermott, B., & Murray, J. (2013). Youth mental illness and the family: Parents' loss and grief. *Journal of Child and Family Studies, 22*, 719–736.

Richmond, M. E. (1917). *Social diagnosis*. New York: Russell Sage Foundation. Retrieved from http://www.historyofsocialwork.org/PDFs/1917,%20Richmond,%20Social%20Diagnosis%20OCR%20C.pdf

Riggs, S., & Riggs, D. S. (2011). Risk and resilience in military families experiencing deployment: The role of the family attachment network. *Journal of Family Psychology, 25*, 675–687.

Riley, J., & Greene, R. R. (1993). Influence of education on self-perceived attitudes about HIV/AIDS among human service providers. *Social Work, 38*, 396–403.

Ringhoff, D., Rapp, L., & Robst, J. (2012). The criminalization hypothesis: Practice and policy implications for persons with serious mental illness in the criminal justice system. *Best Practices in Mental Health, 8*(2), 1–19.

Robert, S. A. (2002). Community context and aging: Future research issues. *Research on Aging, 24*, 579–599.

Robert, S. A., & Lee, K. Y. (2002). Explaining race differences in health among older adults: The contribution of community socioeconomic context. *Research on Aging, 24*, 654–683.

Robert Wood Johnson Foundation. (2011, December 7). *Health care's blind side: Unmet social needs leading to worse health*. Princeton, NJ: Author. Retrieved from http://www.rwjf.org/en/about-rwjf/newsroom/newsroom-content/2011/12/health-cares-blind-side-unmet-social-needs-leading-to-worse-heal.html

Robinson, M. M., Kropf, N. P., & Myers, L. L. (2000). Grandparents raising grandchildren in rural communities. *Journal of Mental Health and Aging, 6*(4), 353–365.

Robinson-Brown, D., & Brandon-Monye, D. (1995). *Midlife and older African Americans as intergenerational caregivers of school-aged children*. Detroit, MI: Wayne State University, Center for Urban Studies.

Rose, S. M., & Moore, V. L. (1995). Case management. In R. L. Edwards (Ed.), *Encyclopedia of social work* (19th ed., pp. 335–340). Washington, DC: NASW Press.

Rosenberg, S. A., & Robinson, C. C. (2004). Out-of-home placement for young children with developmental and medical conditions. *Children and Youth Services Review, 26*, 711–723.

Rothman, J. (1994). *Practice with highly vulnerable clients*. Englewood Cliffs, NJ: Prentice Hall.

Rovner, J. (2013, May 22). Boomer housemates have more fun [Web log post]. *Shots: Health News from NPR*. Retrieved from http://www.npr.org/blogs/health/2013/05/22/183903991/Boomer-Housemates-Have-More-Fun

Rowe, J. (2012). Great expectations: A systematic review of the literature on the role of family carers in severe mental illness, and their relationships and engagement with professionals. *Journal of Psychiatric and Mental Health Nursing, 19*, 70–82.

Rowe, J. W., & Kahn, R. L. (1998). *Successful aging*. New York: Pantheon Books.

RT. (2013, January 15). *U.S. military suicides continue to climb, reaching record in 2012*. Retrieved from http://rt.com/usa/us-army-suicide-rate-025

Rutter, M. (1987). Psychological resilience and protective mechanisms. *American Journal of Ortho-psychiatry, 57*, 316–331.

Sadavoy, J., Meier, R., & Ong, A. Y. M. (2004). Barriers to access to mental health services for ethnic seniors: The Toronto study. *Canadian Journal of Psychiatry, 49*(3), 192–199.

Saltzman, W., Lester, P., Beardslee, W. R., Layne, C. M., Woodward, K., & Nash, W. P. (2011). Mechanisms of risk and resilience in military families: Theoretical and empirical basis of a family-focused resilience enhancement program. *Clinical Child and Family Psychology Review, 14*(3), 213–230.

Sampson, R., Raudenbush, S., & Earls, F. (1997, August 15). Neighborhoods and violent crime: A multilevel study of collective efficacy. *Science, 277*, 918–924.

Sandler, I. (2001). Quality and ecology of adversity as common mechanisms of risk and resilience. *American Journal of Community Psychology, 29*, 19–61.

San Francisco AIDS Foundation. (2012). *Annual report.* San Francisco: Author.

Savin-Williams, R. C. (2001). *Mom, Dad, I'm gay: How families negotiate coming out.* Washington, DC: American Psychological Association.

Sawyer, M. G., Whaites, L., Rey, J. M., Hazell, P. L., Graetz, B. W., & Baghurst, P. (2002). Health-related quality of life of children and adolescents with mental disorders. *Journal of the American Academy of Child & Adolescent Psychiatry, 41*, 530–537.

Scharlach, A. E. (1994). Caregiving and employment: Competing or complementary roles? *Gerontologist, 34*, 378–385.

Schneider, R. L., & Lester, L. (2001). *Social work advocacy: A new framework for action.* Stamford, CT: Thomson Learning.

Schon, D. A. (1983). *The reflective practitioner: How professionals think in action.* New York: Basic Books.

Scott, K. M., Van Korff, M., Alonso, J., Angermeyer, M. C., Bromet, E., Fayyad, J., et al. (2009). Mental-physical co-morbidity and its relationship with disability: Results from the World Mental Health Surveys. *Psychological Medicine, 39*, 33–43.

Sebelius, K. (2011). *Letter to Congress about CLASS.* Retrieved from U.S. Department of Health and Human Services Web site, http://www.hhs.gov/secretary/letter10142011.html

Seretean, T. (Producer). (2000). *Big Mama* [Documentary]. United States: California Newsreel.

Severson, K. (2011, December 9). Thousands sterilized, a state weighs restitution. *New York Times.* Retrieved from http://www.nytimes.com/2011/12/10/us/redress-weighed-for-forced-sterilizations-in-north-carolina.html?pagewanted=all&_r=0

Shankar, J., & Muthuswamy, S. S. (2007). Support needs of family caregivers of people who experience mental illness, and the role of mental health services. *Families in Society, 88*, 302–310.

Shanker, T. (2013, February 11). Partners of gays in service are granted some benefits. *New York Times.* Retrieved from http://www.nytimes.com/2013/02/12/us/partners-of-gay-military-personnel-are-granted-benefits.html

Sheafor, B., Horejsi, C., & Horejsi, G. (2012). *Techniques and guidelines for social work practice* (9th ed.). Boston: Allyn & Bacon.

Shetty, A. K., & Powell, G. (2003). Children orphaned by AIDS: A global perspective. *Seminars in Pediatric Infectious Diseases, 4*(1), 25–31.

Shulman, L. (1999). *Skills in helping individuals, families, groups, and communities.* Belmont, CA: Wadsworth.

Sieben, L. (2011, April 3). Counseling directors see more students with severe psychological problems. *Chronicle of Higher Education.* Retrieved from http://chronicle.com/article/Counseling-Directors-See-More/126990/

Skirboll, B. W., Bennett, L., & Klemens, M. (Eds.). (2006). *Compeer: Recovery through the healing power of friends.* Rochester, NY: University of Rochester Press.

References

Slone, L. B., & Friedman, M. J. (2008). *After the war zone: A practical guide for returning troops and their families*. Philadelphia: Da Capo Press.

Smith, B. (2004). Positive impact: A community-based mental health center for people affected by HIV. *Health & Social Work, 29*, 145–148.

Smith, C., & Beltran, A. (2000). Grandparents raising grandchildren: Challenges faced by these growing numbers of families and effective policy solutions. *Journal of Aging and Social Policy, 12*(1), 7–17.

Social Security Administration. (n.d.). *A summary of the 2013 annual reports*. Retrieved from http://www.socialsecurity.gov/OACT/TRSUM/index.html

Stanley, T. (2005). *Making decisions: Social work processes and the construction of risk(s) in child protection work*. Doctoral thesis, University of Canterbury.

Stanley, T. (2007). Risky world: Child protection practice. *Social Policy Journal of New Zealand, 30*, 163–177.

Steadman, H. J., Davidson, S., & Brown, C. (2001). Law and psychiatry: Mental health courts: Their promise and unanswered questions. *Psychiatric Services, 52*, 457–458.

Stewart, P. (2007). Impact of migration on African American family development and relationships. *Journal of Family History, 32*(1), 45–65.

Strozier, A. L., Elrod, B., Beiler, P., Smith, A., & Carter, K. (2004). Developing a network of support for relative caregivers. *Children and Youth Services Review, 26*, 641–656.

Substance Abuse and Mental Health Services Administration. (n.d.). *What is jail diversion?* Retrieved from http://gainscenter.samhsa.gov/topical_resources/jail.asp

Sullivan, P. M., & Knutson, J. F. (2000). Maltreatment and disabilities: A population-based epidemiological study. *Child Abuse & Neglect, 24*, 1257–1273.

Sun, H. L. (2012, June 20). HIV infection rate skyrockets among some DC women. *Washington Post*. Retrieved from http://www.washingtonpost.com/national/health-science/in-dc-hiv-infection-rate-nearly-doubles-for-some-poor-black-women/2012/06/20/gJQAXIqKrV_story.html

Supiano, K., & Berry, P. H. (2013). Developing interdisciplinary skills and confidence in palliative care social work students. *Journal of Social Work Education, 49*, 387–396.

Surface, D. (2007). HIV/AIDS medication: How social supports works. *Social Work Today, 7*(5), 20.

Sutton, M., Anthony, M. N., Vila, C., McLellan-Lemal, E., & Weidle, P. J. (2010). HIV testing and HIV/AIDS treatment services in rural counties in 10 southern states: Service provider perspectives. *Journal of Rural Health, 26*, 240–247.

Swan, R. W., & Lavitt, M. (1988). Patterns of adjustment to violence in families of the mentally ill. *Journal of Interpersonal Violence, 3*(1), 42–54.

Swann, S. K., & Anastas, J. W. (2003). Dimensions of lesbian identity during adolescence and young adulthood. *Journal of Gay & Lesbian Social Services, 15*(1–2), 109–125.

Talley, A. E., Sher, K. J., & Littlefield, A. K. (2010). Sexual orientation and substance use trajectories in emerging adulthood. *Addiction, 105*, 1235–1245.

Tapper, J. (2013, February 13). Obama announces 34,000 troops to come home. *CNN Politics*. Retrieved from http://www.cnn.com/2013/02/12/politics/obama-sotu-afghanistan-troops

Tavernise, S. (2011, November 24). As fewer Americans serve, growing gap is found between civilians and military. *New York Times*. Retrieved from http://www.nytimes.com/2011/11/25/us/civilian-military-gap-grows-as-fewer-americans-serve.html

Taylor, D. (1995). Effects of a behavioral stress-management program on anxiety, mood, self-esteem, and T-cell count in HIV-positive men. *Psychological Reports, 76*, 451–457.

Tedeschi, R. G., & Calhoun, L. G. (1996). The post traumatic growth inventory: Measuring the positive legacy of trauma. *Journal of Traumatic Stress, 9*, 455–471.

Terkelsen, G. (1980). Toward a theory of the life cycle. In E. A. Carter & M. McGoldrick (Eds.), *The family life cycle: A framework for family therapy* (pp. 21–52). Hawthorne, NY: Aldine de Gruyter.

Tervo, R. C., Azuma, S., Palmer, G., & Redinius, P. (2002). Medical students' attitudes toward persons with disability: A comparative study. *Archives of Physical Medicine and Rehabilitation, 83*, 1537–1542.

Tessler, R. C., & Gamache, G. (2000). *Family experiences with mental illness.* New York: Praeger.

Texas Department of State Health Services. (2012). *Texas State Board of Social Worker Examiners rules-regulations.* Retrieved from http://www.dshs.state.tx.us/socialwork/sw_rules.shtm

Thoits, P. (1995). Stress, coping, and social support processes: Where are we? What next? *Journal of Health and Social Behavior, 35*(Special issue), 53–79.

Thompson, K. (2008). Role theory. In R. R. Greene (Ed.), *Human behavior theory and social work practice.* New Brunswick, NJ: Aldine Transaction Press.

Thompson, M. (2013). Pentagon medics weigh in on the "signature scars of a long war." *Time.* Retrieved from http://nation.time.com/2013/04/25/msmr/

Thompson, M. S. (2007). Violence and the costs of caring for a family member with severe mental illness. *Journal of Health and Social Behavior, 48*, 318–333.

Tomasello, N. M., Manning, A. R., & Dulmus, C. N. (2010). Family-centered early intervention for infants and toddlers with disabilities. *Journal of Family Social Work, 13*(2), 163–172.

Torian, L. V., & Wiewel, E. W. (2011). Continuity of HIV-related medical care, New York City, 2005–2009: Do patients who initiate care stay in care? *AIDS Patient Care & STDs, 25*(2), 79–88.

Trattner, W. I. (1994). *From poor law to welfare state: A history of social welfare in America.* New York: Free Press.

Tucker, C. (2012). New research aimed at mental health: U.S. veterans struggle with pain, stigma of post traumatic stress. *Nation's Health, 42*(3). Retrieved from http://thenationshealth.aphapublica tions.org/content/42/3/1.1.full

United Nations High Commissioner for Refugees. (n.d.). *Internally displaced people figures.* Retrieved from http://www.unhcr.org/pages/49c3646c23.html

Updegraff, J. A., & Taylor, S. E. (2000). From vulnerability to growth: Positive and negative effects of stressful life events. In J. H. Harvey & E. D. Miller (Eds.), *Loss and trauma: General and close rela-tionship perspectives* (pp. 3–28). Philadelphia: Brunner-Routledge.

Urban Coalition for HIV/AIDS Prevention Services. (2011). *Learning Immune Function Enhancement— L.I.F.E. Program: San Francisco.* Retrieved from http://www.uchaps.org/homegrown7.shtml

U.S. Agency for International Development. (2008, September). *Orphans and vulnerable children in high HIV-prevalence countries in sub-Saharan Africa.* Retrieved from http://www.measuredhs .com/pubs/pdf/AS15/AS15.pdf

U.S. Army. (2014). *Comprehensive solider and family fitness.* Retrieved from http://www.army.mil/csf

U.S. Census Bureau. (2009). *American Community Survey.* Retrieved from https://www.census.gov/acs/

U.S. Census Bureau. (2010a, April). *Households and families: 2010.* Retrieved from http://www.census .gov/prod/cen2010/briefs/c2010br-14.pdf

U.S. Census Bureau. (2010b, November). *The older population: 2010.* Retrieved from http://www .census.gov/prod/cen2010/briefs/c2010br-09.pdf

U.S. Department of Defense & U.S. Department of Agriculture. (2014). *Project Youth Extension Ser-vice (Y.E.S!).* Retrieved from http://militaryfamilies.extension.org/yes-intern-program/

U.S. Department of Health and Human Services. (2012, January). *U.S. Department of Health and Human Services recommended actions to improve the health and well-being of lesbian, gay, bisexual, and transgender communities.* Retrieved from http://www.hhs.gov/lgbt/health.html

U.S. Department of Health and Human Services. (2014). *Key indicators for refugee replacement FY 2014.* Retrieved from http://www.acf.hhs.gov/programs/orr/news/key-indicators-for-refugee-placement-fy2014-report-released

References

U.S. Department of Housing and Urban Development. (2012, November). *The 2011 annual homeless assessment report to Congress.* Retrieved from https://www.onecpd.info/resources/documents/2011AHAR_FinalReport.pdf

U.S. Department of Justice. (2002). *Report on minor children who have a mother or father in prison.* Washington, DC: Bureau of Justice Statistics.

U.S. Department of Veterans Affairs. (2011). *One in ten older vets is depressed.* Retrieved from http://www.va.gov/health/NewsFeatures/20110624a.asp

U.S. Department of Veterans Affairs. (2014). Polytrauma/TBI system of care. Retrieved from http://www.polytrauma.va.gov/

U.S. Department of Veterans Affairs, Office of Public and Intergovernmental Affairs. (2011). VA creates women veterans call center [Press release]. Washington, DC: Author.

Valdiserri, R. (2011). Thirty years of AIDS in America: A story of infinite hope. *AIDS Education and Prevention, 23*(6), 479–494.

Van Soest, D., & Garcia, B. (2003). *Diversity education for social justice: Mastering teaching skills.* Alexandria, VA: Council on Social Work Education.

Ventura, S. J., Curtin, S. C., Abma, J. C., & Henshaw, S. K. (2012). Estimated pregnancy rates and rates of pregnancy outcomes for the United States, 1990–2008. *National Vital Statistics Reports, 60*(7), 1–21.

Vourlekis, B., & Greene, R. R. (1992). *Social work case management.* New York: Aldine de Gruyter.

Waldrop, D. P., & Weber, J. A. (2001). From grandparent to caregiver: The stress and satisfaction of raising grandchildren. *Families in Society, 82,* 461–472.

Walsh, F. (1998). *Strengthening family resilience.* New York: Guilford Press.

Wang, P. S., Lane, M., Olfson, M., Pincus, H. A., Wells, K. B., & Kessler, R. C. (2005). Twelve-month use of mental health services in the United States: Results from the National Comorbidity Survey Replication. *Archives of General Psychiatry, 62,* 629–640.

Ward, R. L., Nichols, A. D., & Freedman, R. I. (2010). Uncovering health care inequalities among adults with intellectual and developmental disabilities. *Health & Social Work, 35,* 280–290.

Weick, A. (1993). Reconstructing social work education. In J. Laird (Ed.), *Revisioning social work education: A social constructionist approach* (pp. 11–30). New York: Haworth Press.

Weil, M., & Karls, J. (1985). *Case management in human service practice.* San Francisco: Jossey-Bass.

Weimand, B. M., Hedelin, B., Hall-Lord, M. L., & Sällström, C. (2011). "Left alone with straining but inescapable responsibilities": Relatives' experiences with mental health services. *Issues in Mental Health Nursing, 32,* 703–710.

Weiss, J. A., Dwonch-Schoen, K., Howard-Barr, E. M., & Panella, M. P. (2010). Learning from a community action plan to promote safe sexual practices. *Social Work, 55,* 19–26.

Weissbourd, B. (1994). The evolution of the family resource movement. In S. Kagan & B. Weissbourd (Eds.), *Putting families first: America's family support movement and the challenge of change* (pp. 28–47). San Francisco: Jossey-Bass.

Whitaker, T., Weismiller, T., & Clark, E. (2006). *Assuring the sufficiency of a frontline workforce: A national study of licensed social workers—Executive summary.* Retrieved from the NASW Web site, http://workforce.socialworkers.org/studies/nasw_06_execsummary.pdf

White House Office of National AIDS Policy. (2010, July). *National HIV/AIDS Strategy for the United States.* Retrieved from http://www.whitehouse.gov/sites/default/files/uploads/NHAS.pdf

White, M., & Epston, D. (1990). *Narrative means to therapeutic ends.* New York: W. W. Norton.

Wiener, J. M. (2012). The CLASS Act: Is it dead or just sleeping? *Journal of Aging and Social Policy, 24*(2), 118–135.

Wilkerson, I. (2010). *Warmth of other suns: The epic story of America's great migration.* New York: Random House.

Williamson, V., & Mulhall, E. (2009, January). *Invisible wounds: Psychological and neurological injuries confront a new generation of veterans*. Washington, DC: Iraq and Afghanistan Veterans of America.

Willis, R. (2012). Individualism, collectivism and ethnic identity: Cultural assumptions in accounting for caregiving behaviour in Britain. *Journal of Cross-Cultural Gerontology, 27,* 201–216.

Wood, D. (2012, December 10). Wounded Iraq, Afghanistan troops increase as Pentagon says Afghan war will continue. *World Post.* Retrieved from http://www.huffingtonpost.com/2012/12/10/wounded-troops-iraq-afghanistan_n_2272619.html

Woodworth, R. S. (1996). You're not alone . . . you are one in a million. *Child Welfare, 75,* 619–635.

Woolf, L. (1998). *Gay and lesbian aging.* Retrieved from http://www.webster.edu/~woolfm/oldergay.html

World Health Organization. (2001). *The international classification of functioning, disability and health.* Geneva: Author.

World Health Organization. (2007). *Global age-friendly cities: A guide.* Retrieved from http://www.who.int/ageing/publications/Global_age_friendly_cities_Guide_English.pdf

Yancura, L. (2013). Justifications for caregiving in White, Asian American, and Native Hawaiian grandparents raising grandchildren. *Journal of Gerontology: Psychological Sciences, 68B,* P139–P144.

Yehuda, R., & LeDoux, J. (2007). Response variation following trauma: A translational neuroscience approach to understanding PTSD. *Neuron, 56,* 19–32.

Zarit, S. H., Reever, K. E., & Bach-Peterson, J. (1980). Relatives of the impaired elderly: Correlates of feelings of burden. *Gerontologist, 20,* 649–655.

Zoroya, G. (2009, August 4). Troops' families feel weight of war. *USA Today.* Retrieved from http://usatoday30.usatoday.com/news/military/2009-08-03-broken-families_N.htm

Index

Page numbers in *italics* denote illustrations, figures, or tables.